# Skin of Color

Andrew F. Alexis · Victoria H. Barbosa
Editors

# Skin of Color

## A Practical Guide to Dermatologic Diagnosis and Treatment

Foreword by A. Paul Kelly

Springer

*Editors*
Andrew F. Alexis, MD, MPH
Skin of Color Center
Department of Dermatology
St. Luke's Roosevelt Hospital
New York, NY, USA

Victoria H. Barbosa, MD, MPH, MBA
Department of Dermatology
Millennium Park Dermatology
Rush University
Chicago, IL, USA

ISBN 978-0-387-84928-7 ISBN 978-0-387-84929-4 (eBook)
DOI 10.1007/978-0-387-84929-4
Springer New York Heidelberg Dordrecht London

Library of Congress Control Number: 2012942799



Printed on acid-free paper

Springer is part of Springer Science+Business Media (www.springer.com)

# Foreword

As a history buff with a long-standing interest in the history of dermatology, I have a particular interest in the development of specialized treatment for skin of color. The introduction of slavery into the United States in the early seventeenth century resulted in a variety of skin hues as the races mixed. White doctors of the nineteenth century, while recognizing that darker skin often presented different pathology from lighter skin, either applied standard treatments or, worse, experimental ones based on prejudice, myths, and folktales.

It was African-American medical practitioners of the early twentieth century who pioneered new approaches to treating skin of color. Prominent among many other innovators were Drs. T.K. Lawless, John A. Kenney, Jr., Harold Pierce, and Vernal Cave.

Legally sanctioned segregation and the Civil Rights Movement in the United States led to the establishment of racially and ethnically centered hospital complexes, such as the Martin Luther King, Jr. Multi-Service Ambulatory Care Center, formerly known as Martin Luther King Jr./Drew Medical Center, in Los Angeles, CA; medical colleges at Meharry and Howard Universities; Cook County Hospital, Chicago, IL; Homer G. Phillips Hospital, St. Louis, MO; and many others. By serving large populations of darker-skinned patients, dermatologists were able to hone in on their treatments for skin of color.

In Oman, as a 2010–2011 Fulbright Regional Research Scholar at the College of Medicine & Health Sciences, Sultan Qaboos University, I saw firsthand the racial and ethnic mixtures in the population, the result of close Omani ties with East Africa, along with centuries of seafaring ventures. No wonder keloids, the focus of my research project, are as prevalent in Oman as in the United States.

As the world's population swells, the need for dermatologists skilled in treating a variety of racial and ethnic groups becomes ever more urgent. Advances in DNA research undoubtedly will lead to the redefinition of racial and ethnic mixtures. Still, the fact remains that more darkly pigmented skin reacts or displays differently to many dermatological conditions. *Skin of Color: A Practical Guide to Dermatologic Diagnosis and Treatment* provides the sound medical information dermatologists all over the world are seeking.

The editors, Andrew F. Alexis and Victoria H. Barbosa, are present-day pioneers in improving our knowledge and treatments for skin of color, both in clinical and cosmetic dermatology. The authors of the 21 chapters also break new ground in sharing their experience and treatment options. All leading authorities on dermatology address topics ranging from the basics to skin diseases in children, to cultural considerations in treating different racial and ethnic groups, and to issues related to cosmetic dermatology for skin of color. Written in a clear and concise manner, using a vocabulary familiar to a variety of medical professionals who treat skin of color patients, this book will be an indispensable resource in your daily dermatology practice.

Muscat, Oman A. Paul Kelly, M.D.

# Preface

Demographic projections in the United States and worldwide indicate that a growing proportion of the global population will consist of individuals belonging to the various nonwhite racial and ethnic groups that are characterized as having skin of color. As such, understanding racial and ethnic variations in the epidemiology, clinical presentation, and treatment of skin and hair conditions is of growing importance to providers of dermatologic care. *Skin of Color: A Practical Guide to Dermatologic Diagnosis and Treatment* is intended to serve as a practical, clinically oriented reference for the management of dermatologic disorders that are more prevalent in the rapidly growing, richly pigmented patient population.

This book is designed to be a useful guide for dermatologists, dermatology residents, physician extenders, medical students, and other health-care providers who are involved in the treatment of skin and hair conditions in patients with skin of color. To this end, the chapters provide practical, "how-to" descriptions by world-renowned dermatologists. The content of the book includes a comprehensive range of medical and aesthetic dermatologic conditions that are relevant to the darker-skinned patient. Chapters covering alopecias, pigmentary disorders, keloids, pseudofolliculitis barbae, and inflammatory disorders with unique manifestations in skin of color provide the reader with practical approaches to the common "bread and butter" dermatologic conditions characteristic of skin of color, while chapters on lasers, chemical peels and microdermabrasion, botulinum toxin, soft tissue fillers, and hair transplantation address the nuances of performing cosmetic procedures in nonwhite patients. In addition, chapters on cultural considerations in African-American, Asian, and Latino populations are intended to serve as a useful guide to ensuring cultural competence when treating various racial and ethnic groups with skin of color.

It has been an honor and a pleasure to invite leading authorities in the field of dermatology to share their practical insights into treating darker-skinned patient populations for the completion of this important project. It is our hope that this book will serve as a practical tool that will help clinicians provide optimum dermatologic care for their patients with skin of color.

New York, NY, USA Andrew F. Alexis, MD, MPH
Chicago, IL, USA Victoria H. Barbosa, MD, MPH, MBA

# Contents

# Contributors

**Adedamola Adegbenro, MD** Department of Dermatology, Riverside Family Medicine Residency, Newport News, VA, USA

**Ama Alexis, MD** Department of Pediatrics, NYU Langone Medical Center, New York, NY, USA

**Andrew F. Alexis, MD, MPH** Skin of Color Center, Department of Dermatology, St. Luke's Roosevelt Hospital and Columbia University College of Physicians and Surgeons, New York, NY, USA

**Hilary Baldwin, MD** Clinical Dermatology, State University of New York, Brooklyn, NY, USA

**Victoria H. Barbosa, MD, MPH, MBA** Department of Dermatology, Millennium Park Dermatology, Rush University, Chicago, IL, USA

**Eliot Battle, MD** Cultura Dermatology & Laser Center, Washington, DC, USA

Department of Dermatology, Howard University Hospital, Washington, DC, USA

**Cheryl M. Burgess, MD, FAAD** Department of Dermatology, Georgetown University Medical Center, George Washington University, Washington, DC, USA

Center for Dermatology and Dermatologic Surgery, Washington, DC, USA

**Valerie D. Callender, MD** Callender Dermatology and Cosmetic Center, Glenn Dale, MD, USA

Department of Dermatology, Howard University College of Medicine, Washington, DC, USA

**Carlos A. Charles, MD, FAAD** Department of Dermatology, Weill Medical College of Cornell University, New York, NY, USA

New York Presbyterian Hospital/Cornell, New York, NY, USA

**Marcelyn K. Coley, MD** Department of Dermatology, SUNY Downstate Medical Center, Brooklyn, NY, USA

**Fran E. Cook-Bolden, MD** Skin Specialty Group, New York, NY, USA

Department of Dermatology, The College of Physicians and Surgeons of Columbia University, New York, NY, USA

**Erica C. Davis, MD** Callender Dermatology and Cosmetic Center, Glenn Dale, MD, USA

**Vincent A. DeLeo, MD** Department of Dermatology, St. Luke's-Roosevelt Hospital Center and Columbia University College of Physicians and Surgeons, New York, NY 10025, USA

**Kelli D. Grim, MD** Department of Dermatology, Tulane University Health Science Center, New Orleans, LA, USA

**Rebat M. Halder, MD** Department of Dermatology, Howard University College of Medicine, Washington, DC, USA

**Brooke A. Jackson, MD** Founder and Medical Director, Skin Wellness Center of Chicago, SC, Chicago, IL, USA

Clinical Assistant professor, Department of Dermatology, Northwestern Medical School, Northwestern Memorial Hospital, Chicago, IL, USA

**Elena Jones, MD** Department of Dermatology, St. Luke's Roosevelt Hospital, New York, NY, USA

**Jenna N. Kammer, BA** Drexel University College of Medicine, Philadelphia, PA, USA

**A. Paul Kelly, MD** Division of Dermatology, Charles Drew University of Medicine and Science, Former King/Drew Medical Center, The David Geffen School of Medicine, Burdeck Drive, 94602 Oakland, CA, USA

**Yolanda M. Lenzy, MD, MPH** Department of Dermatology, Boston University School of Medicine, Boston, MA, USA

**Henry W. Lim, MD** Department of Dermatology, Clarence S. Livingood Chair in Dermatology, Detroit, MI, USA

Henry Ford Hospital/Henry Ford Health System, Detroit, MI, USA

**Amy J. McMichael, MD** Department of Dermatology, Medical Center Boulevard, Wake Forest University School of Medicine, Winston-Salem, NC, USA

**So Yeon Paek, MD** 3031 W. Grand Blvd, 8th floor, Detroit, MI, USA

Henry Ford Hospital, Detroit, MI, USA

**Amit G. Pandya, MD** Department of Dermatology, University of Texas Southwestern Medical Center, Dallas, TX, USA

**Jocelyne Papacharalambous, MD** Skin Specialty Group, New York, NY, USA

**Ife J. Rodney, MD** Department of Dermatology and Pathology, Howard University College of Medicine, Washington, DC, USA

**David Rodriguez, MD** Dermatology Associates, Miami, FL, USA

Dermatology and Cutaneous Surgery, University of Miami, Miami, FL, USA

Dermatology Associates and Research, 1301 Ponce de Leon Boulevard, Coral Gables, FL 33134, USA

**Ted Rosen, MD** Department of Dermatology, Baylor College of Medicine, Houston, TX, USA

**Sejal K. Shah, MD** Department of Dermatology, St. Luke's Roosevelt Hospital Center, New York, NY, USA

**Nanette B. Silverberg, MD** Pediatric and Adolescent Dermatology, St. Luke's Roosevelt Hospital Center and Columbia University College of Physicians and Surgeons, New York, NY, USA

**Tanasha Sylvester, MD** Skin Specialty Group, New York, NY, USA

**Susan Taylor, MD** Society Hill Dermatology and Columbia University College of Physicians and Surgeons, Philadelphia, PA, USA

**Chanisada Wongpraparut, MD** Department of Dermatology, Faculty of Medicine Siriraj Hospital, 2 Prannok Street, Bangkok 10700, Thailand

**Heather Woolery-Lloyd, MD** University of Miami Cosmetic Medicine and Research Institute, Miami Beach, FL, USA

# Chapter 1
# Structural, Physiological, Functional, and Cultural Differences in Skin of Color

**Adedamola Adegbenro and Susan Taylor**

Skin of color is defined as non-Caucasian skin types, which by Fitzpatricks' classification comprise skin types III-VI. There is great variability in skin pigmentation among distinct racial and ethnic groups, making it difficult to define skin types simply by ethnicity, race, or culture. Individuals with darker skin comprise a wide range of racial and ethnic groups including Africans, African-Americans, African-Caribbean, Japanese, Chinese, Asians, Latinos, Indians, and Pakistanis, to name just a few (Table 1.1) [1].

The US census indicates that by the year 2056, greater than 50% of the US population will be non-Caucasian [2]. Presently, individuals with pigmented skin comprise 80% of the world population [3]. As expected, demand for health care services by individuals with skin of color will grow substantially as this population grows. This demand will also expand as newer technologies and treatment for skin diseases develop. Therefore, the importance of studying the differences that exist in the structure, physiology, function, and culture of ethnic skin cannot be overemphasized.

Most of the early literature on pigmented skin has produced conflicting results that are difficult to interpret or generalize. This is as a result of small sample sizes, non-standardized approaches and methodologies, varying anatomic sites, and the use of subjective parameters. This chapter will summarize the current data regarding ethnic skin differences. An understanding of structural, physiological, and functional differences in pigmented skin will lead to a better grasp of the pathophysiologic mechanisms of skin diseases particularly those that disproportionately affect the ethnic population.

A. Adegbenro, M.D.
Department of Dermatology, Riverside Family Medicine Residency, Newport News, VA, USA

S. Taylor, M.D. (✉)
Society Hill Dermatology and Columbia University College of Physicians and Surgeons, Philadelphia, PA, USA
e-mail: drstaylor1@aol.com

A.F. Alexis and V.H. Barbosa (eds.), *Skin of Color: A Practical Guide to Dermatologic Diagnosis and Treatment*, DOI 10.1007/978-0-387-84929-4_1,

**Table 1.1** Groups that comprise persons defined as having ethnic skin[a]

| | |
|---|---|
| "Black" | African, people of African descent, including African American, Caribbean-American, and Latin-American persons |
| Latino or Hispanic | Persons of Spanish and indigenous Central/South American descent, including Central Americans, South Americans, and Caribbean-American; persons of Spanish descent, including Cuban, Puerto Rican, and Dominican |
| East Asian | Chinese, Japanese, Korean |
| Southeast Asian and Pacific islander | Filipino, Vietnamese, Cambodian, Thai, Malaysian, Laotian, Burmese, Hmong descent, Polynesian, Micronesian |
| Australoid | Australian aborigine, Melanesian descent (the Republic of Guinea, Papua, Solomon Islands) |
| Native Americans | More than 560 recognized tribes, including Inuit (Native Alaskans) |
| South Asia | Indian, Pakistani, Bangladesh, Sri Lanka |
| Middle Eastern | Iranian, Iraqi, persons from Saudi Arabia and the Arabian Peninsula (including Kuwait, Bahrain, Oman, Qatar, the United Arab Emirates, Yemen), Lebanese, Afghani, Jordanian, Syrian, *Israeli*, Turkish, North African (Egypt, Morocco, Algeria, Libya) |

From Talakoub and Wesley [1], with permission of Elsevier

[a]Traditionally, there are nine geographic races, each with particular genetic similarities. These geographic races include Europeans (which include Middle Eastern and Mediterranean persons), Eastern Indians, Asians, American Indians, Africans, Melanesians, Micronesians, Polynesians, and Australian aborigines. We modify these schema into categories in which ethnic persons share similar anatomic characteristics

## Basic Structure and Function of Skin

### *Stratum Corneum*

The stratum corneum deserves special mention given that, as the outermost layer of the skin, it is the skin's primary protective barrier from the environment. It is also the layer of the skin that has received the most attention in studies on differences between skin types. The stratum corneum is a two-compartment system comprised of disk-like corneocytes embedded in a matrix of lipid-enriched membranes. Individual corneocytes contain keratin filaments and osmotically active molecules such as filaggrin encased in a resistant, flexible cell envelope. Within the intercellular spaces of the corneocytes are lipids which provide the permeability barrier of the skin. The lipids include ceramides, cholesterol, long-chain saturated fatty acids, and other less active constituents. These lipids are elaborately organized into multilamellar structures. The stratum corneum functions primarily to prevent water loss from the interior cell layers of the skin. It serves as the interface barrier between the body and the external environment. Consequently, it protects against mechanical insult, irritant/foreign chemicals, ultraviolet light, and microorganisms.

## *Epidermis*

The other layers of the epidermis are highly cellular and composed mainly of keratinocytes. These layers are divided into the basal layer, stratum spinosum, and stratum granulosum based on the morphology of the cells comprising each layer. The basal layer, which is the innermost layer of the epidermis, contains an actively dividing population of keratinocytes. An important constituent of the basal layer of the epidermis is melanocytes, which are derived from neural crest cells and are responsible for the production of melanin pigment. Melanocytes produce melanin which is packaged into organelles termed melanosomes. The melanosomes are subsequently transferred to adjacent keratinocytes via phagocytosis. It is thought that melanin absorbs radiant energy from the sun and protects the skin from the harmful effects of ultraviolet radiation. The ratios of melanocytes to keratinocytes in the epidermis vary by anatomic sites as a function of the degree of sun exposure.

## *Dermal-Epidermal Junction*

The dermal-epidermal junction (DEJ) is an undulating basement membrane zone where the epidermis and dermis adhere to each other. It is composed of two layers known as the lamina lucida and lamina densa. The lamina lucida is an electron-lucent region beneath the basal cell layer. Anchoring filaments from the hemidesmosomes of the basal cells above cross into the lamina lucida below. In turn, anchoring fibrils extend down from the lamina densa into the papillary dermis. Beneath the lamina densa are fingerlike projections of the papillary dermis termed rete ridges. The DEJ is thus a highly irregular junction that greatly increases the surface area over which oxygen, nutrients, and waste products are exchanged between the dermis and the avascular epidermis [4].

## *Dermis*

The primary function of the dermis is to sustain and support the epidermis. The dermis is a more complex structure and is composed of two layers, the more superficial papillary dermis and the deeper reticular dermis. It is made up of collagen, elastic fibers, fibroblasts, blood vessels, lymphatics, and various glands all surrounded by a gel-like ground substance. The fibroblast is the major cell type of the dermis producing mainly collagen and sparse elastic fibers. Although elastic fibers constitute less than 1% of the weight of the dermis, they play an enormously important functional role by resisting deformational forces and returning the skin to its resting shape [4]. Sebaceous glands, eccrine sweat glands, and apocrine glands are epidermal appendages embedded deep within the dermis.

## Structural and Physiological Differences

### *Biophysical Properties: Transepidermal Water Loss, Water Content, and pH*

Currently, literature defines transepidermal water loss (TEWL) as the total amount of water vapor lost through the skin and appendages, under non-sweating conditions. TEWL remains the most studied biophysical property in defining differences between various skin types. The data obtained from all previous studies does not lead to consistent conclusions. An in vitro study by Wilson et al. [5] demonstrated that TEWL was 1.1 times greater in Black compared to White skin. In other studies, in vivo evaluation of baseline TEWL showed higher values in Blacks and Asians compared with Whites, but this was after treatment with methyl nicotinate [6, 7]. This led to the conclusion that Black and Asian subjects have a more compromised epidermal barrier function (discussed later in this chapter) that would most likely be more susceptible to irritants.

In contrast, several in vivo studies conducted by Berardesca et al. demonstrated no significant differences in TEWL and water content (WC) between Black, Hispanic, and White skin at baseline [8–10]. However, in these studies, Blacks had higher TEWL than Whites after application of sodium lauryl sulfate, a water soluble irritant, to preoccluded skin. Yet another study using a larger sample size found TEWL in Blacks to be significantly lower on the cheeks and legs compared with that of Whites [11]. This study also found a lower TEWL in the volar forearms of Black compared to White skin, but this difference was not significant. Importantly, these studies have varied in the anatomic sites used with studies using the back and inner thighs demonstrating a greater TEWL in Blacks compared with Whites, while studies of the cheeks and legs found TEWL to be lower in Blacks. One might conclude that inconsistencies in study results may be due to variation in anatomic sites for a particular skin type or to differences in measurement parameters. TEWL is known to be inversely proportional to water content [12].

Water content (WC), a measure of hydration of the skin, has also been studied extensively. WC is measured as a factor of skin resistance, capacitance, conductance, and impedance with the use of skin electrodes. A review of early data on WC demonstrated conflicting results and the use of varying methodologies in assessing ethnic skin differences. One recent study on water content measured by skin electric capacitance found no significant differences between Black, African/Carribean mixed-race, and Caucasian women [13]. Anatomic site variation, skin microrelief, sweat production, and artifacts from topical agents may modify the quality of electrode contact and serve as confounding factors in these studies [14]. This idea is further substantiated by a recent study of a large sample of Chinese individuals that demonstrated SC hydration changes with age, gender, and anatomic site [15]. More recently, a large-scale study using new skin capacitance imaging technique to compare skin WC among African-American, Chinese, Caucasian, and Mexican subjects in Chicago found that with age, African-American and Caucasian women exhibit lower WC than Chinese and Mexican women [16]. These findings are yet to be validated using the new imaging technique.

Ethnic differences in stratum corneum pH have been explored and deserve some mention. Recent studies have shown that pH regulates homeostasis in epidermal permeability [17]. The most recent study examining pH of the cheek, forehead, and arm did not find any differences among African-Americans, Asian Indians, Caucasians, East Asians, and Latinos [18]. A prior study found a significantly lower pH in Black women compared to Caucasian women only after three tape strippings [19]. Moreover, there were no significant differences in pH with further tape strippings suggesting pH is similar in both races within deeper layers of the skin. Another study by Warrier et al. demonstrated a lower baseline pH on the cheeks in Blacks but not on the legs [11]. The overall results of these studies trend toward the hypothesis that Black skin has a lower pH compared to Whites with some variations according to body sites and depth of skin layers.

## *Corneocyte Variability and Cell Layers*

Differences in the thickness, density, and compactness of the stratum corneum have been studied. Various studies have found that there is no significant difference in thickness of the stratum corneum (SC) between Black and White skin. A comparative study found that in Black subjects, a greater number of tape strippings were required for complete removal of the SC when compared to Whites [20]. Microscopically, Black skin demonstrated higher average numbers of stratum corneum layers than White skin. This led to the conclusion that the stratum corneum is more compact and cohesive in Blacks accounting for the higher number of layers.

Differences in corneocyte surface area have also been examined. A comparative study among African-Americans, White Americans, and Asians of Chinese descent demonstrated no difference in corneocyte surface area, but there was a significant increase in spontaneous corneocyte desquamation by a factor of 2.5 in the Black group [21]. This was attributed to a difference in the composition of the lipids of the stratum corneum. However, another study showed a higher desquamation index of corneocytes on the cheeks and forearms of White subjects [11]. Corcuff et al., in the former study, examined the upper outer arm whereas Warrier et al., in the later study, examined the cheeks, forearms, and lower legs. A recent study using the forehead and volar forearm found no differences in desquamation index among Black, African/Carribean mixed-race, and Caucasian women [13]. Given that corneocyte surface area is believed to vary by anatomic sites in Caucasians, it is possible that corneocyte desquamation also varies by site and not necessarily by race.

## Stratum Corneum Lipid Composition

Studies have shown that the intercellular matrix composition of the stratum corneum may vary among ethnic groups. The earliest in vitro studies on epidermal lipid content demonstrated that Black skin has higher lipid content than White skin [22]. However, this study had a small sample size (two Black and four White subjects) and compared skin from both living and cadaveric subjects at different body sites. One experiment demonstrated the lowest levels of ceramide in Blacks followed by Whites, Hispanics, and Asians [12]. This is partially confirmed by another study which reported lower ceramide levels in African-Americans but similar levels for Asians and Caucasians [18]. Lower ceramide levels correlate with higher TEWL and lower water content, suggesting that alterations in the composition and organization of the lipids may have an effect on transepidermal water loss (TEWL) [12].

Of note, a recent study evaluating racial differences in dandruff found no differences in scalp SC lipid content between UK and Thai subjects during the wet season regardless of the presence or absence of dandruff [23]. In the dry season, the Thai subjects had higher levels of free SC lipids. However, this study failed to characterize the specific ethnic groups to which these subjects belonged. Overall, there seems to be some ethnic differences in lipid composition and probably in lipid content as well but current data is inconclusive.

## Melanin/Melanosomes

It has been confirmed in various studies that melanin protects the skin from damage by UV light, and it is the source of skin pigmentation [24–26]. There is strong evidence from various studies demonstrating no significant difference in the total number of melanocytes across racial groups [27, 28]. However, studies have shown that melanosomes, the melanin-containing organelles assembled in melanocytes, are more numerous in Africans, African-Americans, and Australian aborigines [25]. Heredity appears to play a role in skin pigmentation, distribution of melanocytes, melanin content, and melanin activity [29]. Variations in melanosome quantity, size, type, and arrangement within melanocytes are deemed responsible for the differences in skin color [28].

Darker skin types have larger, non-aggregated melanosomes that are degraded more slowly than lighter skin types who have smaller, aggregated melanosomes [30]. More recent studies by Alaluf et al. showed an increasing size of melanosomes across ethnicities with Africans having the largest melanosomes followed by Indians, Mexicans, Chinese, and Europeans [31, 32]. Another recent study using electron microscopy confirms that African-Americans have predominantly individual melanosomes (88.9%), Caucasians have predominantly clustered melanosomes (84.5%), while Asians have a combination of individual (62.6%) and clustered (37.4%) melanosomes [33]. This study also found that dark-skinned Africans have larger non-aggregated melanosomes while light-skinned Africans have smaller, aggregated melanosomes. This is consistent with the premise that variations in aggregation and size of melanosomes exist within individual ethnic groups.

The degree of sun exposure correlates with aggregation of melanosomes as demonstrated by a study of Asian skin showing that anatomic sites with less sun exposure have more aggregated melanosomes than more sun-exposed sites [34]. Epidermal distribution of melanosomes varies across races. A contributing factor may be the differences that exist in the rate of degradation of melanosomes. Melanosomes in Black skin are distributed throughout the epidermis with increased numbers in the basal layer, whereas in White skin, they are confined to the basal layer (in fewer numbers) and absent in the upper layers [35, 36]. After transfer of mature melanosomes into the keratinocytes in the basal layer, the keratinocytes become terminally differentiated and migrate to the SC, where the melanosomes are generally degraded [37]. As demonstrated in a recent study, the pattern of degradation of melanosomes in the stratum corneum may vary among ethnic groups given that Black skin had higher numbers of melanosomes in the SC followed by Asian skin and White skin in whom melanosomes are almost absent [33].

Research has also shown a greater rate of melanogenesis and higher melanin content in darker skin types. Lighter skin types (European, Chinese, and Mexican) have approximately half as much epidermal melanin as the most darkly pigmented skin types (African and Indian) as demonstrated in various studies [30, 31]. In vitro cultures of melanocytes from Black skin produce more melanin than those from White skin [38]. The rate of melanogenesis may be determined by intracellular pH of melanocytes. In Black skin, the pH of melanocytes was found to be closer to a neutral pH and optimal for melanin synthesis. A recent study showed that decreased intracellular pH in Whites compared with Blacks correlated with reduced melanogenesis [37]. In contrast to these findings, a recent study analyzing the effects of stratum corneum pH on barrier function demonstrated that vesicular organelles that correspond to melanosomes in darkly pigmented melanocytes (SPT 1V-V) are significantly more acidic than those in their counterparts (SPT I-II) [39]. These findings are yet to be validated by other studies.

In another recent study, rates of melanogenesis following UV insult were found to vary among racial groups [40]. Seven days after a single UV dose, this study found that only darker and more UV-resistant skin types demonstrated significant increase in melanin content. A study by De Winter et al. [41] demonstrated increased and higher p53 immunoreactivity in the epidermis after UV exposure in darker-skinned individuals. p53 is a tumor suppressor gene that upregulates DNA repair enzymes following DNA damage. This would suggest that no skin type is immune to photodamage, but it also suggests more efficient repair system against UV damage of the skin in Black subjects compared with Whites. Further details will be discussed later in this chapter.

## Dermal Structure

There appears to be no difference in thickness of the dermis across ethnic groups. A recent study by Bernard et al. using modern imaging studies of the skin of female subjects shows no significant difference in papillary dermis thickness across four ethnic groups (African-Americans, Mexicans, Caucasians, and Chinese) [42].

However, this study demonstrated an increased thickness of the dermal-epidermal junction in African-Americans compared to Caucasians. Also, the subepidermal nonechogenic band (SENEB), a marker of skin aging, was lower in African-Americans than Caucasians with intermediate thickness in Mexicans and Chinese [42]. A more recent study also found no difference in superficial dermis thickness between African and Caucasian skin [43]. This study found that the DEJ in African skin was increased about threefold and more convoluted than in Caucasian skin. Another study on facial skin found more dermal papillae in African-Americans and Hispanics than Caucasians and Asians [44].

Pertaining to the cellular composition of the dermis, studies have shown that the dermis in Black subjects is more compact with smaller, more closely stacked collagen fiber bundles; more numerous fiber fragments; larger and greater number of fibroblasts; and more macrophages compared to White subjects [35, 45]. One of these studies also found no differences in the size and number of mast cells. However, there were greater numbers of and larger melanophages in Black skin as compared to White skin. A more recent study demonstrated that mast cells in African-American skin contained larger granules, increased parallel linear striations (PLS) and increased tryptase levels localized to the PLS in Black compared to White skin [46]. Black skin is known to have a higher predisposition to keloidal scarring, and other early studies suggested the participation of mast cells in aberrant fibrosis seen in these disorders [47–49]. Given the higher levels of tryptase found in Blacks, the investigators in this study suggested involvement of tryptase in the development of keloidal and hypertrophic scars. These differences may also account for more pruritus experienced in Black skin compared to White skin [46].

## Functional Differences

### *Percutaneous Absorption and Barrier Function*

Variations in permeability and barrier function of the skin are dependent on epidermal thickness, stratum corneum structure, density of cutaneous appendages, and several other factors [50–52]. Studies of interracial differences in percutaneous absorption of the skin have been contradictory. Most of these studies have used TEWL as a measure of the skin's permeability to water. Although inconclusive, dark skin is thought by some to display superior epidermal barrier function because darkly pigmented subjects typically require more tape strippings to disrupt the epidermal barrier. A study in Black, White, and Asian subjects evaluating TEWL and LDV after irritant exposure showed an increase in TEWL in Asians and Blacks compared to Whites [6]. Another study by Reed et al. showed that darker skin types (SPT V-VI) have a faster recovery back to baseline TEWL than light skin (SPT II-III) after tape stripping [53]. However, a more recent study found no differences in TEWL when comparing Black, African/Caribbean mixed-race, and Caucasians [13].

Studies have suggested that pigment type (not ethnicity, race, or gender) seems to determine differences in barrier function. Reed et al. demonstrated that neither the number of tape strippings required to perturb the barrier nor the rates of barrier recovery were significantly different in White versus Asian subjects or in female versus male subjects [53]. However, patients with skin types II/III required only 29.6 +/– 2.4 tape strippings to perturb the barrier, while the skin type V/VI group required 66.7 +/– 6.9 tape strippings. This was confirmed by another more recent study showing that subjects with darkly pigmented skin (SPT IV-V) have an enhanced epidermal barrier than lightly pigmented skin types (SPT II-III) [39]. The investigators also demonstrated that these differences are secondary to differences in epidermal lipid content and pH-regulated enzymatic mechanisms. Skin surface temperature differences may also contribute to differences in TEWL, which may be a confounding factor in attempts to assess TEWL as a measure of epidermal barrier function.

Racial differences in the skin's rate of absorption of different chemicals have been studied extensively, albeit with inconclusive evidence. This is probably due to the use of several different methodologies and varying techniques for assessing barrier function in these studies. Though it is difficult to make comparisons across studies, there seems to be a trend toward greater permeability to chemicals in White skin compared to Black skin. Studies by Stoughton et al. and Berardesca et al. show less absorption of fluocinolone and nicotinate respectively in Black skin compared to White skin [54, 55]. The study by Berardesca et al. showed no difference in absorption between White and Hispanic skin although the researchers applied nicotinate after skin structure had been altered by stripping or lipid removal. Earlier studies by Wickrema et al. and Guy et al. found no differences in radiolabeled excretion of diflorasone and absorption of methyl nicotinate respectively in Black and White skin [56, 57].

## *Blood Vessel and Skin Reactivity*

Differences in skin reactivity to irritants, sometimes measured by cutaneous blood flow among different ethnic groups, have been studied with inconclusive evidence of differences [58]. Interobserver variability in evaluation of subclinical degrees of irritancy and subjective assessment of erythema as a function of degree of irritation in pigmented skin poses a major challenge in attempts to make comparisons across these studies. There are some recent studies using new objective techniques like laser Doppler velocimetry (LDV) and photoplethysmography (PPG) to assess blood vessel reactivity as a measure of skin irritancy, but they have also produced conflicting results. Consequently, there is no consensus about the relationship between propensity to develop irritant dermatitis and ethnicity.

Earlier studies using erythema as a measure of skin reactivity demonstrated that Black men showed less erythema in reaction to various chemicals [29]. Furthermore, another study showed that White subjects with the lightest complexions were most susceptible to erythema as a measure of skin irritation [59]. However, given the difficulties in assessing erythema in darker skin, these studies are likely unreliable. Other subsequent studies assessed skin reactivity through its effects on SC integrity and used objective measures such as TEWL, WC, and microcirculation via LDV.

Several studies by Berardesca et al. using these measures demonstrated that Black and Hispanic skin displays a stronger irritant reaction than Whites, whereas Hispanic and White subjects have similar erythematous reactions, albeit more erythema than Black subjects [8–10]. One of these studies by Berardesca show higher TEWL in Blacks and Hispanics after irritant exposure compared to Caucasians, but this was only significant after 0.5% SLS was applied to preoccluded skin [9]. There were no differences in TEWL, WC, and microcirculation of untreated skin after application of sodium lauryl sulfate (SLS) in Blacks, Whites, and Hispanics. However, in another study by Berardesca et al. on racial differences in irritation induced by topical corticosteroid, Blacks showed a decrease in baseline blood vessel reactivity as measured by LDV compared with Whites [60].

Yet another study evaluating skin irritation to 2% SLS as measured by TEWL showed no differences in fair-skinned Chinese, darker-skinned Malaysians, and very dark Indians [61]. Studies in Asian subjects have also been contradictory. One study found increased reactivity to octanoic acid, SLS, acetic acid, and decanol in Asian subjects compared to Caucasians [62]. A study by Foy et al. reported that irritation responses were greater in Japanese women when compared to Caucasian women [63]. However, another study by Aramaki et al. reported no differences in reactivity after an SLS challenge in Japanese and German (Caucasian) subjects [64].

## *Photoprotection*

It is well documented that melanin, by absorbing and deflecting rays of UV light, helps protect the skin from the damaging effects of UV light [24]. A study found that five times more UV light reaches the upper dermis of White skin compared to Black skin [26]. The melanin content and distribution of melanosomes can impact the degree of photoprotection across racial groups. Studies by Szabo et al. [65] and Kaidbey et al. [26] have shown that larger, individually dispersed stage-IV melanosomes (predominantly in Black skin) have a higher melanin content and absorb more UV light than aggregated, smaller melanosomes with less melanin content (predominantly in White skin).

In 1968, Mitchell observed that the Australoid subjects with non-aggregated, large melanosomes were protected from UV-light-induced skin cancers [25]. Australians of European descent, on the other hand, had a high incidence of skin malignancies. Studies have found that rates of basal/squamous carcinomas and melanomas in the USA are 50 and 13 times higher respectively in White skin than in Black skin [66, 67]. An earlier study attempting to explain these differences demonstrated that the main site of UV filtration in fair-skinned subjects is the stratum corneum, whereas in Black subjects, it is the malpighian layer of the epidermis [26]. This study also found that the protection afforded against sunburn in Black epidermis was on average equivalent to a sun-protective factor (SPF) of 13.4. Also, a study in Japanese women comparing skin color and minimal erythema dose (MED) shows that greater melanin content as evidenced by darker complexion correlated with less severe reaction to the sun [68].

A more recent study demonstrated a higher rate of melanin increase in darker and more UV-resistant skin types 7 days after a single UV dose [40]. However, this study found that neither melanin content nor ethnic groups correlated with the efficiency of DNA damage removal. In contrast, another study by Yamaguchi showed that melanin content correlated inversely with cyclobutane pyrimidine dimers (CPD markers of DNA damage) [69]. This study demonstrated that the correlation coefficient was significantly higher in the lower epidermis compared to the upper epidermis in dark skin. In contrast, fair skin demonstrated similar CPD levels in both the upper and lower epidermis [69]. One prior study demonstrated that changes in the distribution of melanin from the lower layers upward to the middle layer of the skin were more pronounced in Black skin 1 week after UV exposure than in White skin [70]. Rijken et al. recently compared the responses of Black and White skin to solar-simulating radiation and found that subjects with skin of color did not show an increase in neutrophils, active proteolytic enzymes, or diffuse keratinocyte activation unlike Caucasians [71]. The authors suggested that this may explain why Black skin is less predisposed to sunburn and photoaging.

De Winter et al. demonstrated increased p53 (a tumor suppressor gene) immunoreactivity in the epidermis after a single UV exposure, and the levels were higher in darker-skinned individuals [41]. Conversely, another recent study found more p53 protein in nuclei of White skin than Black skin after UV exposure. However, in this study, phosphorylated p53, which actively mediates apoptosis of damaged DNA, was absent in White skin compared to Black skin which also contained a greater number of apoptotic cells [72]. The investigators concluded that UV-induced apoptosis is less frequent in White skin after low dose of UV although it is significant in Black skin, suggesting that Black skin removes UV-damaged cells by apoptosis more effectively. Taken together, these studies suggest that Black skin possesses more efficient mechanisms including facilitating apoptosis of damaged DNA, thus conferring better protection against UV-induced photodamage than White skin. These mechanisms may or may not be independent of melanin content or melanosome distribution. Notably, there are very few studies comparing Asian skin to Black or Caucasian skin.

## *Vitamin D Production*

In the study of human evolution, a number of authors have suggested that lighter skin developed to optimize the production of vitamin D [73, 74]. However, a review of these studies demonstrates equivocal evidence for the theory that populations with lighter skin types maintained selective survival in higher latitudes as a function of vitamin D production [75]. Vitamin D is initiated in the skin at the optimal UVB wavelengths of 297 nm by conversion of 7-dehydrocholesterol to cholecalciferol, also termed vitamin D3 [76]. It has been documented that UVA does not participate in the initiation of vitamin D production but rather breaks it down in the skin [77, 78]. Vitamin D deficiency was originally known to cause rickets, osteomalacia, and osteoporosis. However, many recent papers have suggested that vitamin D deficiency may correlate with higher rates of cancer, infections, hypertension, cardiovascular disease, and autoimmune diseases [79].

Vitamin D insufficiency is far more common in Blacks than Whites as demonstrated in current literature. Data from the Third National Health and Nutrition Examination Survey showed that in the winter months, 53–76% of non-Hispanic Blacks compared with 8–33% of non-Hispanic Whites had vitamin D levels below 50 nmol/l [80]. The lower cholecalciferol levels in individuals with darker skin may be due to greater pigmentation reducing UV radiation and, hence, vitamin D photosynthesis in the skin. Given sufficient UV exposure, darker skin can produce adequate vitamin D levels as demonstrated in one study [81]. This study further demonstrated that Black and White skin has similar capacity to produce cholecalciferol, but, at usual levels of sun exposure, vitamin D synthesis is less efficient among Blacks.

However, under normal conditions at most latitudes in North America, even young, black, healthy African-Americans do not attain optimal levels of vitamin D at any time of the year [82]. One study shows that children with darker complexions are at risk for suboptimal vitamin D levels [83]. Low dietary intake may contribute to this deficiency of vitamin D in Blacks as demonstrated in several studies [84]. Blacks have a higher prevalence of the medical conditions that have been seen to correlate with vitamin D deficiency. In light of these findings, clinicians should be encouraged to promote improved vitamin D status among Blacks.

## *Cutaneous Appendages*

The eccrine, apocrine, and apoeccrine sweat glands and sebaceous glands are four separately recognized cutaneous appendages contained in the dermis. Race is believed to have evolved as a function of adaptation to variable environmental conditions in a continuum from cold climates to hot and humid climates. This leads to the speculation that differences should exist in sweat gland quantity, structure, and activity among various ethnic groups and race. There are a few inconclusive studies analyzing the differences among sweat glands from various ethnic groups.

A majority of evidence demonstrates no significant racial differences between the quantity and structure of eccrine sweat glands [85, 86] but does suggest differences in the function of these glands. One author found that in response to physical labor and cholinergic stimulation, White Europeans had a higher sweating rate than either Black Africans or Asian Indians [87, 88]. These studies also found that after cholinergic stimulation by pilocarpine, Black Africans had significantly lower concentrations of sodium chloride in their sweat compared to White Europeans or Asian Indians, thus suggesting that Black skin has a more efficient electrolyte conservation system [87–89]. Other electrophysiology studies that correlate skin resistance with sweat activity consistently demonstrate a higher skin resistance in Black subjects compared to White subjects [58]. One of the studies found that Hispanic and Spanish subjects had an intermediate skin resistance falling between Black and White subjects [90]. However, a couple of studies found no significant differences in onset of sweating and quantity of sweat in Black and White skin [58].

There are a few very early observational studies that suggest that Black subjects have larger apocrine glands and in greater numbers than Caucasians and Chinese [91–93]. However, the small-scale nature and lack of investigator-blinded assessment preclude definitive conclusions. One of these studies noted that Black subjects secreted more turbid fluid with a different odor from their apocrine glands compared to White subjects [93]. The apoeccrine gland which develops at puberty from eccrine glands is localized in the axilla, perianal regions, and nasal skin. It is larger and produces secretions at a rate 10× the rate of eccrine gland secretions. One study showed no differences in the average number of apoeccrine glands among racial groups but did demonstrate high interindividual variability [35]. In contrast, another study found that apoeccrine glands occur in greater numbers in Black versus White female facial skin [94].

Literature analyzing differences in sebaceous glands has produced conflicting results. One study suggests the presence of larger glands with higher sebum production in Black compared to White subjects [95]. However, another study found a higher sebum production on the forehead of Black men compared to White men but an opposite finding in Black compared to White women [96]. In yet another study, no significant difference was seen in sebum excretion of Whites, Blacks, and Asians [97]. A recent study also found no significant difference in sebum quantity among Black, African/Carribean mixed-race, and Caucasian women [13]. The most recent study on facial skin shows greater facial pore area and pore size in African-Americans compared to Asians [43]. This study also found that Hispanics and Caucasians have similar pore area and size as African-American skin. Of note, facial pores correspond to enlarged openings of pilosebaceous units which consist of hair shaft, hair follicle, arrector pili, and sebaceous gland.

The literature contains very few studies on racial differences in sebum composition. One study found that the sebum of both Japanese and Caucasian subjects contains more straight chain fatty acids than branched chain fatty acids [98]. However, Japanese skin had a greater number of C16 isobranched chain fatty acids and greater sebaceous gland activity than Caucasian skin [98]. This study also demonstrated that sebum levels consistently decline with age.

## Cultural Differences

Cultural practices and cosmetic needs vary among racial and ethnic groups. These factors may play a role in presentation and predisposition to dermatologic diseases and other conditions in certain ethnic groups. Practices unique to some ethnic groups include but are not limited to the use of skin-lightening agents, unique hair grooming practices and styles, henna use by Africans and Middle Easterners, and dietary differences such as chili peppers in Hispanic diet. It also includes alternative medicine practices such as cupping, moxibustion, and Cao gio as practiced by Southeast Asians. Dermatologists should be knowledgeable of these practices so as to provide culturally sensitive care to their ethnic patients.

The misuse and excessive use of skin-lightening agents in ethnic populations, particularly of African descent, has been widely reported in literature [99–101]. Several of the products used in the United States are often purchased from the internet or beauty supply stores that cater to the cosmetic needs of African, Caribbean, and Asian communities. Some of these over-the-counter products contain hydroquinone or potent topical steroids such as clobetasol [58]. Potential adverse side effects of these practices have also been studied, and they include exogenous ochronosis, irritant and allergic contact dermatitis, extensive striae, skin atrophy, and adrenal insufficiency [99, 100].

In one study, 33 out of 35 subjects reported that they make mixtures of a superpotent topical steroid diluted with skin-lightening creams, some of which contained hydroquinone concentrations as high as 4–16% [100]. This study also found a distinctive late stage of exogenous ochronosis termed *pigmented colloid milium* in 11% of Africans living in Paris, who reported current or past use of skin-bleaching creams. Another study on the use of skin-lightening products in pregnant women in Senegal found a higher rate of low birth weight and small placentas in those who reported using highly potent steroid creams [102]. These reports underscore the need for dermatologists to increase public awareness and assess for the use of these OTC agents by their ethnic patients.

Due to the unique properties of ethnic hair, African, African-American, African-Caribbean, and Hispanic women use hairstyles and techniques that may lead to temporary or permanent traction alopecia [58]. These hairstyles and techniques include braids with extensions, cornrows, microbraids, twists, hot combing, and curl ironing. Also, hair pomades, which contain mixtures of comedogenic agents like petrolatum and lanolin, are more frequently used in Black and Hispanic populations. The waxy nature of these pomades helps alleviate dry scalp and itching associated with seborrheic dermatitis and also aids in coating and protecting the hair shafts [58, 102]. Adverse events include pomade acne, comedogenic acne involving the forehead and temples.

Henna is a natural dye made from a shrub indigenous to Africa and the Middle East, known as *Lawsonia alba* [102]. When the dry leaves of this shrub are soaked, it produces various colors. This dye is then applied to the skin, hair, and nails for decorative purposes during certain ceremonies and rituals such as circumcisions. However, there have been reported cases of hemolysis and neonatal hyperbilirubinemia secondary to the oxidizing effect of *L. alba* on red blood cells, especially those that are G6PD-deficient [103]. Capsaicin dermatitis is a contact dermatitis caused by chile peppers which is more commonly used by Hispanics as a condiment in their diet [2]. These chile peppers can produce irritation, burning pain, and erythema when handled, and patients should be advised to wear gloves prior to coming into contact with these peppers.

Traditional healing practices common to the Asian population include Cao gio (also termed coining), cupping, and moxibustion. These practices are used on various parts of the body such as the back, chest, shoulders, forehead, and arms for treatment of flu-like symptoms, febrile illnesses, and headaches [104]. They are believed to bring bad blood to the surface and cause bad or excessive wind to escape from the body, thereby restoring balance [105]. Cao gio involves application of an analgesic ointment such as "Tiger balm" or "Monkey balm" to the area to be abraded, after which the skin is firmly rubbed or pinched with the smooth edge of a metal object such as a spoon or coin. This procedure results in erythema, streaks of petechiae, and ecchymosis that eventually disappear in a few days [104–106]. Care must be taken to avoid interpreting these lesions as physical or child abuse.

Cupping is another healing practice that makes use of cups or jars with bell-like suction applied to the skin which pulls the involved skin into the cup or jar for brief moments. This produces circular and ecchymotic lesions that also resolve after a few days. Moxibustion on the other hand results in circular burns from skin contact with heated stick and embers from burning incense [58]. Again, dermatologists should be aware of these presentations in order not to associate them with physical abuse.

## References

1. Talakoub L, Wesley NO. Differences in perceptions of beauty and cosmetic procedures performed in ethnic patients. Semin Cutan Med Surg. 2009;28(2):115–29.
2. US Census Bureau. Population projections of the US by age, sex, race and Hispanic origin: 1995–2050. Current population report: 25–1130. Washington, DC: US Government Press; 2002.
3. Halder RM, Nootheti PK. Ethnic skin disorders overview. J Am Acad Dermatol. 2003;48(6):S143–8. Supplement 1.
4. Carlson BM. Integumentary, skeletal, and muscular systems. In: Carlson BM, editor. Human embryology and developmental biology. 1st ed. St. Louis: Mosby; 1994. p. 153–8.
5. Wilson D, Berdardesca E, Maiback HI. In vitro transepidermal water loss: differences between Black and White skin. Br J Dermatol. 1988;119:647–52.
6. Kompaore F, Marty JP, Dupont C. In vivo evaluation of the stratum corneum barrier function in Blacks, Caucasians and Asians with two non-invasive methods. Skin Pharmacol. 1993;6:200–7.
7. Kompaore F, Marty JP, Dupont C. In vivo evaluation in man by two noninvasive methods of the stratum corneum barrier function after physical and chemical modifications. Int J Cosmetic Sci. 1991;13(6):293–302.
8. Berardesca E, Maibach HI. Racial differences in sodium lauryl sulfate induced cutaneous irritation: Black and White. Contact Dermatitis. 1988;18:65–70.
9. Berardesca E, Maibach HI. Sodium-lauryl-sulphate-induced cutaneous irritation comparison of White and Hispanic subjects. Contact Dermatitis. 1988;19:136–40.
10. Berardesca E. Racial differences in skin function. Acta Derm Venereol. 1994;185(suppl):44–6.
11. Warrier AG, Kligman AM, Harper RA, Bowman J, Wickett RR. A comparison of Black and White skin using noninvasive methods. J Soc Cosmetic Chem. 1996;47:229–40.
12. Sonia Badreshia-Bansal, Taylor SC. The structure and function of skin of color. In: Kelly PA, Kelly AP, Taylor SC, editors. Dermatology for skin of color. 1st ed. New York: McGraw-Hill; 2009. p. 71–7.
13. Fotoh C, Elkhyat A, et al. Cutaneous differences between Black, African or Caribbean mixed-race and Caucasian women: biometrological approach of the hydrolipidic film. Skin Res Technol. 2008;14(3):327–35.

14. Wesley NO, Maibach HI. Racial (ethnic) differences in skin properties: the objective data. Am J Clin Dermatol. 2003;4(12):843–60.
15. Man MQ, Sin XJ, et al. Variation of skin surface pH, sebum content and stratum corneum hydration with age and gender in a large Chinese population. Skin Pharmacol Physiol. 2009;22(4):190–9.
16. Diridollou S, Rigal J, et al. Comparative study of the hydration of the stratum corneum between four ethnic groups: influence of age. Int J Dermatol. 2007;46 Suppl 1:11–4.
17. Hachem J, Crumrine D, et al. pH directly regulates epidermal permeability barrier homeostasis, and stratum corneum integrity/cohesion. J Invest Dermatol. 2003;121:345–53.
18. Hellemans L, et al. Characterization of stratum corneum properties in human subjects from a different genetic background. J Invest Dermatol. 2005;124:371.
19. Berardesca E, Pirot F, Singh M, et al. Differences in stratum corneum pH gradient when comparing White Caucasian and Black African-American skin. Br J Dermatol. 1998;139:855–7.
20. Weigand DA, Haygood C, Gaylor JR. Cell layers and density of Negro and Caucasian stratum corneum. J Invest Dermatol. 1974;62:563–8.
21. Corcuff P, Lotte C, Rougier A, et al. Racial differences in corneocytes: a comparison between Black, White, and oriental skin. Acta Derm Venereal. 1978;70:355–7. (Stockh) 1991; 71: 146–8.
22. Reinerston RP, Wheatley VR. Studies on the chemical composition of human epidermal lipids. J Invest Dermatol. 1959;32:49–59.
23. Harding CR, Moore AE, et al. Dandruff: a condition characterized by decreased levels of intercellular lipids in scalp stratum corneum and impaired barrier function. Arch Dermatol Res. 2002;294:221–30.
24. Olson RL, Gaylor J, Everett MA. Skin color, melanin, and erythema. Arch Dermatol. 1973;108:541–4.
25. Mitchell R. The skin of the Australian aborigines: a light and electron microscopical study. Aust J Dermatol. 1968;9:314.
26. Kaidbey KH, Agin PP, Sayre RM, Kligman A. Photoprotection by melanin – a comparison of Black and Caucasian skin. J Am Acad Dermatol. 1979;1:249–60.
27. Szabo G. Pigment cell biology. In: Gordon M, editor. Mitochondria and other cytoplasmic inclusions. New York: Academic; 1959.
28. Starkco RS, Pinkush H. Quantitative and qualitative data on the pigment cell of adult human epidermis. J Invest Dermatol. 1957;28:33.
29. Lehman AL, Silvers WK, et al. The underwhite (uw) locus acts autonomously and reduces the production of melanin. J Invest Dermatol. 2000;115(4):601–6.
30. Smit NPM, Kolb RM, Lentjes EGWM, Noz KC, van der Meulen H, Koerten HK, et al. Variations in lelanin formation by cultured melanocytes from different skin types. Arch Dermatol Res. 1998;290:342–9.
31. Alaluf S, Heath A, Carter N, et al. Variation in melanin content and composition in type V and VI photoexposed and photoprotected human skin: the dominant role of DHI. Pigment Cell Res. 2001;14:337–47.
32. Alaluf S, Atkins D, Barrett K, Blount M, Carter N, Heath A. Ethnic variation in melanin content and composition in photoexposed and photoprotected human skin. Pigment Cell Res. 2002;15:112–8.
33. Thong Y, Jee SH, et al. The patterns of melanosome distribution in keratinocytes of human skin as one determining factor of skin colour. Br J Dermatol. 2003;149(3):498–505.
34. Toda K, Patnak MA, Parrish A, Fitzpatrick TB. Alteration of racial differences in melanosome distribution in human epidermis after exposure to ultraviolet light. Nat New Biol. 1972;236:143–4.
35. Montagna W, Carlisle K. The architecture of Black and White facial skin. J Am Acad Dermatol. 1991;24:929–37.
36. Herzberg AJ, Dinehart SM. Chronologic aging in Black skin. Am J Dermatopathol. 1989;11:319–28.

37. Ancans J, Tobin DJ, Hoogduijn MJ, Smit NP, Wakamatsu K, Thody AJ. Melanosomal pH controls rate of melanogenesis, eumelanin/phaeomelanin ratio and melanosome maturation in melanocytes and melanoma cells. Exp Cell Res. 2001;268:26–35.
38. Yohn JJ, Lyons BM, et al. Cultured human melanocytes from Black and White donors have different sunlight and ultraviolet A radiation sensitivities. J Invest Dermatol. 1992;99(4):454–9.
39. Gunathilake R, Schurer N, et al. pH-regulated mechanisms account for pigment-type differences in epidermal barrier function. J Invest Dermatol. 2009;129:1719–29.
40. Tadokoro T, Kobayashi N, Zmudzka BZ, et al. UV induced DNA damage and melanin content in human skin differing in racial/ethnic origin. J Fed Am Soc Exp Biol. 2003;17:1177–9.
41. De Winter S, Vink AA, Roza L, Pavel S. Solar-simulated skin adaptation and its effect on subsequent UV-induced epidermal DNA damage. J Invest Dermatol. 2001;117:678–82.
42. Querleux B, Baldeweck T, et al. Skin from various ethnic origins and aging: an in vivo cross-sectional multimodality imaging study. Skin Res Technol. 2009;15:306–13.
43. Girardeau S, et al. The Caucasian and African skin types differ morphologically and functionally in their dermal component. Exp Dermatol. 2009;18:704–11.
44. Sugiyama-Nakagiri Y, et al. Ethnic differences in the structural properties of facial skin. J Dermatol Sci. 2009;53:135–9.
45. Johnson Jr BL. Differences in skin type. In: Johnson Jr BL, Moy RL, White GM, editors. Ethnic skin: medical and surgical. St. Louis: Mosby; 1998. p. 3–5.
46. Sueki H, Whitaker-Menezes D, Kligman AM. Structural diversity of mast cell granules in Black and White skin. Br J Dermatol. 2001;144:85–93.
47. Ketchum LD, et al. Hypertrophic and keloidal scars. Plast Reconstr Surg. 1974;53:140–54.
48. Oluwasanmi JO. Keloidal scars in the African. Clin Plast Surg. 1974;1:179–95.
49. Kischer CW, Bunce H, Sheltar MR. Mast cell analysis in hypertrophic scars, hypertrophic scars treated with pressure and mature scars. J Invest Dermatol. 1978;70:355–7.
50. Malkinson FD, Gehlman L. Factors affecting percutaneous absorption. In: Drill VA, Lazar P, editors. Cutaneous toxicology. New York: Academic; 1977.
51. Scheuplein RJ, Blank IH. Permeability of the skin. Physiol Rev. 1971;51:702.
52. Marzulli FN. Barriers to skin penetration. J Invest Dermatol. 1962;39:387.
53. Reed JT, Ghadially R, Elias PM. Effect of race gender, and skin type of epidermal permeability barrier function. J Invest Dermatol. 1994;102:537.
54. Stoughton RB. Bioassay methods for measuring percutaneous absorption. In: Montagna W, Stoughton RB, van Scott EJ, editors. Pharmacology of the skin. New York: Appleton; 1969. p. 542–4.
55. Berardesca E, Maibach HI. Racial differences in pharmacodynamic responses to nicotinates in vivo in human skin: Black and White. Arch Derm Venereol. 1990;70:63–6.
56. Wickrema-Sinha WJ, Shaw SR, Weber OJ. Percutaneous absorption and excretion of tritium-labelled diflorasone diacetate: a new topical corticosteroid in the rat, monkey and man. J Invest Dermatol. 1978;7:372–7.
57. Guy RH, Tur E, Bjerke S, Maibach H. Are there age and racial differences to methyl nicotinate-induced vasodilatation in human skin? J Am Acad Dermatol. 1985;12:1001–6.
58. Taylor S. Understanding skin of colour. J Am Acad Dermatol. 2002;46(Suppl):S41–2.
59. Frosch RJ, Kligman AM. The chamber scarification test for assessing irritancy of topically applied substances. In: Drill VA, Lazar P, editors. Cutaneous toxicology. New York: Academic; 1977. p. 150.
60. Berardesca E, Maibach HI. Cutaneous reactive hyperemia: racial differences induced by corticoid application. Br J Dermatol. 1989;129:787–94.
61. Goh CL, Chia SE. Skin irritability to sodium-lauryl sulphate-as measured by skin water vapour loss – by sex and race. Clin Exp Dermatol. 1988;13:16–9.
62. Robinson MK. Population differences in acute skin irritation response: race, sex, sensitive skin and repeat subject comparisons. Contact Dermatitis. 2002;46:86–93.
63. Foy V, Weinkauff R, Whittle E, Basketter DA. Ethnic variation in the skin irritation response. Contact Dermatitis. 2001;45:346–9.

64. Aramaki J, Kawana S, Effendy I, Happle R, Loffler H. Differences of skin irritation between Japanese and European women. Br J Dermatol. 2002;146:1052–6.
65. Szabo G, Gerald AB, Patnak MA, Fitzpatrick TB. Racial differences in the fate of melanosomes in humane epidermis. Nature. 1969;222:1081–2.
66. Halder RM, Bridgeman-Shah S. Skin cancer in African Americans. Cancer. 1995;75:667–73.
67. English DR, Armstrong BK, Kricker A, Fleming C. Sunlight and cancer. Cancer Causes Control. 1997;8:271–83.
68. Abe T, Arai S, Mimura K, Hayakawa R. Studies of physiological factors affecting skin susceptibility to ultraviolet light irradiation and irritants. J Dermatol. 1983;10:531–7.
69. Yamaguchi Y, Takahashi K, et al. Human skin responses to UV radiation: pigment in the upper epidermis protects against DNA damage in the lower epidermis and facilitates apoptosis. FASEB J. 2006;20:1486–8.
70. Tadokoro T, Yamaguchi Y, Batzer J, Coelho SG, Zmudzka BZ, Miller SA, et al. Mechanisms of skin tanning in different racial/ethnic groups in response to ultraviolet radiation. J Invest Dermatol. 2005;124:1326–32.
71. Rijken F, Brunijnzeel PLB, van Weedlden H, Kiekens RCM. Responses of Black and White skin to solar simulating radiation: differences in DNA photodamage, infiltrating neutrophils, proteolytic enzymes induced, keratinocyte activation and IL-10 expression. J Invest Dermatol. 2004;122:1448–55.
72. Yamaguchi Y, Beer J, et al. Melanin mediated apoptosis of epidermal cells damaged by ultraviolet radiation: factors influencing the incidence of skin cancer. Arch Dermatol Res. 2008;30:S43–50.
73. Jablonski NG, Chaplin G. The evolution of human skin coloration. J Hum Evol. 2000;39(1):57–106.
74. Loomis WF. Skin-pigment regulation of vitamin-D biosynthesis in man. Science. 1967;157(788):501–6.
75. Aoki K. Sexual selection as a cause of human skin color variation: Darwin's hypothesis revisited. Ann Hum Biol. 2002;29(6):589–608.
76. Lips P. Vitamin D physiology. Prog Biophys Mol Biol. 2006;92(1):4–8.
77. Webb AR, Holick MF. The role of sunlight in the cutaneous production of vitamin D3. Annu Rev Nutr. 1988;8:375–99.
78. Webb AR, DeCosta BR, Holick MF. Sunlight regulates the cutaneous production of vitamin D3 by causing its photodegradation. J Clin Endocrinol Metab. 1989;68(5):882–7.
79. Yuen AW, Vitamin NG. Vitamin D: in the evolution of human skin colour. Med Hypotheses. 2010;74(1):39–44.
80. Looker AC, Dawson-Hughes B. Seasonal changes in plasma 25-hydroxyvitamin D status of adolescents and adults in two seasonal subpopulations from NHANES III. Bone. 2002;30:771–7.
81. Brazerol WF, McPhee AJ, et al. Serial UVB exposure and serum 25 hydroxyvitamin D response in young adult Americans Black and Whites. J Am Coll Nutr. 1988;7:111–8.
82. Harris SS, Dawson-Hughes B. Seasonal changes in plasma 25-hydroxyvitamin D concentrations of young American Black and White women. Am J Clin Nutr. 1998;67:1232–6.
83. Cornish DA, Maluleke V, Mhlanga T. An investigation into a possible relationship between vitamin D, parathyroid hormone, calcium and magnesium in a normally pigmented and an albino rural Black population in the Northern Province of South Africa. Biofactors. 2000;11:35–8.
84. Harris SS. Vitamin D and African Americans. Am Soc Nutr. 2006;136:1126–9.
85. Johnson LG, Landon MM. Eccrine sweat gland activity and racial differences in resting skin conductance. Psychophysiology. 1965;1:322–9.
86. Montagna W, Parakkal PF. The structure and function of skin. 3rd ed. New York: Academic; 1974.
87. McCance RA, Purohit G. Ethnic differences in response to the sweat glands to pilocarpine. Nature. 1969;221:378–9.
88. McCance RA, Rutishauser IHE, Knight HC. Response to sweat glands to pilocarpine in the Bantu of Uganda. Lancet. 1968;1:663–5.

89. Calhoun DA, Oparil S. Racial differences in the pathogenesis of hypertension. Am J Med Sci. 1995;310:S86–90.
90. Homma H. On apocrine sweat glands in White and Negro men and women. Bull Johns Hopkins Hosp. 1956;38:365.
91. Schiefferdecker P. Die Hautdruisen des Menschen und der Saugetiere, ihre biologische und rassenanatomische Bedeutung, sowie die Muscularis sexualis. Zoologica. 1922;27:1–154.
92. Homma H. On apocrine sweat glands in White and Negro men and women. Bull Johns Hopkins Hosp. 1926;38:365.
93. Hurley HJ, Shelley WB. The physiology and pharmacology of the apocrine sweat gland. In: Hurley HJ, Shelley WB, editors. The human apocrine sweat gland in health and disease. Springfield: Charles Thompson; 1960.
94. Goldsmith LA. Biology of eccrine and apocrine sweat glands. In: Freedberg IM, Eisen AZ, Wolff K, Austen KF, Goldsmith LA, et al., editors. Fitzpatrick's dermatology in general medicine, vol. 1. New York: McGraw-Hill; 1999.
95. Kligman AM, Shelley WB. An investigation of the biology of the sebaceous gland. J Invest Dermatol. 1958;30:99–125.
96. Pochi P, Strauss JS. Sebaceous gland activity in Black skin. Dermatol Clin. 1988;6:349.
97. Abedeen SK, Gonzalez M, Judodihardjo H, Gaskell S, Dykes P. Racial variation in sebum excretion rate. Program and abstracts of the 58th annual meeting of the American Academy of Dermatology; March 10–15. San Francisco; 2000. Abstract #559.
98. Yamamoto A, Serizawa S, Ito M. Effect of aging on sebaceous gland activity and on the fatty acid composition of wax eaters. Invest Dermatol. 1987;89:507.
99. del Guidice P, Yves P. The widespread use of skin lightening creams in Senegal: a persistent public health problem in West Africa. Int J Dermatol. 2002;41(2):68–72.
100. Petit A, Cohen-Ludmann C, Clevenbergh P, Bergmann JF, Dubertret L. Skin lightening and its complications among African people living in Paris. J Am Acad Dermatol. 2006;55:873–8.
101. Holloway V. Ethnic cosmetic products. Dermatol Clin. 2003;21:743–9.
102. Mahe A, et al. The cosmetic use of skin-lightening products pregnancy in Dakar, Senegal: a common and potentially hazardous practice. Trans R Soc Trop Med Hyg. 2007;101:183–7.
103. Sir Hazsnim M. Poisoning from henna dye and paraphenylenediamine mixture in children in Khartoum. Ann Trop Paediatr. 1992;12:3–6.
104. Zinkham WH, Oski FA. Henna: a potential cause of oxidative hemolysis and neonatal hyperbilirubinemia. Pediatrics. 1996;97:707–9.
105. Look KM, Look RM. Skin scraping, cupping, and moxibustion that may mimic physical abuse. J Forensic Sci. 1997;42:103–5.
106. Davis RE. Cultural health care or child abuse? The Southeast Asian practice of Caogio. J Am Acad Nurse Pract. 2000;12(3):89–95.

# Chapter 2
# Acne and Rosacea in Skin of Color

**Sejal K. Shah and Andrew F. Alexis**

Acne vulgaris (AV) and rosacea are among the most common skin disorders treated by dermatologists. While both conditions can affect individuals of all racial and ethnic backgrounds, variations in clinical presentation and approaches to treatment exist. This chapter will review the epidemiology, clinical features, and management of AV and rosacea in darkly pigmented patient populations.

## Acne Vulgaris

### *Clinical Features*

Acne vulgaris (AV) in skin of color shares many of the clinical features typically seen in lighter skin types. However, concomitant postinflammatory hyperpigmentation (PIH) is a key distinguishing feature of acne in the darker-skinned patient (Fig. 2.1). PIH is often of equal or greater concern to patients with skin of color as the acne itself. Patients frequently refer to the lesions of PIH as *scars,* and the cosmetic disfigurement caused by PIH adds to the psychological distress associated with acne. While pigmentary alterations can occur without manipulation of acne lesions, they tend to be more severe and of longer duration in excoriated lesions (e.g., in patients with acne excoriee). Excoriated lesions typically appear as hypopigmented macules with hyperpigmented borders (Fig. 2.2).

S.K. Shah, M.D.
Department of Dermatology, St. Luke's-Roosevelt Hospital Center,
1090 Amsterdam, Suite 11D, New York, NY 10025, USA

A.F. Alexis, M.D., MPH (✉)
Skin of Color Center, Department of Dermatology, St. Luke's Roosevelt Hospital
and Columbia University College of Physicians and Surgeons,
New York, NY, USA
e-mail: alexisderm@yahoo.com

A.F. Alexis and V.H. Barbosa (eds.), *Skin of Color: A Practical Guide to Dermatologic Diagnosis and Treatment*, DOI 10.1007/978-0-387-84929-4_2,

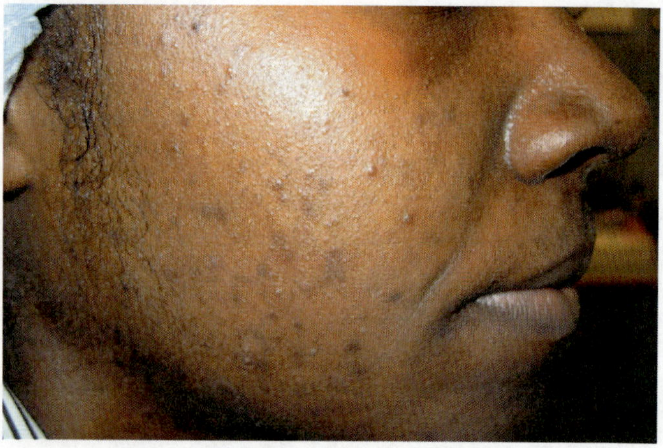

**Fig. 2.1** Acne vulgaris with postinflammatory hyperpigmentation

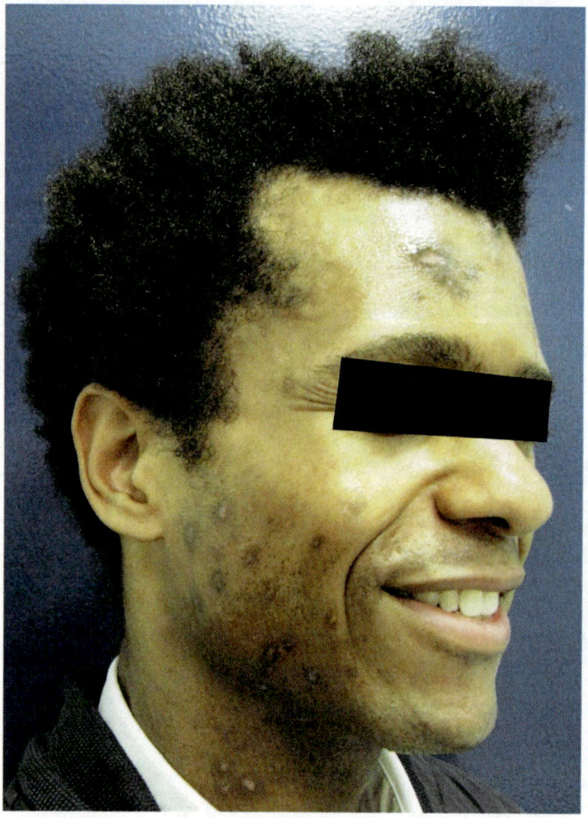

**Fig. 2.2** Acne excoriee with severe postinflammatory pigment alteration

**Table 2.1** Factors that may exacerbate AV in SOC

| |
|---|
| *Hair pomades* |
| – May contain any of the following: petroleum jelly, mineral oil, wax, beeswax, olive oil |
| Corticosteroid-containing skin bleaching products (e.g., Movate®, Lemonvate®, Le Gel®, Fashion Fair®, Dermavate®, Topsone®) |
| *Occlusive skin products* |
| – Cocoa butter |
| – Comedogenic makeups (e.g., when used to mask hyperpigmentation) |

Cultural skin and hair care practices may play a role in the development of acne and affect clinical presentation (Table 2.1). *Pomade acne*, which consists predominantly of comedonal lesions along the hairline, occurs secondary to the use of pomade and other thick, occlusive hair products. Corticosteroid-containing skin bleaching agents, which may be used by some dark-skinned patients to improve hyperpigmentation or lighten complexion, can induce steroid acne. When such non-prescription (and in many cases illegally sold over the counter) bleaching creams are used, patients are frequently unaware that they contain corticosteroids (which are commonly potent or superpotent). As such, when examining a patient who has clinical features of steroid acne, it is prudent to inquire specifically about skin lightening or "fade" creams and have the patient bring in all products that are being used so that the ingredient list can be reviewed. By taking these steps, misuse of potent/superpotent corticosteroids can be discontinued and the patient can be educated on the importance of avoiding the use of such agents without a prescription and the guidance of their physician. In addition, thick, comedogenic cosmetic cover-ups often used to mask hyperpigmentation may induce or exacerbate acne.

A lower incidence of nodulocystic acne has been reported in African-Americans compared to both Caucasians and Hispanics [1]. However, the development of keloids on the trunk as a result of nodulocystic acne is a potential long-term sequela that is more commonly seen in patients with skin of color, especially those of African descent.

Acne is a disorder of the pilosebaceous unit that is caused by four key pathogenic factors: excess sebum production, follicular epithelial hyperproliferation and plugging, *Propionibacterium acnes* (*P. acnes*) colonization, and inflammation. There is not adequate data to suggest racial/ethnic differences in these etiologic factors. However, Halder et al. [2] found marked polymorphonuclear cell infiltration in biopsies of each type of acne lesions including comedones (i.e., clinically noninflammatory lesions) in a study involving 30 black female subjects. It has been hypothesized that this subclinical inflammation may contribute to an increased susceptibility to developing postinflammatory hyperpigmentation (PIH) in black patients.

## *Epidemiology*

Published studies suggest that AV is one of the most common dermatologic disorders among patients with skin of color as it is in the general population. A recent practice survey conducted by Alexis et al. found it to be the most common diagnosis

**Table 2.2** Treatment pearls for acne in SOC

*Reduce inflammation*
- Initiate effective and appropriately aggressive treatment early in disease course
- Include topical BPO and topical retinoid in treatment regimen
- Low threshold to initiate oral antibiotics when indicated

*Minimize irritation*
- Treatment regimen must be well tolerated
- Appropriate selection of vehicle, concentration, and dosing
- Gradual change of vehicle, concentration, and dosing as tolerated

*Eliminate exacerbating factors (see Table 2.1)*
- Use silicone-based hair products and noncomedogenic cosmetics (e.g., mineral makeups) and moisturizers
- Apply hair products at least 1 in. behind hairline or limit application to distal hair shafts

*Educate patient about PIH*
- Difference between active acne lesions and PIH
- Establish realistic expectation regarding treatment outcome (e.g., length of treatment, potential need for adjunctive treatments for PIH)
- Importance of sun protection

in both black and Caucasian patients at a New York City teaching hospital [3]. Likewise, Halder et al. [4] and Child et al. [5] reported it as the most common diagnosis in black patients, accounting for 27.7% and 13.7% of dermatoses, respectively [4, 5]. Data in other ethnic populations is limited. Among adult Asian patients at one clinic in Singapore, acne was reported as the second most common diagnosis with a prevalence of 10.9% [6]. It was reported as the most commonly diagnosed skin condition among Arab-Americans, and data on Hispanic/Latino patients suggest that it is the most common diagnosis in this group as well [7, 8].

## *Management*

Although treatments for acne are similar in all skin types, nuances in selection, dosing, timing, and combination of treatments exist for the safe and effective management of AV in skin of color. In patients with darkly pigmented skin, the increased risk of PIH is a key consideration. The selected regimen must be aggressive enough to clear the acne lesions and prevent the development of new lesions but also nonirritating so that PIH is not induced. Utilizing agents that improve PIH is also a necessary aspect of the treatment regimen as PIH itself is often the presenting complaint in patients with skin of color.

Treatment pearls for managing AV in skin of color are outlined in Table 2.2.

### Topical Therapy

Topical therapies for AV include retinoids and antimicrobials. Topical retinoids remain first-line treatment for AV and should be considered for every patient because they target hyperkeratinization and comedogenesis and possess anti-inflammatory and antifibrotic properties [1, 9]. Thus, they reduce both inflammatory and noninflammatory acne lesions. Retinoids are also capable of reducing hyperpigmentation by inhibiting tyrosinase, inhibiting melanosome transfer, dispersing epidermal melanin, and promoting desquamation which leads to removal of epidermal melanin [10–14].

The topical retinoids currently available in the USA – tretinoin, adapalene, and tazarotene – have been shown to be safe and effective in the treatment of patients with skin of color [10–12, 15]. As noted above, minimizing irritation that may inadvertently result in pigment alteration is essential. Tolerability depends on concentration, dosing, and vehicle, all of which must be taken into account when selecting a retinoid. When using tazarotene or generic tretinoin, the current authors recommend initiating treatment with a cream vehicle rather than an alcohol-based gel, as creams are less likely to cause drying and irritation. However, newer aqueous gel vehicles, microsphere formulations, and crystalline formulations are generally well tolerated and are also appropriate vehicles for first-line therapy in skin of color patients. Short contact application or alternate-night application is appropriate in patients who cannot tolerate nightly application; application time is gradually increased as tolerated. The concentration can also be increased as tolerated, usually after at least 4–6 weeks of treatment with the lower strength. For retinoid-naive patients, the current author (AFA) typically begins with any of the following retinoids depending on patient tolerability, severity of acne, and cost considerations: adapalene 0.1% gel or cream, tretinoin 0.025% or 0.05% cream (when generic is used) or 0.05% aqueous gel (when a branded product is used) or 0.04% gel (when a branded microsphere formulation is used), or tazarotene 0.05% cream. Over the course of treatment, changes can be made in the strength or the specific retinoid prescribed depending on efficacy and tolerability. In addition, patients should be advised to use gentle cleansers and moisturizers with sunscreen and discontinue all harsh and potentially irritating skin products, especially astringents and exfoliating treatments that may increase their sensitivity to topical retinoids.

Benzoyl peroxide (BPO) and topical antibiotics are also important in the management of AV. Similar to retinoids, the primary consideration when selecting an antimicrobial agent is maximizing efficacy while minimizing irritation and the potential for pigment alteration. One advantage of BPO is that it is bactericidal and helps to prevent the development of antibiotic-resistant strains of *P. acnes*; therefore, it should be included in all antibiotic regimens for AV.

The safety and efficacy of topical products containing benzoyl peroxide have been evaluated in several studies. In an 8-week, community-based trial of 5% benzoyl peroxide-1% clindamycin gel, no racial/ethnic differences in efficacy were observed [16, 17]. In skin of color patients, it is appropriate to add a topical retinoid, especially to treat PIH. A study comparing three different regimens consisting of BPO 5%-clindamycin 1% gel plus either tretinoin microsphere (RAM) 0.04% gel, RAM 0.1% gel, or adapalene 0.1% gel for the treatment of acne and PIH reported better results with BPO 5%-clindamycin 1% gel plus RAM 0.04% gel [18]. While benzoyl peroxide is safe and effective in patients with skin of color, caution is advised to minimize irritation – which could result in postinflammatory pigment alteration.

With this in mind, utilizing benzoyl peroxide in concentrations of 5% or less is preferred for the face, with a lower risk of dryness and irritation with decreasing concentrations (e.g., 2.5% benzoyl peroxide tends to be less irritating or drying than 5% and therefore should be considered in a patient with sensitive and/or dry skin). In the author's (AFA) experience, the fixed combination clindamycin-benzoyl peroxide formulations (in aqueous gels) are less drying and better tolerated than erythromycin 3%-benzoyl peroxide 5% gel (the vehicle of which contains 20% alcohol).

When topical antibiotics are used, every attempt is made to use benzoyl peroxide concurrently to minimize the development of antibiotic resistance. This is best achieved with the fixed combination products mentioned above but can also be done with separate agents when desired (e.g., for cost reasons). When this approach is taken, the current authors prescribe clindamycin phosphate 1% (in a lotion for patients with dry or sensitive skin and gel for those with oily skin) in combination with a benzoyl peroxide wash. A recently approved fixed combination retinoid-benzoyl peroxide formulation containing adapalene 0.1% and benzoyl peroxide 2.5% in an aqueous gel has also been studied in subjects with skin of color and is an appropriate treatment option for this population when combination treatment is required [19].

Azelaic acid 20% cream has also been found to successfully treat acne. It has been reported to be as effective as tretinoin 0.05% cream, BPO 5% gel, erythromycin 2% ointment, and clindamycin 1% gel [20, 21]. It is not only an anti-inflammatory but also reduces *P. acnes* proliferation and normalizes keratinization. Like BPO, *P. acnes* resistance to azelaic acid has not been reported [21]. Azelaic acid is well tolerated and relatively mild, so it is a suitable option for individuals with sensitive skin [9]. It appears to have an inhibitory effect on melanocyte proliferation and melanogenesis, so it can potentially reduce hyperpigmentation [1, 9]. It is an especially useful treatment option for skin of color patients with PIH who cannot tolerate retinoids. Azelaic acid can be combined with other acne therapies to improve efficacy [1, 21]. Greater efficacy and patient satisfaction have been reported with various topical combination regimens containing azelaic acid compared to monotherapy. Another study reported a greater reduction in lesion counts, both inflammatory and noninflammatory, and tolerability with azelaic acid plus BPO 4% gel compared to erythromycin 3%-BPO 5% gel [21]. In this author's (AFA) experience, the efficacy of azelaic acid (as monotherapy) in the treatment of acne tends to be less than that observed with topical benzoyl peroxide formulations or retinoids; as such, it is reserved as a second-line agent.

Topical dapsone 5% gel is a sulfone in aqueous gel that has been recently approved in the USA for the treatment of AV. Clinical trial data [22] and clinical experience suggest that dapsone 5% gel is well tolerated and no racial/ethnic differences in safety have been identified. Therefore, topical dapsone should also be considered an appropriate therapeutic option in the topical management of AV in skin of color patients.

## Oral Therapy

For patients with moderate-to-severe acne, systemic therapy may be required to achieve satisfactory results. Oral treatments consist of antibiotics, retinoids, and hormonal modulators. In skin of color patients, a lower threshold to initiate oral treatment is recommended in order to reduce inflammation at an earlier stage, thus reducing the risk of PIH and scarring.

## Procedural Therapies

In-office procedures are often utilized as adjunctive therapeutic options for AV.

Two well-established and widely used procedures are comedone extraction and intralesional corticosteroids. Their key advantages are that they do not require any anesthesia, do not have any associated "downtime" or significant post-procedure care, and quickly lead to resolution of targeted lesions. Comedone extraction, or acne surgery, reduces comedones, both open and closed, by pushing out the follicular plug. Topical retinoids may make the lesions more amenable to extraction, and a 6–8-week course prior to the procedure is recommended in skin of color patients to help reduce trauma and PIH [9]. Intralesional corticosteroids (e.g., triamcinolone acetonide 2.5–5.0 mg/cc) can be used to treat inflammatory lesions. Improvement is usually noted within 2–5 days. These "quick fix" treatments are often beneficial in patients with skin of color to prevent progression to larger lesions or the development of negative sequelae.

Superficial chemical peels can be used to treat both acne and PIH, but deep chemical peels are not recommended in patients with skin of color as they are associated with a greater risk of scarring and PIH. Superficial chemical peels include salicylic acid 20–30%, glycolic acid 20–70%, trichloroacetic acid 10–35%, and Jessner's peel [9]. In this author's (AFA) experience, salicylic acid peels are the preferred choice for patients with both acne and PIH. Grimes [23] investigated the safety and efficacy of 20–30% salicylic acid peels performed every 2 weeks in 25 patients (skin types V and VI) with various conditions including acne and PIH. A series of five peels resulted in moderate to significant improvement in eight of the nine patients with acne and in all five patients with PIH. Only transient (≤14 days duration) crusting, dryness, and dyschromia were reported [23]. However, a recent split-face study (n = 10) – in which one half of the face was treated with five salicylic acid peels (two 20% peels followed by three 30% peels) while the contralateral side remained untreated – failed to show a significant difference in PIH reduction on the treatment side compared to the untreated side as measured by blinded investigators' assessment (using a visual analog scale) [24]. Further studies (that are larger and of longer duration) are needed to substantiate the use of peels in the management of PIH secondary to AV. To minimize adverse effects, peels should be initiated at the lowest concentration and titrated up as tolerated and performed at a minimum of 4-week intervals. If the patient is also being treated with a retinoid, it should be discontinued 7 days prior to each peel. Discontinuation of benzoyl peroxide containing agents

1–2 days prior to peels is optional and, in this author's experience (AFA), is not usually necessary. Pre- and posttreatment with a hydroquinone-containing product is often added to reduce the risk of treatment-associated PIH, but this is also optional and usually not necessary in this author's (AFA) opinion – as long as careful technique and appropriate peeling agents are used to minimize the extent of epidermal injury.

Light, laser, and photodynamic treatments have not been well studied in skin of color patients. However, published studies using intense pulsed light (IPL) [25], IPL-photodynamic therapy (PDT) [25, 26], infrared lasers [27–29], blue light [30], red light [1, 31], aminolevulinic acid (ALA)-PDT [1, 31], ALA alone [1, 31], and methyl aminolevulinate (MAL)-PDT [32] have included a limited number of patients with skin types IV and greater and show promise in treating this patient population [1, 25–32].

### *Sequelae of Acne Vulgaris in Skin of Color*

Individuals with skin of color have an increased tendency to develop long-term sequelae secondary to acne, namely, PIH and keloids. Furthermore, in this population, PIH is often the presenting complaint and may be of equal or greater concern than the acne itself; accordingly, it must be thoroughly addressed and managed. Explaining to the patient the difference between active acne and PIH as well as establishing that resolution of both issues is the treatment goal helps to strengthen the physician-patient relationship and leads to greater adherence to the treatment regimen.

## Rosacea

Rosacea is a chronic inflammatory skin disorder that is characterized by flushing, telangiectasias, papules, and pustules predominantly in a centrofacial distribution. Its clinical presentation can be quite variable, making diagnosis rather challenging. In addition, it is often difficult to detect in darker-pigmented populations. Therefore, this section will focus on the clinical variants and approaches in skin of color.

### *Epidemiology*

Rosacea is more common in fair-skinned individuals of Western and Northern European descent. In one epidemiological study based in Sweden, a prevalence of 10% was reported among a nonselected population of office employees [33].

**Table 2.3** Acne vulgaris versus rosacea: key distinguishing feature

| Acne vulgaris | Rosacea |
|---|---|
| Comedones | Absence of comedones |
| Background erythema unusual | Background erythema typical |
| Absence of telangiectasias | Telangiectasias |
| Papules usually irregular +/– tenderness | Papules more uniform, nontender |
| Cystic lesions | Absence of cystic lesions |
| Involvement of face, shoulders/uppers arms, back and/or chest | Involvement typically limited to face, specifically central face/facial convexities |
| Skin sensitivity within the range of normal | Stinging/burning or intolerance of many topical agents |

Epidemiologic data regarding rosacea in nonwhite patient populations is limited [34]; among patients of color, its incidence is most likely highest in Asians and lowest in darkly pigmented racial/ethnic groups [35]. However, this observation may be based on easier disease recognition in Asians due to lighter skin type. Adler reported that African, Latino, or Asian patients comprise approximately 4% of rosacea patients [36, 37]. Several clinic-based studies investigating the epidemiology of skin diseases in black adult patients have not reported rosacea among the most common diagnoses [3–5, 38, 39]. In addition, an incidence of 0% and <0.1% was reported in Ghana and Kenya, respectively [40, 41]. Similarly, rosacea was not listed among the most common dermatologic diagnoses recorded in 3,000 Latino patients treated in a private- and hospital-based clinic [8]. However, a recent 5-year longitudinal cohort study of rosacea patients enrolled in North Carolina Medicaid and prescribed at least one topical prescription for rosacea found 16.27% of the patients to be African-American and 10.98% of "other race," suggesting that the prevalence of rosacea in nonwhite populations may be higher than previously reported. Overall, the limited data pertaining to rosacea in skin of color may reflect a truly lower prevalence or rather may be due to challenges in recognizing the disease in these populations [34].

## *Clinical Features*

The primary clinical features of rosacea include erythema, telangiectasias, papules, and pustules affecting the convexities of the face: cheeks, chin, nose, and central forehead. Secondary features include burning or stinging, plaques, dry appearance, edema, ocular involvement, nonfacial involvement, and phymatous changes [42]. There are four major subtypes of rosacea: erythematotelangiectatic, papulopustular, phymatous, and ocular. In addition, a granulomatous variant has been described. Clinical differences between acne vulgaris and rosacea are listed in Table 2.3.

Erythematotelangiectatic rosacea (ETR) is characterized by persistent facial flushing, usually greater than 10 min, that may extend to the neck and upper chest [43]. Initially, transient episodes of flushing may occur but with time the erythema becomes permanent and telangiectasias begin to form [35]. Triggers, such as alcohol, spicy foods, exercise, hot or cold weather, and emotional stress, may be reported [43]. Symptoms of burning or stinging are often experienced during episodes of flushing. These patients are typically more sensitive to topical products (e.g., cosmetics, sunscreens, medications) and may note worsening of symptoms after application. Scaling or "dryness" may also be reported and may be a result of irritation rather than the disease process [42]. In skin of color, the characteristic erythema of ETR may be more difficult to recognize; thus, the diagnosis may rest more on history – episodes of facial stinging and burning, especially in response to common triggers, and inability to tolerate various topical products. In addition, patients with this form of rosacea usually do not have a history of acne [43]. Diagnostic challenges notwithstanding, ETR is considered uncommon in darker-skinned racial/ethnic groups.

Patients with papulopustular rosacea (PPR), "classic rosacea," present with prominent erythema, papules, and pustules of the central face. This is the most common subtype observed in skin of color patients. Although similar in appearance to acne vulgaris (AV), one key distinction is the absence of comedones in rosacea. Edema may be associated with episodes of PPR, and external triggers are not a consistent feature [43]. Additionally, the inflammatory lesions in rosacea may be a deeper red compared to those of acne; this difference, likely related to increased vasoreactivity in rosacea, may be more difficult to appreciate in skin of color [35]. Distinguishing this variant from adult acne is often a challenge in skin of color patients. A history of trigger factors, a central distribution of papules/pustules and erythema, and an absence of comedones are helpful in making this diagnosis (Fig. 2.3). A history of stinging/burning and/or intolerance to many topical agents is a helpful clue in the diagnosis (especially when erythema is less apparent in a darker-skinned patient) [34].

Phymatous rosacea is characterized by significant skin thickening and irregular surface nodularities, which can affect the nose, chin, forehead, ears, and eyelids [43]. Papules, pustules, and erythema may also be present. This form of rosacea can markedly distort facial features. Reports of phymatous rosacea in nonwhite patients are exceedingly rare [44, 45].

Ocular rosacea has a variety of manifestations, most commonly blepharitis and conjunctivitis [43]. It may precede, occur concurrently, or present after cutaneous signs and symptoms. In a patient in whom the diagnosis of rosacea is unclear, ocular symptoms favor the diagnosis and warrant appropriate evaluation and management.

Features of granulomatous rosacea include yellow, brown, or red monomorphic papules or nodules in a periorificial distribution [43]. Unlike the primary subtypes, patients with this variant often lack flushing and persistent erythema and may have unilateral disease that is not limited to the central face but rather perioral, and often periocular, areas. It has been suggested that black patients have a tendency to develop this variant [46, 47]. Facial Afro-Caribbean childhood eruption (FACE syndrome) is considered a variant of granulomatous rosacea that is seen in African-American and Afro-Caribbean children [48].

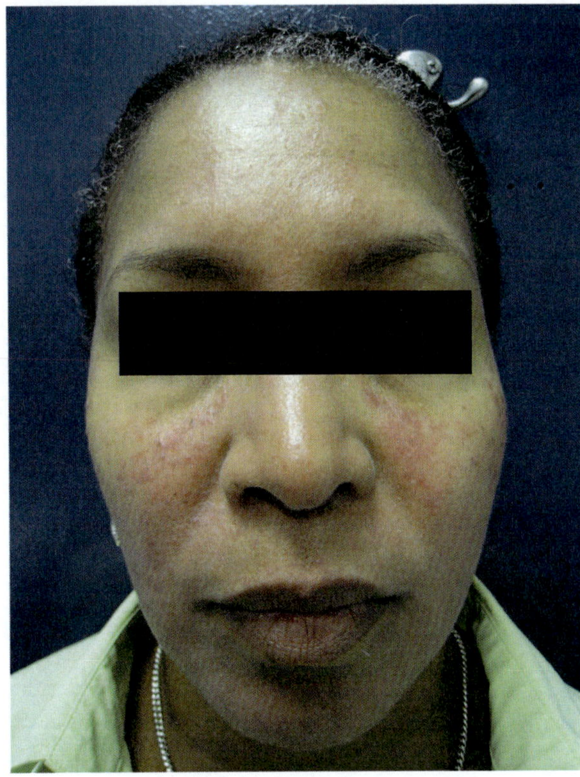

**Fig. 2.3** Rosacea in an African-American woman with Fitzpatrick skin type 4. Note papules, pustules and centrofacial erythema (without scale)

## *Management*

The treatment selected is based on the predominant variant of rosacea present and severity of disease. Studies investigating the treatment of rosacea in skin of color populations are sparse. Similar to treatment selection for AV, judicious selection of an efficacious treatment must be balanced with limiting the risks of pigment alteration and scarring in these patients. In addition to avoidance of triggers, treatment regimens consist of topical, oral, laser, and light therapies and surgical interventions. There is some treatment overlap between rosacea and AV as the two conditions share some clinical features.

Besides prescription products, there are several nonprescription elements that may comprise an effective treatment regimen. Because patients often exhibit a low tolerance to topical products, they should be advised to avoid harsh or irritating products. Soap-free cleansers; gentle emollients, especially as a base for other products; and cosmetics containing protective silicones are often beneficial [49]. Lastly, several redness-reducing cosmetic cover-ups and moisturizers are now readily available.

## Topical Therapy

Multiple topical agents have demonstrated efficacy in the management of rosacea, and no racial/ethnic differences in safety or efficacy have been reported. These agents include metronidazole [50–52], azelaic acid [53, 54], sodium sulfacetamide and sulfur [51], retinoids [49, 55], calcineurin inhibitors [56], benzoyl peroxide [57, 58], and topical antibiotics [49]. Of these, only the first three have been approved by the US Food and Drug Administration (FDA) for the treatment of papules, pustules, and erythema associated with rosacea. In this author's (AFA) experience, all of the above therapies are safe and effective options for rosacea in patients with skin of color; whereas metronidazole, azelaic acid, and sodium sulfacetamide are first-line topical agents, the others listed are alternative or adjunctive therapies to be considered for treatment failures. Tolerability may vary between the various topical agents; one study found metronidazole gel 1% (which has an aqueous vehicle containing niacinamide) to have a lower cumulative irritation potential than metronidazole gel 0.75%, which in turn had less irritation potential than azelaic acid gel 15% [59]. Sensitivity to topical retinoids and benzoyl peroxide is common among rosacea patients and should be used with caution.

## Oral Therapy

Oral treatments for rosacea include oral antibiotics, usually tetracyclines, and isotretinoin (typically used at lower doses than in acne patients – e.g., 0.5 mg/kg or less) [60]. Anti-inflammatory (or subantimicrobial) dose doxycycline (a once-daily 40-mg capsule consisting of 30 mg immediate-release and 10 mg delayed-release doxycycline beads) is the only FDA-approved oral therapy for rosacea. This formulation has demonstrated significantly greater improvement in inflammatory lesions compared to placebo [61]. Other tetracycline antibiotics have long been used off-label in the management of rosacea. However, growing concerns regarding the development of antibiotic-resistant bacteria are a major limitation. As with treatment regimens for AV, the oral medications may be combined with topical treatments.

Oral macrolides (i.e., erythromycin, azithromycin) and metronidazole are alternatives to the tetracyclines. These antibiotics may be used in the setting of tetracycline allergy or intolerance, failure to respond to tetracyclines, and contraindications to tetracyclines (e.g., pregnancy).

Isotretinoin has been shown to improve several rosacea variants, but there are only a few small studies investigating its efficacy [60, 62, 63]. It should be reserved for cases where conventional therapies have failed or as a nonsurgical treatment option for phymatous rosacea.

## Physical Modalities

Physical modalities include laser- and light-based treatments and more invasive surgical procedures. Laser and light therapies are increasingly being used to treat rosacea, especially ETR which is often resistant to topical and oral medication. Various laser- and light-based therapies have been studied, but as noted above, they have not been well studied in skin of color patients, and review of the literature did not reveal published data specifically for the treatment of rosacea in skin types IV–VI with these modalities. Vascular lasers are primarily used in the treatment of ETR and include pulsed dye laser (PDL), potassium-titanyl-phosphate (KTP) laser, and diode-pumped frequency-doubled laser [49]. In the past, it has been noted that the vascular lasers are relatively contraindicated in darker skin types because their wavelengths are absorbed not only by hemoglobin but also by epidermal melanin, thereby increasing the risk of side effects such as dyschromias [64]. However, both the 585- and 595-nm PDL have been shown to be safe and effective for the treatment of various vascular lesions in darker skin types. Dyspigmentation, usually hyperpigmentation, is a common adverse effect of PDL in darker skin, but it is usually transient and can be reduced by the use of skin cooling techniques [65]. Intense pulsed light has also been shown to be safe and effective in the treatment of vascular lesions in patients with darker skin [65, 66]. Advanced-stage phymatous rosacea which can cause significant disfigurement requires more invasive approaches including electrocautery, dermabrasion, laser ablation, and excision [49]. As these procedures are relatively aggressive, there is an increased risk of permanent pigment alteration and scarring in skin of color patients. Radiofrequency is a newer nonablative technique that is safe for all skin types and has shown promise in the treatment of phymatous rosacea [65, 67].

## Conclusion

Acne vulgaris and rosacea are common dermatological conditions that affect all racial and ethnic groups. Although the basic pathophysiology involved in the development of both diseases is likely similar in all skin types, variations in the clinical presentation are seen in skin of color. The dermatologist treating a patient with darkly pigmented skin must be cognizant of the propensity to develop PIH and keloidal scarring in this population and choose treatment regimens appropriately. In patients with darker skin types, the need for early aggressive interventions must be balanced with the risk of irritation. When performing procedural therapies, measures must be taken to limit cutaneous injury given the increased risk of PIH and scarring. Newer laser and light modalities are a promising development in the management of acne and rosacea; however, more data is needed to elucidate optimal treatment parameters in skin of color patients.

## References

1. Hongcharu W, Taylor CR, Chang Y, Aghassi D, Suthamjariya K, Anderson RR. Topical ALA-photodynamic therapy for the treatment of acne vulgaris. J Invest Dermatol. 2000;115(2): 183–92.
2. Halder RM, Holmes YC, Bridgeman-Shah S, Kligman A. A clinical pathological study of acne vulgaris in black females. J Invest Dermatol. 1996;106:888.

3. Alexis AF, Sergay AB, Taylor SC. Common dermatologic disorders in skin of color: a comparative practice survey. Cutis. 2007;80(5):387–94.
4. Halder RM, Grimes PE, McLaurin CI, Kress MA, Kenney Jr JA. Incidence of common dermatoses in a predominantly black dermatologic practice. Cutis. 1983;32(4):388–90.
5. Child FJ, Fuller LC, Higgins EM, Du Vivier AW. A study of the spectrum of skin disease occurring in a black population in south-east London. Br J Dermatol. 1999;141(3):512–7.
6. Goh CL, Akarapanth R. Epidemiology of skin disease among children in a referral skin clinic in Singapore. Pediatr Dermatol. 1994;11(2):125–8.
7. El-Essawi D, Musial JL, Hammad A, Lim HW. A survey of skin disease and skin-related issues in Arab Americans. J Am Acad Dermatol. 2007;56(6):933–8.
8. Sanchez MR. Cutaneous diseases in Latinos. Dermatol Clin. 2003;21(4):689–97.
9. Callender VD. Acne in ethnic skin: special considerations for therapy. Dermatol Ther. 2004;17(2):184–95.
10. Grimes P, Callender V. Tazarotene cream for postinflammatory hyperpigmentation and acne vulgaris in darker skin: a double-blind, randomized, vehicle-controlled study. Cutis. 2006;77(1):45–50.
11. Halder RM. The role of retinoids in the management of cutaneous conditions in blacks. J Am Acad Dermatol. 1998;39(2 Pt 3):S98–103.
12. Jacyk WK. Adapalene in the treatment of African patients. J Eur Acad Dermatol Venereol. 2001;15 Suppl 3:37–42.
13. Bulengo-Ransby SM, Griffiths CE, Kimbrough-Green CK, Finkel LJ, Hamilton TA, Ellis CN, et al. Topical tretinoin (retinoic acid) therapy for hyperpigmented lesions caused by inflammation of the skin in black patients. N Engl J Med. 1993;328(20):1438–43.
14. Gupta AK, Gover MD, Nouri K, Taylor S. The treatment of melasma: a review of clinical trials. J Am Acad Dermatol. 2006;55(6):1048–65.
15. Kawashima M, Harada S, Loesche C, Miyachi Y. Adapalene gel 0.1% is effective and safe for Japanese patients with acne vulgaris: a randomized, multicenter, investigator-blinded, controlled study. J Dermatol Sci. 2008;49(3):241–8.
16. Fernandez-Obregon A, Davis MW. The BEST study: evaluating efficacy by selected demographic subsets. Cutis. 2003;71(2 Suppl):18–26.
17. Shavin J, Weiss J. Implications of the BEST study. Cutis. 2003;71(2 Suppl):35–6.
18. Taylor SC. Utilizing combination therapy for ethnic skin. Cutis. 2007;80(1 Suppl):15–20.
19. Callender VD, Preston N, Osborn C, Johnson L, Gottschalk RW. A meta-analysis to investigate the relation between Fitzpatrick skin types and tolerability of Adapalene-benzoyl peroxide topical gel in subjects with mild or moderate acne. J Clin Aesthet Dermatol. 2010;3(8):15–9.
20. Gollnick HP, Graupe K, Zaumseil RP. Azelaic acid 15% gel in the treatment of acne vulgaris. Combined results of two double-blind clinical comparative studies. J Dtsch Dermatol Ges. 2004;2(10):841–7.
21. Webster G. Combination azelaic acid therapy for acne vulgaris. J Am Acad Dermatol. 2000;43(2 Pt 3):S47–50.
22. Draelos ZD, Carter E, Maloney JM, Elewski B, Poulin Y, Lynde C, et al. Two randomized studies demonstrate the efficacy and safety of dapsone gel, 5% for the treatment of acne vulgaris. J Am Acad Dermatol. 2007;56(3):439 e1–10.
23. Grimes PE. The safety and efficacy of salicylic acid chemical peels in darker racial-ethnic groups. Dermatol Surg. 1999;25(1):18–22.
24. Joshi SS, Boone SL, Alam M, Yoo S, White L, Rademaker A, et al. Effectiveness, safety, and effect on quality of life of topical salicylic acid peels for treatment of postinflammatory hyperpigmentation in dark skin. Dermatol Surg. 2009;35(4):638–44. discussion 44.
25. Yeung CK, Shek SY, Bjerring P, Yu CS, Kono T, Chan HH. A comparative study of intense pulsed light alone and its combination with photodynamic therapy for the treatment of facial acne in Asian skin. Lasers Surg Med. 2007;39(1):1–6.
26. Rojanamatin J, Choawawanich P. Treatment of inflammatory facial acne vulgaris with intense pulsed light and short contact of topical 5-aminolevulinic acid: a pilot study. Dermatol Surg. 2006;32(8):991–6. discussion 6-7.

27. Jih MH, Friedman PM, Goldberg LH, Robles M, Glaich AS, Kimyai-Asadi A. The 1450-nm diode laser for facial inflammatory acne vulgaris: dose–response and 12-month follow-up study. J Am Acad Dermatol. 2006;55(1):80–7.
28. Paithankar DY, Ross EV, Saleh BA, Blair MA, Graham BS. Acne treatment with a 1,450 nm wavelength laser and cryogen spray cooling. Lasers Surg Med. 2002;31(2):106–14.
29. Wang SQ, Counters JT, Flor ME, Zelickson BD. Treatment of inflammatory facial acne with the 1,450 nm diode laser alone versus microdermabrasion plus the 1,450 nm laser: a randomized, split-face trial. Dermatol Surg. 2006;32(2):249–55. discussion 55.
30. Tzung TY, Wu KH, Huang ML. Blue light phototherapy in the treatment of acne. Photodermatol Photoimmunol Photomed. 2004;20(5):266–9.
31. Pollock B, Turner D, Stringer MR, Bojar RA, Goulden V, Stables GI, et al. Topical aminolaevulinic acid-photodynamic therapy for the treatment of acne vulgaris: a study of clinical efficacy and mechanism of action. Br J Dermatol. 2004;151(3):616–22.
32. Wiegell SR, Wulf HC. Photodynamic therapy of acne vulgaris using 5-aminolevulinic acid versus methyl aminolevulinate. J Am Acad Dermatol. 2006;54(4):647–51.
33. Berg M, Liden S. An epidemiological study of rosacea. Acta Derm Venereol. 1989;69(5):419–23.
34. Alexis AF. Rosacea in patients with skin of color: uncommon but not rare. Cutis. 2010;86(2): 60–2.
35. Webster G. Rosacea and related disorders. In: Bolognia J, Jorizzo J, Rapini R, editors. Dermatology. 2nd ed. Philadelphia: Mosby Elsevier; 2008. p. 509–16.
36. Adler M. Rosacea in patients with darker skin types. Rosacea Acne Brief. 2002;1(4):1–7.
37. Halder R, Brooks H, Callender V. Acne in ethnic skin. Dermatol Clin. 2003;21(4):609–15.
38. Kenney Jr JA. Management of dermatoses peculiar to Negroes. Arch Dermatol. 1965;91:126–9.
39. Taylor SC. Epidemiology of skin diseases in ethnic populations. Dermatol Clin. 2003;21(4):601–7.
40. Doe PT, Asiedu A, Acheampong JW, Rowland Payne CM. Skin diseases in Ghana and the UK. Int J Dermatol. 2001;40(5):323–6.
41. Verhagen AR, Koten JW, Chaddah VK, Patel RI. Skin diseases in Kenya. A clinical and histopathological study of 3,168 patients. Arch Dermatol. 1968;98(6):577–86.
42. Wilkin J, Dahl M, Detmar M, Drake L, Feinstein A, Odom R, et al. Standard classification of rosacea: report of the national rosacea society expert committee on the classification and staging of rosacea. J Am Acad Dermatol. 2002;46(4):584–7.
43. Crawford GH, Pelle MT, James WD. Rosacea: I. Etiology, pathogenesis, and subtype classification. J Am Acad Dermatol. 2004;51(3):327–41. quiz 42–4.
44. Koffi-Aka V, Kouassi AA, D'Horpock FA, Boka NJ, Ehouo F. Rhinophyma in a black African. Rev Laryngol Otol Rhinol (Bord). 2002;123(2):109–10.
45. Khoo CT, Saad MN. Rhinophyma in a Negro: case report. Br J Plast Surg. 1980;33(2):161–3.
46. Culp B, Scheinfeld N. Rosacea: a review. Phys Ther. 2009;34(1):38–45.
47. Rosen T, Stone MS. Acne rosacea in blacks. J Am Acad Dermatol. 1987;17(1):70–3.
48. Williams HC, Ashworth J, Pembroke AC, Breathnach SM. FACE–facial Afro-Caribbean childhood eruption. Clin Exp Dermatol. 1990;15(3):163–6.
49. Pelle MT, Crawford GH, James WD. Rosacea: II. Therapy. J Am Acad Dermatol. 2004;51(4): 499–512. quiz 3–4.
50. Korting HC, Schollmann C. Current topical and systemic approaches to treatment of rosacea. J Eur Acad Dermatol Venereol. 2009;23(8):876–82.
51. van Zuuren EJ, Gupta AK, Gover MD, Graber M, Hollis S. Systematic review of rosacea treatments. J Am Acad Dermatol. 2007;56(1):107–15.
52. Yoo J, Reid DC, Kimball AB. Metronidazole in the treatment of rosacea: do formulation, dosing, and concentration matter? J Drugs Dermatol. 2006;5(4):317–9.
53. Thiboutot D, Thieroff-Ekerdt R, Graupe K. Efficacy and safety of azelaic acid (15%) gel as a new treatment for papulopustular rosacea: results from two vehicle-controlled, randomized phase III studies. J Am Acad Dermatol. 2003;48(6):836–45.

54. Elewski BE, Fleischer Jr AB, Pariser DM. A comparison of 15% azelaic acid gel and 0.75% metronidazole gel in the topical treatment of papulopustular rosacea: results of a randomized trial. Arch Dermatol. 2003;139(11):1444–50.
55. Ertl GA, Levine N, Kligman AM. A comparison of the efficacy of topical tretinoin and low-dose oral isotretinoin in rosacea. Arch Dermatol. 1994;130(3):319–24.
56. Goldman D. Tacrolimus ointment for the treatment of steroid-induced rosacea: a preliminary report. J Am Acad Dermatol. 2001;44(6):995–8.
57. Leyden JJ, Thiboutot D, Shalita A. Photographic review of results from a clinical study comparing benzoyl peroxide 5%/clindamycin 1% topical gel with vehicle in the treatment of rosacea. Cutis. 2004;73(6 Suppl):11–7.
58. Ozturkcan S, Ermertcan AT, Sahin MT, Afsar FS. Efficiency of benzoyl peroxide-erythromycin gel in comparison with metronidazole gel in the treatment of acne rosacea. J Dermatol. 2004;31(8):610–7.
59. Colon LE, Johnson LA, Gottschalk RW. Cumulative irritation potential among metronidazole gel 1%, metronidazole gel 0.75%, and azelaic acid gel 15%. Cutis. 2007;79(4):317–21.
60. Erdogan FG, Yurtsever P, Aksoy D, Eskioglu F. Efficacy of low-dose isotretinoin in patients with treatment-resistant rosacea. Arch Dermatol. 1998;134(7):884–5.
61. Del Rosso JQ, Webster GF, Jackson M, Rendon M, Rich P, Torok H, et al. Two randomized phase III clinical trials evaluating anti-inflammatory dose doxycycline (40-mg doxycycline, USP capsules) administered once daily for treatment of rosacea. J Am Acad Dermatol. 2007;56(5):791–802.
62. Baldwin HE. Systemic therapy for rosacea. Skin Therapy Lett. 2007;12(2):1–5. 9.
63. Hoting E, Paul E, Plewig G. Treatment of rosacea with isotretinoin. Int J Dermatol. 1986;25(10):660–3.
64. Battle Jr EF, Hobbs LM. Laser therapy on darker ethnic skin. Dermatol Clin. 2003;21(4):713–23.
65. Bhatt N, Alster TS. Laser surgery in dark skin. Dermatol Surg. 2008;34(2):184–94. discussion 94–5.
66. Clementoni MT, Gilardino P, Muti GF, Signorini M, Pistorale A, Morselli PG, et al. Intense pulsed light treatment of 1,000 consecutive patients with facial vascular marks. Aesthetic Plast Surg. 2006;30(2):226–32.
67. Erisir F, Isildak H, Haciyev Y. Management of mild to moderate rhinophyma with a radiofrequency. J Craniofac Surg. 2009;20(2):455–6.

# Chapter 3
# Contact Dermatitis

**Ama Alexis and Vincent A. DeLeo**

Contact dermatitis is a common dermatologic disorder manifesting as an eczematous skin eruption following exposure to a noxious agent. It is the second most common occupational illness and therefore affects a wide range of patients [1]. Its development may be influenced by a myriad of variables, including age, gender, preexisting skin conditions, skin sensitivity, occupation, as well as the ethnicity and race of the patient. Although contact dermatitis affects patients irrespective of skin color, the clinical presentation, irritant response, as well as exposure patterns to allergens and irritants may differ significantly between racial groups. The gold standard in diagnosing contact dermatitis is patch testing, which can be performed safely in all skin types. Familiarity with ethnic/race-specific presentation and exposure patterns to allergens and irritants may be beneficial in elucidating the etiology of contact dermatitis.

## Epidemiology

The diagnosis of contact dermatitis is one of five leading conditions for dermatologic visits in white, black, and Hispanic patients in the USA [2–4]. The overall prevalence of contact dermatitis as well as access to health care professionals providing patch testing is similar between black and white patients in the USA [5–7]. However, there are reports of slightly decreased access to patch testing when comparing patients from the Indian subcontinent to white Europeans in the UK [8].

A. Alexis, M.D. (✉)
Department of Pediatrics, NYU Langone Medical Center,
250 West 57th Street, Suite 1231, New York, NY 10107, USA
e-mail: AmaalexisMD@gmail.com

V.A. DeLeo, M.D.
Department of Dermatology, St. Luke's-Roosevelt Hospital Center
and Columbia University College of Physicians and Surgeons,
New York, NY 10025, USA
e-mail: VDeleo@chpnet.org

A.F. Alexis and V.H. Barbosa (eds.), *Skin of Color: A Practical Guide to Dermatologic Diagnosis and Treatment*, DOI 10.1007/978-0-387-84929-4_3,

**Table 3.1** Most common sensitizers in patch testing in skin of color

| Study (year) | Patient race (origin) | Number tested | Most common sensitizers |
|---|---|---|---|
| DeLeo (2002) | Black (USA) | N = 1,014 | Nickel sulfate (17.3%)<br>Neomycin sulfate (12.2%)<br>Cobalt chloride (11.1%) |
| Dickel (2001) | Black (Ohio, USA) | N = 114 | Nickel sulfate (10.6%)<br>*p*-Phenylenediamine (10.6%) |
| Bilcha (2009) | Black (Ethiopia) | N = 181 | Nickel<br>Fragrance mix<br>Butylphenol formaldehyde |
| Fairhurst (2008) | Indian subcontinent (UK) | N = 50 | Nickel sulfate (22%)<br>*p*-Phenylenediamine (10%)<br>Methylchloro- and methylisothiazolinone (5.9%) |
| Bajaj (2007) | Indian (Allahabad, North India) | N = 1,000 | *Parthenium* (14.6%)<br>Nickel sulfate (12.9%)<br>Potassium dichromate (11.1%)<br>Neomycin (7%) |
| Singhal (2000) | Indian (Delhi, India) | N = 75 | *Parthenium* (20%)<br>Potassium dichromate (16%)<br>*Xanthium* (13%) |
| Lam (2008) | Chinese (Hong Kong, China) | N = 2,585 | Nickel sulfate (24.4%)<br>Fragrance mix (13.7)<br>Cobalt chloride (8.7%)<br>*p*-Phenylenediamine (6%) |
| Lee (1996) | Chinese (Hong Kong, China) | N = 490 | Nickel sulfate (19.5%)<br>Cobalt chloride (11.3%)<br>Fragrance mix (7.3%) |
| Collazo (2008) | Hispanic (Puerto Rico) | N = 59 | Carba mix (18.7%)<br>Nickel sulfate (17.0%)<br>Thiuram mix (10.2%)<br>Paratertiary butylphenol formaldehyde resin (8.5%)<br>*p*-Phenylenediamine (8.5%) |
| Boonchai (2008) | Asian-Pacific (Bangkok, Thailand) | N = 323 | Potassium dichromate (27%)<br>Nickel sulfate (26.6%)<br>Fragrance mix (20.7%)<br>Cobalt chloride (16.4%) |
| Al-Sheikh (1996) | (Riyadh, Saudi Arabia) | N = 271 | Nickel sulfate (39.5%)<br>Potassium dichromate (32.9%)<br>Cobalt chloride (30.9%) |

When comparing patch test results between different racial patient populations, distinct sensitization patterns to specific allergens among these groups become evident (Table 3.1). The cause of this may be multifactorial and may be a reflection of regional, cultural, or ethnic-specific practices as well as differences between white, black, Asian, and Hispanic patients in their response to specific allergens [9].

## Clinical Presentation

The most common presentation of contact dermatitis follows an eczematous reaction pattern consisting of erythematous, papular, and then vesicular lesions in patients with Fitzpatrick skin types I to IV. The presentation of allergic contact dermatitis (ACD) may differ in dark-skinned patients, who may present more frequently with lichenified and hyperpigmented lesions [5] or with follicular papules. Moreover, in dark-skinned patients who undergo patch testing, the skin presents more often with glazing, wrinkling, and dryness [10] as compared to lighter-skinned patients. In addition, in patients with dark-colored skin, erythema may be harder to appreciate, making the diagnosis of ACD more challenging [5, 10]. The most common site of disease presentation in black patients as well as Caucasian patients is the hand, followed by the face [6]. In patients of Chinese, Hispanic, as well as Indian descent, the hand is also the most common site of presentation [8, 11, 12].

## Specific Differences

### *Skin Structure and Physiology*

#### Black Skin

Structurally, black skin has been shown to differ from white skin in several aspects. For a more extensive review, please see Chap. 1, "Structural, Physiologic, Functional, and Cultural Differences." Briefly, while the stratum corneum in blacks has been found to be of equal thickness compared to whites, it contains more cell layers that are arranged more compactly [13]. In addition, black skin holds increased intracellular lipid content [14], decreased amount of ceramides [15], larger mast cell granules [16], and significantly higher transepidermal water loss (TEWL) when compared to white skin [17, 18]. TEWL is used as a surrogate for stratum corneum barrier function, suggesting that despite contradictory early evidence, black skin may be more susceptible to irritation than white skin.

#### Asian Skin

There is evidence that Asian skin may be more sensitive to irritants than white skin possibly due to higher TEWL after tape stripping [19], thinner stratum [19], and lower ceramide content [15] suggesting a weaker barrier function and increased permeability [19]. However, other studies have reported no structural differences between white and Asian skin [20]. How these aforementioned structural and functional differences translate into different physiologic responses to irritants and environmental factors is in some measures more complex.

## *Specific Sensitization: Skin Irritants and Allergens*

It has been proposed that there are differences in response to irritants between different racial groups. While it is recognized that there is wide interindividual variability, there are some tendencies that should be noted. However, there is only a limited number of studies comparing the reactivity of Caucasian, Asian, Hispanic, and black skin to different irritants. Most studies show conflicting data and are challenging to compare because of small patient sample sizes and a multitude of study confounders. Only few reach statistical significance, making it challenging to make definite conclusions regarding racial differences.

### Black Skin

Initial studies demonstrated that upon cutaneous exposure to irritants, such as mustard gas, significantly more Caucasians than black patients developed erythema [13, 21]. However, by only using erythema as an endpoint, the sensitivity of black patients may have been underestimated. When utilizing more objective measurements, the results are controversial. While evidence of reduced susceptibility to irritants in black skin remains when utilizing more objective measurements including reflectance confocal microscopy, transepidermal water loss, and routine histology [22], contradictory results have also been found: black skin was found to be more sensitive upon exposure to sodium lauryl sulfate in one study [18], while other studies demonstrated no statistically significant differences using multiple irritants [23, 24].

Patch testing has been utilized to elucidate differences in sensitization between black and Caucasian skin. Sensitization with allergens like dinitrochlorobenzene (DNCB) and nitrosodimethylaniline showed that black skin was less sensitive when compared to white skin [25, 26]. Other studies have shown no significant sensitization differences to multiple other allergens [5, 6, 27].

### Asian Skin (Chinese/Japanese)

There is conflicting evidence whether Asian patients are more susceptible to contact dermatitis when compared with Caucasian patients. Although some studies fail to demonstrate objective differences as measured by TEWL and laser Doppler between Japanese and European women [28] as well as permeability to topical methyl nicotinate [23] or benzoic acid [24], indicating no difference in skin barrier function, the majority of studies demonstrate an increased objective response to irritants [29–31]. There is also evidence of increased subjective sensitivity to irritants [28] as well as greater perception of skin reactivity [32] when compared to Caucasian patients.

### Hispanic Skin

There is very limited data suggesting that the skin of Hispanic patients may be more sensitive than Caucasian skin [33]. More studies are needed to confirm these findings.

## Patch Testing and Allergens

The gold standard in elucidating the etiology of contact dermatitis is patch testing. Only limited data is available which includes patients of various racial backgrounds. Patch testing can be performed safely in all skin types; however, the results may be more challenging to interpret in patients of color because erythema may be difficult to appreciate [34]. In a large North American multicenter study, no significant differences in the prevalence of contact dermatitis and response rates to allergens were identified while evaluating about 10,000 patients (89.5% white and 10.5% black). In this study, black patients had highest rates of sensitization to nickel sulfate, neomycin sulfate, and cobalt chloride. There were significantly higher rates of sensitization to *p*-phenylenediamine (PPDA) and thioureas in black patients when compared to white patients. In a similar North American study, nickel sulfate and *p*-phenylenediamine (both 10.6%) were most prevalent among black patients, whereas nickel sulfate and thiomersal (both 8%) were the most common sensitizers among white patients [7]. *p*-Phenylenediamine was statistically significantly elevated ($P = .00599$), when comparing the sensitization rates in blacks (10.6%) to whites (4.5%). The four most common sensitizers in a group of 2,585 patients of Chinese descent were nickel sulfate, fragrance mix, cobalt chloride, and *p*-phenylenediamine [12]. In a cohort of 50 patients with suspected ACD from the Indian subcontinent residing in the UK, the most common allergens were nickel and *p*-phenylenediamine, as compared to nickel and cobalt in the white population [8]. Hispanic patients from Puerto Rico were mostly affected by Carba mix and nickel sulfate. Further patch test results within different racial groups are described in Table 3.1.

As it is difficult to draw definite conclusions about racial differences affecting skin sensitivity and response to irritants, the focus shifts toward exposure to allergens. The results of these patch tests may reflect specific exposure patterns to allergens and irritants within different ethnic/racial groups.

While nickel sulfate and potassium dichromate are common sensitizers among all patients, there are certain sensitizers that seem to be elevated among specific ethnic groups. For example, the increased prevalence of *p*-phenylenediamine (PPDA) in darker-skin-type patients [5–7, 12] is hypothesized to reflect increased exposure to this allergen through dark-colored hair dye. The darker the color of the dye, the higher the concentration of PPDA, which is thought to lead to a higher sensitization rate in patients of color [6]. A possible cross-sensitization to other chemically related substances like thiazide diuretics and oral hypoglycemic agents has been proposed, which should have led to wider sensitization in black patients, whom these drugs are frequently prescribed to. However this hypothesis has not been proven [6].

In both Chinese patch test groups (Table 3.1), the European standard series was used to test patients [12, 35]. When adding locally important allergens to the patch test selection, topical Chinese (17%) and Western medicine (9%) lead to a high number of positive reactions [35].

Also of interest is the increased sensitization to *Parthenium* among Indians. *Parthenium* is a weed, which is known to cause airborne contact dermatitis and photodermatitis in India and Australia [36]. This observation is not replicated in Indians living in the UK, who are not exposed to this weed. This may be evidence that exposure and environment, while influenced by culture and ethnicity, may be more important than genetic factors when considering exposure to allergens and irritants in patients of color.

## References


1. http://www.cdc.gov/niosh/topics/skin/#contact. Accessed 22 Jan 2010.
2. Alexis AF, Sergay AB, Taylor SC. Common dermatologic disorders in skin of color: a comparative practice survey. Cutis. 2007;80:387–94.
3. Halder RM, Grimes PE, McLaurin CI, Kress MA, Kenney Jr JA. Incidence of common dermatoses in a predominantly black dermatologic practice. Cutis. 1983;32:388–90.
4. Sanchez MR. Cutaneous diseases in Latinos. Dermatol Clin. 2003;21:689–97.
5. Fisher AA. Contact dermatitis in black patients. Cutis 1977;20:303, 308–9, 316 passim.
6. Deleo VA, Taylor SC, Belsito DV, et al. The effect of race and ethnicity on patch test results. J Am Acad Dermatol. 2002;46:S107–12.
7. Dickel H, Taylor JS, Evey P, Merk HF. Comparison of patch test results with a standard series among white and black racial groups. Am J Contact Dermat. 2001;12:77–82.
8. Fairhurst DA, Shah M. Comparison of patch test results among white Europeans and patients from the Indian subcontinent living within the same community. J Eur Acad Dermatol Venereol. 2008;22:1227–31.
9. Modjtahedi SP, Maibach HI. Ethnicity as a possible endogenous factor in irritant contact dermatitis: comparing the irritant response among Caucasians, blacks, and Asians. Contact Dermatitis. 2002;47:272–8.
10. Peters L, Marriott M, Mukerji B, et al. The effect of population diversity on skin irritation. Contact Dermatitis. 2006;55:357–63.
11. Collazo MH, Figueroa LD, Sanchez JL. Prevalence of contact allergens in a Hispanic population. P R Health Sci J. 2008;27:333–6.
12. Lam WS, Chan LY, Ho SC, Chong LY, So WH, Wong TW. A retrospective study of 2585 patients patch tested with the European standard series in Hong Kong (1995–99). Int J Dermatol. 2008;47:128–33.
13. Weigand DA, Haygood C, Gaylor JR. Cell layers and density of Negro and Caucasian stratum corneum. J Invest Dermatol. 1974;62:563–8.
14. La Ruche G, Cesarini JP. Histology and physiology of black skin. Ann Dermatol Venereol. 1992;119:567–74.
15. Sugino K, Imokawa G, Maibach H. Ethnic differences of stratum corneum lipid in relation to stratum corneum function. J Invest Dermatol. 1993;100:587 [abstract].
16. Sueki H, Whitaker-Menezes D, Kligman AM. Structural diversity of mast cell granules in black and white skin. Br J Dermatol. 2001;144:85–93.
17. Wilson D, Berardesca E, Maibach HI. In vitro transepidermal water loss: differences between black and white human skin. Br J Dermatol. 1988;119:647–52.

18. Berardesca E, Maibach HI. Racial differences in sodium lauryl sulphate induced cutaneous irritation: black and white. Contact Dermatitis. 1988;18:65–70.
19. Kompaore F, Marty JP, Dupont C. In vivo evaluation of the stratum corneum barrier function in blacks, Caucasians and Asians with two noninvasive methods. Skin Pharmacol. 1993;6:200–7.
20. Reed JT, Ghadially R, Elias PM. Effect of race, gender and skin type on epidermal permeability barrier function. J Invest Dermatol. 1994;102:537 [abstract].
21. Marshall EK Jr LV, Smith HW. On dichloroethylsulphide (mustard gas). II. Variations in susceptibility of the skin to dichloroethylsulphide. J Pharmacol Exp Ther. 1918;12:291–301.
22. Hicks SP, Swindells KJ, Middelkamp-Hup MA, Sifakis MA, Gonzalez E, Gonzalez S. Confocal histopathology of irritant contact dermatitis in vivo and the impact of skin color (black vs. white). J Am Acad Dermatol. 2003;48:727–34.
23. Gean CJ, Tur E, Maibach HI, Guy RH. Cutaneous responses to topical methyl nicotinate in black, oriental, and Caucasian subjects. Arch Dermatol Res. 1989;281:95–8.
24. Lotte C, Wester RC, Rougier A, Maibach HI. Racial differences in the in vivo percutaneous absorption of some organic compounds: a comparison between black, Caucasian and Asian subjects. Arch Dermatol Res. 1993;284:456–9.
25. Rostenberg Jr A, Kanof NM. Studies in Eczematous sensitization. J Invest Dermatol. 1941;4:505–16.
26. Epstein WL, Kligman AM. The interference phenomenon in allergic contact dermatitis. J Invest Dermatol. 1958;31:103–8.
27. Leyden JJ, Kligman AM. Allergic contact dermatitis: sex differences. Contact Dermatitis. 1977;3:333–6.
28. Aramaki J, Kawana S, Effendy I, Happle R, Loffler H. Differences of skin irritation between Japanese and European women. Br J Dermatol. 2002;146:1052–6.
29. Robinson MK. Population differences in acute skin irritation responses. Race, sex, age, sensitive skin and repeat subject comparisons. Contact Dermatitis. 2002;46:86–93.
30. Rapaport MJ. Patch testing in Japanese subjects. Contact Dermatitis. 1984;11:93–7.
31. Foy V, Weinkauf R, Whittle E, Basketter DA. Ethnic variation in the skin irritation response. Contact Dermatitis. 2001;45:346–9.
32. Jourdain R, de Lacharriere O, Bastien P, Maibach HI. Ethnic variations in self-perceived sensitive skin: epidemiological survey. Contact Dermatitis. 2002;46:162–9.
33. Berardesca E, Maibach HI. Sodium-lauryl-sulphate-induced cutaneous irritation. Comparison of white and Hispanic subjects. Contact Dermatitis. 1988;19:136–40.
34. Sherertz EF, Schwartz S. Patch test interpretation of black skin. Am J Contact Dermatitis. 1993;4:247–8.
35. Lee TY, Lam TH. Patch testing of 490 patients in Hong Kong. Contact Dermatitis. 1996;35:23–6.
36. Sharma VK, Sethuraman G. Parthenium dermatitis. Dermatitis. 2007;18:183–90.

# Chapter 4
# Inflammatory Disorders with Unique Clinical Features

**Kelli D. Grim and Ted Rosen**

## Atopic Dermatitis

Atopic dermatitis (AD) is a common disorder, affecting 10–20% of the pediatric population and 1–3% of adults, characterized by an intensely pruritic, papulovesicular rash with development of excoriations and lichenification from chronic scratching and rubbing [1, 2]. Aside from lichenification, post-inflammatory dyschromia can be significant in chronic eczema occurring in skin of color.

AD is categorized by infantile, childhood, and adult types (Table 4.1). Less than 20% of adults with AD have onset after adolescence [2]. A personal and/or family history of atopy (allergic rhinoconjunctivitis, asthma, AD) may exist in up to two-thirds of atopics. Exacerbations of atopic dermatitis typically occur during winter, due to both lower ambient humidity and exposure to indoor heat leading to cutaneous xerosis. Atopics can also worsen in the summer from increased heat, humidity, and perspiration.

A prominent feature of AD in skin of color is the development of close-set, small, pruritic follicular papules, particularly during the early course of the disease (Fig. 4.1). These findings should alert the physician to the diagnosis of AD in a child with skin of color, even before typical flexural eczematous patches appear. Extensor involvement and ichthyosis vulgaris are also more common in atopics with skin of color [3–5]. Additionally, people of African descent may present with a lichen planus-like atopic dermatitis, a violaceous, papular, lichenoid rash primarily on the

K.D. Grim, M.D. (✉)
Department of Dermatology, Tulane University Health Science Center, New Orleans, LA, USA
e-mail: kdgrim@gmail.com

T. Rosen, M.D.
Department of Dermatology, Baylor College of Medicine, 2815 Plumb Street, Houston, TX 77005, USA
e-mail: vampireted@aol.com

A.F. Alexis and V.H. Barbosa (eds.), *Skin of Color: A Practical Guide to Dermatologic Diagnosis and Treatment*, DOI 10.1007/978-0-387-84929-4_4,

**Table 4.1** Distribution and morphology of atopic dermatitis by type

| Type | Distribution | Morphology |
|---|---|---|
| Infantile (before 2 years of age) | • Scalp, cheeks, forehead, chin, trunk, and extensor surfaces<br>• Sparing of diaper area | • Erythematous papules, vesicles, and patches<br>• Weeping, scaling, crusting, exudative |
| Childhood (2 years of age to puberty) | Neck, periorbital, perioral, flexor surfaces, wrists, ankles, hands, and feet | • Less weeping<br>• More lichenification and excoriations<br>• Follicular accentuation in skin of color on trunk<br>• Post-inflammatory hyper- or hypopigmentation |
| Adult (after puberty) | Face, upper arms, flexor surfaces, back, wrists, dorsa of hands and feet, fingers and toes | • Less weeping<br>• Large lichenified plaques with scaling<br>• Prurigo papules<br>• Post-inflammatory hyper- or hypopigmentation |

Data adapted from Wasserbauer and Ballow [2] and Peterson and Chan [13]

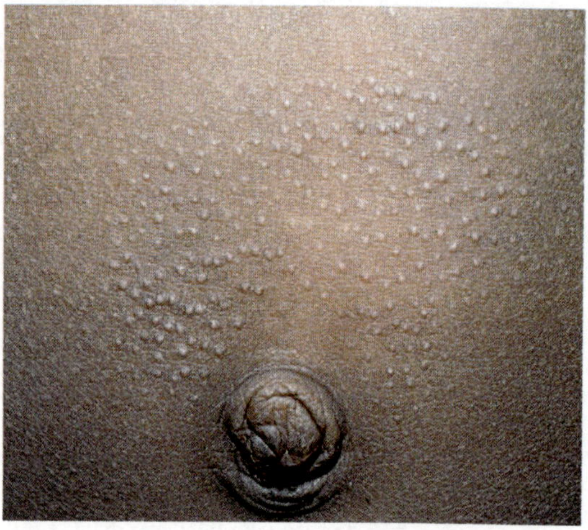

**Fig. 4.1** Close-set pruritic follicular papules: early atopic dermatitis in skin of color

extensor aspects of the arms and legs [3, 6, 7]. Erythema may be less notable in atopics with heavily pigmented skin. This characteristic may lead to a faulty assessment of severity and delay in appropriate therapy [8]. Asian populations may show sandpaper-like skin lesions of the extensor surfaces, ventral wrist dermatitis, and itchy hyperkeratotic papules in association with AD [5]. Unfortunately, development of disfiguring post-inflammatory dyschromia is common and more conspicuous in people with skin of color. Therefore, the physician should assume an aggressive therapeutic approach.

## Epidemiology

Incidence of AD in blacks is probably equal to that of AD in whites. However, there have been reports of increased incidence in blacks [9]. There may also be a higher incidence in Asian populations, particularly people of Chinese descent [10]. There is no gender predilection.

## Pathophysiology

AD is caused by a complex interplay between environmental and genetic factors. AD is characterized by epidermal barrier dysfunction with increased transepidermal water loss leading to xerosis [11]. Mutation of filaggrin, a protein involved in the arrangement of keratin intermediate filaments, has been associated with AD and found to be predictive of the development of asthma in people with AD, also known as the atopic march [11]. Abnormal activity of proteases, antigen-presenting cells, and T-cell lymphocytes has also been implicated [11, 12]. AD may have a biphasic course, with TH2 activity more prominent in the acute phase and TH1 activity more prominent during the chronic phase [12].

Due to a faulty epidermal barrier, atopics are hypersensitive to environmental allergens, such as pollens, molds, animal dander, dust mites, and certain foods. Infectious colonization with *Staphylococcus aureus* and *Malassezia* sp. may elicit strong inflammatory reactions and trigger recurrent eczematous flares [2, 11].

## Histopathology

Acute and chronic phases of AD show varying degrees of hyperkeratosis, psoriasiform epidermal hyperplasia, epidermal spongiosis, perivascular inflammatory infiltrate with mononuclear cells, and epidermal exocytosis of mononuclear cells. Follicular AD shows epidermal hyperkeratosis and parakeratosis at the follicular orifice, with a perifollicular, lymphocytic inflammatory infiltrate.

## Laboratory

Laboratory findings may include increased serum IgE levels and increased skin and serum levels of histamine. It is not known whether these play an etiologic role or represent epiphenomena.

**Table 4.2** Differential diagnosis of atopic dermatitis

| |
|---|
| Psoriasis |
| Seborrheic dermatitis |
| Irritant/allergic contact dermatitis |
| Dermatophytosis |
| Scabies |
| Nutritional deficiency |
| Zinc, niacin, pyridoxine, essential fatty acid |
| Dermatitis herpetiformis |
| Immunodeficiency syndromes |
| Wiskott-Aldrich |
| Severe combined immunodeficiency |
| Ataxia-telangiectasia |
| Netherton's syndrome |

Adapted from Wasserbauer and Ballow [2], with permission

### *Differential Diagnosis*

Table 4.2 gives the differential diagnosis for atopic dermatitis.

### *Treatment*

Therapy for AD is multifaceted and includes topical/systemic corticosteroids, topical calcineurin inhibitors, oral antihistamines, prophylaxis against (*S. aureus*) and treatment of superinfection, allergen avoidance, and liberal application of emollients (Table 4.3) [13]. Severe AD may require administration of immunosuppressives (e.g., methotrexate or cyclosporine).

## Lichen Planus

Lichen planus (LP) is a papulosquamous disorder with an incidence of less than 1% in the USA [14, 15], although the prevalence may be greater in geographical locations with endemic viral hepatitides, such as India and Africa [16]. LP is characterized by 6 Ps: *p*ruritic, *p*urple, *p*lanar, *p*olygonal *p*apules, and *p*laques with an overlying, lacy white reticular pattern known as Wickham's striae [14]. Sites of predilection include the flexural surfaces of the forearms and wrists, sides of the neck, lumbosacral area, ankles, oral and genital mucosa, nails, and scalp (lichen planopilaris). Nail changes include dystrophy, longitudinal ridging, splitting, pterygium formation, destruction of the matrix, and thinning of the nail plate [17, 18]. Scarring alopecia may be present in the scalp. The Koebner phenomenon may be noted in both cutaneous and oral lichen planus (OLP), such as following dental procedures [19].

**Table 4.3** Therapy for atopic dermatitis

| Topical and systemic steroids | Ointment = gel > cream > lotion > foam |
|---|---|
| Topical calcineurin inhibitors | Pimecrolimus 1% cream and tacrolimus 0.03% and 0.1% ointments applied twice daily to affected areas. Should be avoided in patients less than 2 years of age. Tacrolimus 0.1% should be avoided in people < 16 years of age |
| Antihistamine agents | Diphenhydramine, hydroxyzine, cyproheptadine, doxepin |
| Allergen and trigger avoidance | • Animal dander, cockroach, dust mites, molds, pollens, cigarette smoke, laundry detergents, wool, synthetic fibers<br>• Sweating, winter months, emotional stress<br>• Cow milk, eggs, peanuts, soy, tree nuts, wheat |
| Treatment of superinfection | • *S. aureus* – first-generation cephalosporin and/or mupirocin 2% ointment/cream<br>• Eczema herpeticum – oral acyclovir<br>• Eczema molluscatum – imiquimod 5% cream |
| Emollients | Aquaphor®, Vaseline®, Vanicream™, CeraVe®, Eucerin®, Lac-Hydrin®, Keri Lotion® |
| Miscellaneous | • Immunomodulators (cyclosporine, azathioprine)<br>• Phototherapy (PUVA, broadband UVB/UVA, broadband UVA, broadband UVB, narrowband UVB, UVA-1) |

Information adapted from Peterson and Chan [13], with permission

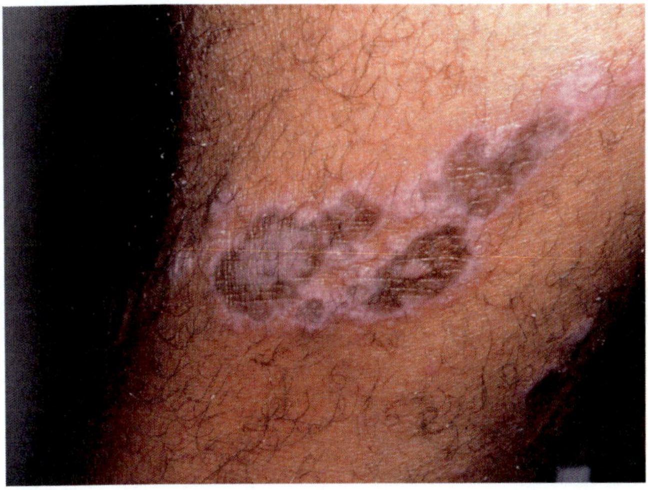

**Fig. 4.2** Annular lesions of lichen planus are more common in skin of color

Unique to skin of color, a deeper hue of LP papules and plaques may be noted due to greater amounts of melanin displaced into the dermis. Annular LP lesions with a central grayish hue are considerably more frequent in darkly pigmented skin [16] (Fig. 4.2). Hypertrophic LP, consisting of markedly thickened, hyperpigmented plaques, most typically on the shins, is also more common in blacks. Bullous

**Table 4.4** LP associations

| |
|---|
| Alopecia areata |
| Autoimmune disorders |
| Hepatitis C virus |
| Dermatomyositis |
| Diabetes mellitus |
| HIV infection |
| Morphea |
| Myasthenia gravis |
| Primary biliary cirrhosis |
| Renal stones |
| Thymoma |
| Ulcerative colitis |
| Vitiligo |

From Marshman [17], with permission

and erosive/ulcerative LP of the plantar surface of the foot is a more common manifestation in blacks compared to whites. In contrast, OLP is less common in blacks than whites, but more common in Asians than whites [20].

## *Epidemiology*

Lichen planus is most prevalent in the fifth to seventh decades of life with a slight female predominance [17]. Men, however, tend to develop LP earlier than women [17]. There seems to be no racial predilection [17], although an Asian predominance has been reported [20].

## *Pathophysiology*

Current pathogenesis of LP is unknown. Cytotoxic CD8+ T lymphocytes represent the major effector cell type for damage to and resultant liquefactive necrosis of the epidermal basal cell layer keratinocytes [21].

## *Other Associations*

LP is associated with a variety of systemic illnesses (Table 4.4). LP, particularly ulcerated OLP, is associated with HCV [22]. Although the incidence is low, malignant transformation to in situ or invasive squamous cell carcinoma is of particular concern in OLP and vulvovaginal LP [22]. Lichenoid drug eruptions (LDE) are also well documented (Table 4.5).

**Table 4.5** Drugs and contactants associated with LDE

| |
|---|
| Angiotensin-converting enzyme inhibitors |
| Antimalarials (quinine, quinacrine, chloroquine) |
| Beta blockers |
| Calcium channel blockers |
| Dental amalgams (mercury, copper, gold) |
| Lithium |
| Methyldopa |
| NSAIDs |
| Penicillamine |
| Phenylenediamine (color photography-developing chemicals) |
| Quinidine |
| Sulfonylureas (chlorpropamide, tolazamide) |

Data from Ellgehausen et al. [15] and Sontheimer [21]

**Table 4.6** Differential diagnosis of LP[a]

| |
|---|
| Granuloma annulare (with annular lesions) |
| Lichenoid drug eruption |
| Lichen simplex chronicus (with hypertrophic lesions) |
| Pityriasis lichenoides chronica |
| Pityriasis lichenoides et varioliformis acuta |
| Psoriasis (particularly guttate) |
| Scabies |
| Syphilis |

[a]Depth of pigment in dark skin may obscure the correct diagnosis

## *Histopathology*

Liquefactive degeneration of the basal cell layer keratinocytes with a band-like, interface lymphocytic infiltrate in the upper dermis is the hallmark of LP. Colloid, or Civatte, bodies are composed of hyalinized keratinocytes and are found in the lower epidermis [15, 17]. Wickham's striae correlate to an increased granular layer [17]. In pigmented skin, considerable melanin may be found within the upper dermal macrophages. Manifestations of erosive LP are from subepidermal bulla. Hypertrophic LP shows irregular, extensive acanthosis, dermal fibrosis, and marked hyperkeratosis [17].

## *Differential Diagnosis*

Table 4.6 gives the differential diagnosis for lichen planus.

### Treatment

- Topical or systemic corticosteroids
- Topical calcineurin inhibitors
- Systemic retinoids
- Cyclosporine (3–5 mg/kg/d)
- Other less common agents: dapsone, griseofulvin, thalidomide, PUVA therapy

## Lupus Erythematosus

Lupus erythematosus is a chronic, autoimmune disorder, and 4 out of the 11 American Rheumatologic Association(ARA) criteria for diagnosis of systemic lupus erythematosus (SLE) are mucocutaneous manifestations (Table 4.7) [23, 24]. The major categories of LE-specific cutaneous disease are acute cutaneous LE (ACLE), subacute cutaneous LE (SCLE), and discoid or chronic cutaneous LE (DLE/CCLE). While any race can be affected by cutaneous LE, the focus of this topic will be on DLE due to its unique presentation in skin of color. DLE is the most frequently encountered form of CCLE, and discoid type lesions are present in 20% of patients with systemic disease (Table 4.8) [25, 26]. DLE lesions begin as one or more discrete, erythematous macules or papules with a superficial scale; the papule increases in size to develop into a disk-shaped, erythematous, edematous plaque with follicular hyperkeratosis and scaling [26]. Eventually, the lesion involutes, yielding a hyperpigmented, peripheral border and an atrophied, depressed, telangiectatic hypopigmented center [25, 26]. This results in striking contrast between normal skin and lesional skin, particularly so in skin of color (Fig. 4.3). Lesions may

**Table 4.7** ARA diagnostic criteria for SLE

| | |
|---|---|
| Malar rash | Flat or raised, malar erythema that typically spares the nasolabial folds |
| Discoid rash | Erythematous raised plaques with adherent hyperkeratotic scale and follicular plugging |
| Photosensitivity | Photodistributed erythematous rash |
| Oral ulcers | Oral or nasopharyngeal ulceration |
| Arthritis | Nonerosive, involving two or more joints |
| Serositis | Pleuritis (pleuritic pain, rub on physical examination, or pleural effusion) *OR* pericarditis (by EKG, rub on physical examination, or pericardial effusion) |
| Renal disorder | Persistent proteinuria > 9.5 g/day or 3+ on urine dipstick *OR* cellular casts (red cell, granular, tubular, etc.) |
| Hematologic disorder | Hemolytic anemia with reticulocytosis *OR* leukopenia (<4,000/mm$^3$) *OR* lymphopenia (<1,500/mm$^3$) *OR* thrombocytopenia (<100,000/mm$^3$) |
| Immunologic disorder | Positive antiphospholipid Ab titer *OR* positive anti-DNA Ab titer *OR* positive anti-SM Ab titer *OR* false-positive nonspecific treponemal test, confirmed negative by FTA-ABS |
| Neurological disorder | Seizures *OR* psychosis |
| Antinuclear antibody | Positive ANA |

From Tan et al. [23] and Hochberg [24], with permission

**Table 4.8** LE-specific skin disorders and morphology

| | |
|---|---|
| ACLE | • Diffuse, photosensitive, edematous erythema with an overlying, fine scale<br>• May be localized (butterfly distribution of malar eminences of the face and bridge of the nose) *OR* generalized (face, upper trunk, and/or extremities)<br>• Parallels activity of underlying SLE<br>• Spares nasolabial folds, MCP, PIP, and DIP joints |
| SCLE | • Erythematous, scaly macules and papules that evolve into papulosquamous or annular plaques with typical photodistribution<br>• Annular plaques have erythematous borders with central clearing<br>• Papulosquamous plaques are psoriasiform with well-defined borders and adherent, hyperkeratotic scale<br>• Predominantly found in Caucasians<br>• Other variants: exanthematous, follicular erythematous, pityriasiform, and exfoliative erythroderma |
| CCLE | Classic DLE. *Early:* disk-shaped, erythematous plaques with follicular plugging and scaling. *Late*: hypopigmented, atrophied depressed plaques with hyperpigmented borders and central telangiectasias<br>Hypertrophic (verrucous) DLE – hyperkeratotic plaques on face, upper back, extensor surfaces of arms and legs, and palms and soles<br>LE profundus (panniculitis) – firm, mobile subcutaneous nodules with adherent, depressed overlying skin<br>Lupus tumidus – erythematous, indurated, urticarial plaques from mucin deposition in the dermis<br>Chilblain lupus – erythematous to violaceous patches and plaques in acral areas developing upon exposure to cold temperatures and damp climates |

Adapted from McCauliffe [25] and Rothfield et al. [26], with permission

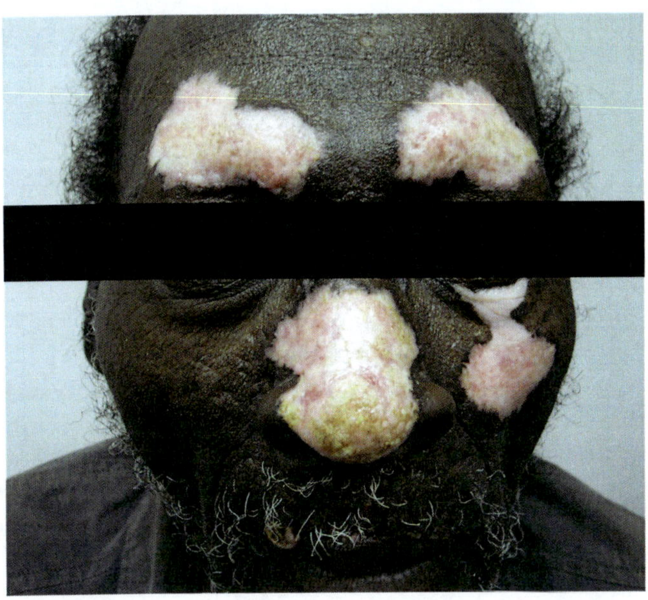

**Fig. 4.3** Strikingly hypopigmented plaques with scarring and follicular plugging in DLE

converge and produce large, disfiguring plaques [26]. Hyperkeratotic, adherent scales are often present, particularly on the conchae of the ear. The typical distribution of DLE includes the face (excluding the nasolabial folds), scalp (producing a scarring alopecia), external ear, neck, and extensor surfaces of the arms [26]. DLE lesions can develop in non-photosensitive areas and may undergo Koebnerization following trauma [26]. In addition, DLE has been associated with destructive, metastatic secondary squamous cell carcinoma in black patients [27].

Nail changes may include leukonychia striata, pitting, onycholysis, erythema or telangiectasia of the proximal nail fold, and development of DLE lesions in the nail bed [25, 26, 28]. Individuals of African descent may show dark, blue-black nail dyschromia [25].

## *Epidemiology*

Women are more commonly affected by lupus of all types, the female to male ratio in DLE being approximately 3:1 [28]. LE typically occurs in the fourth to fifth decades of life [28]. African Americans have among the highest prevalence rates of SLE in the world [29], and DLE is also more common among them [25].

## *Pathophysiology*

The cause of SLE and cutaneous LE is unknown and heterogeneous. Possible etiology is due to a genetic susceptibility, particularly from HLA type, leading to autoimmune induction, loss of self-tolerance, and resultant end-organ damage due to autoantibody production and immune complex deposition [26]. There is evidence that DLE in certain African Americans families may be associated with genetic locus 11p13 [30].

## *Histopathology*

Typical findings include orthohyperkeratosis, liquefactive degeneration of the epidermal basal layer, follicular hyperkeratosis, and perivascular, perifollicular, and dermal-epidermal infiltrate of mononuclear cells (macrophages and T lymphocytes) [26]. Epidermal basement membrane thickening and melanin pigment incontinence may also be present [26, 28]. Older lesions may show epidermal atrophy with ectasia of the superficial blood vessels [28].

**Table 4.9** Differential diagnosis for DLE

| |
|---|
| Sarcoidosis |
| Leishmaniasis |
| Inflammatory dermatophytosis |
| Psoriasis |
| Seborrheic dermatitis |
| Vitiligo leukoderma |
| Phenolic compound-related leukoderma |
| Acne rosacea (rarely found in blacks) |
| Lymphocytoma cutis |
| Mycosis fungoides |
| Granuloma faciale |
| Polymorphous light eruption |

From McCauliffe [25], with permission

## Laboratory

In DLE, ANA-positive titer $\geq$ 1:160 is present in less than 10% of patients [25]. Single-stranded DNA(ss-DNA) antibodies occur in one-fifth of DLE patients and typically indicate widespread and progressive disease [28]. Anti-Ro/SS-A antibodies have been found to be associated with photosensitivity in LE [28]. Patients with SCLE or DLE and ANA titers $\geq$ 1:160 are at greater risk of developing or already having SLE [25]. Direct immunofluorescence may help to differentiate DLE from other conditions, since over 80% of lesional skin will have immunoglobulin and/or complement protein deposition at the dermal-epidermal junction [25].

## Differential Diagnosis

The lesions of DLE are very striking and unique. However, early lesions may be more difficult to diagnose and resemble other erythematous papulosquamous cutaneous disorders (Table 4.9) [25].

## Treatment

Table 4.10 offers therapeutic options for cutaneous lupus erythematosus. Antimalarials (hydroxychloroquine, chloroquine, quinacrine) are the most useful systemic therapy. Retinopathy is the most concerning side effect for hydroxychloroquine and chloroquine therapy and occurs in 3% and 10% of treated patients, respectively [28]. These agents should not be used together due to additive effects on retinal damage. Periodic ophthalmologic examination, hematologic, and hepatic

**Table 4.10** Therapeutic options for cutaneous LE

- Photoprotection (avoidance, broad-spectrum sunscreens with UVB photoprotection and SPF>30, UV light-blocking films for home and automobile windows)
- Topical corticosteroids (can be given under occlusion)
  - Medium potency: triamcinolone acetonide 0.1%
  - High potency: clobetasol propionate 0.05%, betamethasone dipropionate 0.05%, diflorasone diacetate 0.05%, amcinonide 0.1%
- Intralesional corticosteroids
- Aminoquinoline antimalarials[a]
  - Hydroxychloroquine 200–400 mg/day
  - Quinacrine 100–200 mg/day
  - Chloroquine 250–500 mg/day
- Dapsone 100–200 mg/day
- Other agents

  Oral steroids, retinoids (isotretinoin or acitretin 0.5–1 mg/kg/day), clofazimine 100 mg/day, thalidomide 100–200 mg/day, cytotoxic immunosuppressive agents (azathioprine, methotrexate, cyclophosphamide, cyclosporine), and gold

Adapted from McCauliffe [25], Rothfield et al. [26], and Fabbri et al. [28], with permission

[a]Hydroxychloroquine 200–400 mg/day divided in 2 doses for 2–3 months; if no signs of clinical improvement, can add quinacrine 100 mg/day. If response remains inadequate after another 4–6 weeks, chloroquine can be substituted for hydroxychloroquine. Chloroquine and hydroxychloroquine should not be used as combined therapy due to retinal toxicity.

functioning tests are required while on antimalarial agents [28]. Topical or intralesional corticosteroids may be used for localized lesions [26, 28]. Oral steroids can be a beneficial therapy while waiting for antimalarial agents to take effect or for lesions refractory to antimalarials [26, 28]. Thalidomide is useful for refractory lesions [26]. Thalidomide may stimulate regrowth of hair in LE-related alopecia and effluvium [28].

## Pityriasis Rosea

Pityriasis rosea (PR) is a common, self-limited, papulosquamous eruption. Classically, the rash is heralded by the development of a pink macule or papule, typically on the trunk, that expands over a few days to become a 2–10-cm, salmon-colored, oval plaque with slightly raised borders and a collarette of scale, known as the herald patch [31, 32]. A prodrome consisting of headache, general malaise, loss of appetite, arthralgias, and low-grade fever may occur in 5% of cases [31]. After about 10 days, secondary lesions erupt and consist of round to ovoid, 5–10-mm, salmon-colored, scaling patches with long axes following the lines of cleavage across the trunk; these lesions erupt in successive crops over the following 1–3 weeks [32]. Spontaneous resolution occurs in 2–14 weeks. Lesions may be intensely pruritic. Other less common variants of PR exist (Table 4.11).

**Table 4.11** Pityriasis rosea variants

| |
|---|
| *Variants in distribution* |
| Inverse (face and distal extremities) |
| Unilateralis (does not cross midline) |
| Irritata (wrists and feet) |
| *Variants in morphology* |
| Giganta (fewer, larger papules and plaques) |
| Circinata et marginata (large, coalescent plaques) |
| Pustular |
| Purpuric (may be associated with hematologic malignancies) |
| Papular |
| Vesicular |
| Urticarial |

Information adapted from González et al. [31], with permission

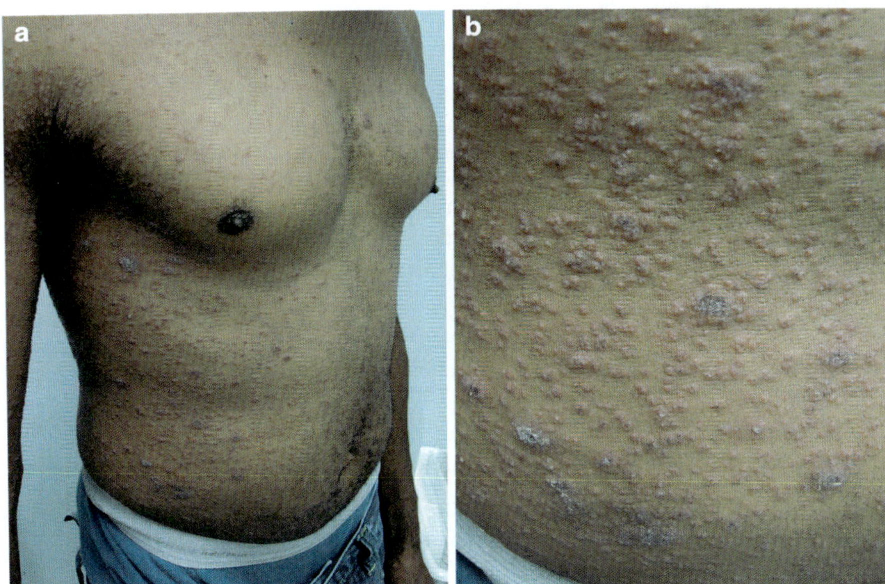


**Fig. 4.4** (**a**) Pityriasis rosea presents as edematous papules, papulovesicles, and plaques. (**b**) Close-up of prior image. Note atypical indurated lesions

Most notably in skin of color, the classically described "salmon-pink"-colored lesions of PR are typically a dull, reddish-brown to deep brown hue, which may obscure the diagnosis for some clinicians. PR more commonly presents as a generalized eruption with associated lymphadenopathy in blacks compared to whites [31]. Moreover, the eruption may consist of edematous papules or papulovesicles, rather than as flat, scaly patches [31, 33] (Fig. 4.4a, b). These papular lesions still tend to orient along lines of cleavage and may undergo post-inflammatory hypo- or hyperpigmentation, particularly when located on the face [33]. People of African descent may also be more likely to present with scalp, facial, and oral lesions than other populations [31, 33]. PR lesions resolve without scarring, although persistent post-inflammatory dyschromia is common in skin of color.

## Epidemiology

PR typically presents between the ages of 10 and 35 in 75% of the cases [31]. PR is uncommon in the very young and the elderly, although reported cases have ranged in age from 3 months old to 83 years old [31]. There is no gender or racial predilection. In temperate zones, such as the United States, PR has a seasonal distribution, being highest in autumn and spring; this difference is not reported in Africa.

## Etiology

PR is most likely caused by a viral agent, due to its seasonal variation, low risk of recurrence, increased risk of recurrence in immunodeficient states, association with a prodromal illness, reported clustering of cases, and, most importantly, programmed sequence of events [31, 34]. Current focus is on human herpesviruses 6 and 7 [31, 34–36].

## Histopathology

Nonspecific findings include patchy parakeratosis, slight acanthosis, mild spongiosis, reduced granular cell layer, and a dermal, perivascular infiltrate of lymphocytes, histiocytes, and occasional eosinophils [31]. Extravasation of papillary dermal red blood cells may be particularly prominent in purpuric PR [31]. Dyskeratotic cells of the upper dermis and multinuclear giant cells of the epidermis may also be found [31, 35].

## Differential Diagnosis

Table 4.12 gives the differential diagnosis of pityriasis rosea. PR can often be confused with the papulosquamous rash of secondary syphilis. There are also a number of drugs associated with a pityriasiform eruption (Table 4.13).

**Table 4.12** Differential diagnosis of pityriasis rosea

| |
|---|
| *Herald patch* |
| Tinea corporis |
| Granuloma annulare |
| *Secondary lesions* |
| Secondary syphilis (especially if palms and soles involved) |
| Guttate psoriasis |
| Nummular eczema (diffuse) |
| Parapsoriasis |
| Lichen planus |
| Erythema dischromicum perstans |
| Tinea versicolor |
| Drug associated (Table 4.3) |

Data adapted from González et al. [31] and Stulberg and Wolfrey [32], with permission

**Table 4.13** Drugs associated with pityriasiform eruptions

| |
|---|
| Arsenic compounds |
| Barbiturates |
| Bismuth |
| Calmette-Guerin bacillus vaccine |
| Captopril |
| Clonidine |
| D-penicillamine |
| Diphtheria toxoid vaccine |
| Gold |
| Hepatitis B vaccine (Recombivax-HB) |
| Hydroxychloroquine |
| Imatinib mesylate (Gleevec) |
| Interferon |
| Isotretinoin |
| Ketotifen (Zaditor) |
| Levamisole |
| Metronidazole |
| Omeprazole |
| Terbinafine |

Data adapted from González et al. [31] and Stulberg, Wolfrey [32]

## *Treatment*

Patients should be reassured that PR will resolve without therapeutic intervention, and any therapy is geared only toward symptomatic relief. Options include oral antihistamines, topical steroids, and soothing lotions (containing zinc oxides, menthol, phenol, and oatmeal) [31]. Severe cases may be treated with intramuscular corticosteroids, systemic corticosteroids, or oral dapsone. Although exposure to ultraviolet irradiation is effective, this modality is not recommended in skin of color as it may worsen post-inflammatory hyperpigmentation.

## Psoriasis

Psoriasis is a chronic, systemic inflammatory disorder without a permanent cure. Psoriasis presents with typical clinical features that include:

- Well-demarcated, erythematous plaques with an overlying, thick silvery scale
- Nail dystrophy (pits, oil spots, and subungual keratotic debris)
- Scalp involvement with scaling plaques
- Potential for the development of exfoliative erythroderma, localized or generalized pustular psoriasis, and debilitating psoriatic arthritis

Eruptive, guttate psoriasis is typically seen in children recovering from an upper respiratory infection and is notable for 2–10-mm, discrete, inflammatory papules, scattered across the trunk, face, and scalp with sparing of the palms and soles [37]. These lesions typically resolve in a few weeks, but may become recurrent and evolve into chronic, plaque psoriasis [37]. Pustular psoriasis lesions may be localized, generalized, or form annular plaques. Certain triggers may exacerbate psoriasis (Table 4.14) [38].

The scant literature on the subject of psoriasis in skin of color suggests that both nail dystrophy and severe skin manifestations are relatively uncommon compared to whites. From a clinical and morphological standpoint, the severity of psoriasis in heavily pigmented skin, similar to atopic dermatitis, may be difficult to evaluate since erythema is less easily noted [8]. Instead, psoriasis in patients with heavily pigmented skin may present as bluish-black, minimally scaly, flattened plaques without erythema. In obscure cases, biopsy may be needed to secure the diagnosis.

### *Epidemiology*

Psoriasis currently affects 2–3% of the world's population [39]. However, there is significant racial variability. Psoriasis is most common among Caucasians, less common among Asian and African populations, and least common among Native Americans [39].

**Table 4.14** Psoriasis triggers

| |
|---|
| Infections (viral, streptococcal) |
| Medications |
| ACE inhibitors |
| Antimalarials |
| Beta blockers |
| Lithium |
| Stress |
| Sunburn |
| Surgery |
| Trauma (Koebner phenomenon) |

Data adapted from Leder and Farber [38], and Kormeili et al. [39]

**Table 4.15** Age variation in psoriasis

| Type | Age (years) | Severity | Genetic link |
|---|---|---|---|
| Early onset | 16–22 | Generalized, severe | Yes |
| Late onset | 57–60 | Localized, mild | No |

Information adapted from Kormeili et al. [39], with permission

While once thought to be a rare disorder in African Americans, psoriasis may actually occur in approximately 1% of African Americans [40]. A higher psoriasis prevalence is reported for Bantu peoples of eastern Africa (2.4%) than for non-Bantu peoples of western Africa (<1%); the incidence among African Americans is more similar to that found in western Africans likely due to a common ancestry [38]. The age of onset shows a bimodal distribution in the second and sixth decades (Table 4.15). Childhood psoriasis is rare in African Americans. There is no gender predominance.

## *Pathophysiology*

The exact etiology of psoriasis remains elusive and is most likely due to a complex interaction between the environment and genetics. Psoriasis is characterized by hyperproliferative, poorly differentiated keratinocytes and extreme inflammation, the therapeutic targets of oral retinoids [41]. Several HLA alleles have been proposed as psoriasis susceptibility genes. However, HLA alleles that confer increased risk of psoriasis in Caucasians may not confer the same risk for African populations with the same HLA alleles [38]. The immunology of psoriasis is characterized by an overactivity of proinflammatory TH1 response (IL-2, IL-12, IFN-$\gamma$) with resulting increased macrophage activation and overproduction of TNF-$\alpha$, which has also become the target of recent biologic therapies [39, 42].

## *Histopathology*

- Marked parakeratosis, epidermal hyperplasia with thickened and elongated rete ridges, increased mitosis of keratinocytes, edematous and elongated dermal papillae, and decreased granular layer may be noted on microscopic examination [37].
- Microabscesses of Munro, composed of degenerated polymorphonuclear cells, may be noted in the epidermis [37].
- Dilated capillaries are present in the dermal papillae (clinically leading to Auspitz sign) with a variable amount of mononuclear and polymorphonuclear inflammatory infiltrate.

### *Differential Diagnosis*

Atopic dermatitis, drug eruptions, lichen planus, seborrheic dermatitis, tinea corporis, secondary syphilis, contact dermatitis, and cutaneous T-cell lymphoma should all be considered.

### *Treatment*

Therapeutic options are based upon the severity of psoriasis. Therapy is designed to control acute flares and to provide maintenance suppression. As a general rule, topical therapy should not be used as monotherapy if the patient has greater than 20% body surface area (BSA) involvement [43, 44]. Both topical and systemic therapies are available (Tables 4.16, 4.17, and 4.18). Systemic therapies have a number of side effects and may require frequent laboratory monitoring. Combinational, rotational, and sequential therapy may be helpful in reducing adverse effects while maintaining efficacy [44].

## Sarcoidosis

Sarcoidosis is a noncaseating granulomatous disorder of undetermined etiology that can involve almost any organ system. Sarcoidosis most commonly involves the lungs and lymphatic system but may also involve the skin, liver, spleen, eyes, nervous system, parotid and lacrimal glands, and bones [45, 46]. Cutaneous involvement occurs in about 25% of systemic cases but can occur without evidence of systemic involvement [47, 48]. Sarcoidosis shows a wide array of cutaneous manifestations and has been appropriately called the "great imitator"; these lesions can develop during any stage of systemic disease, and their prognostic significance remains controversial [46, 47].

**Table 4.16** Topical versus systemic/phototherapy for psoriasis

| Topical | Systemic/phototherapy |
|---|---|
| • Used for mild, localized psoriasis<br>• Never use as monotherapy if >20% BSA affected<br>• Generally safer<br>• May stain skin and clothing (tar, anthralin), cause skin irritation (tazarotene, calcipotriene, tar, anthralin), or have an unpleasant odor (tar) | • Used for severe (>10% BSA), widespread psoriasis<br>• Generally more side effects than topical therapies<br>• Useful if failed response to topical treatments or diminished quality of life |

Data adapted from Lebwohl [44], with permission

**Table 4.17** Topical agents for psoriasis

| Agent | Formulation | Efficacy | Side effects |
|---|---|---|---|
| Corticosteroids | Ointment = gel > cream > lotion > foam (classes 1–7) | Effective, thinning of plaques, decreased symptoms in first 2 weeks | Atrophy, striae, rosacea, telangiectasias, acneiform eruption, contact dermatitis, systemic absorption |
| Vitamin D3 analogs | Dovonex® (calcipotriene 0.005%) cream, ointment, scalp solution<br>Taclonex® (calcipotriene 0.005%, betamethasone dipropionate 0.064%) ointment and scalp solution | • As effective as class 2 corticosteroids<br>• Response observed in first 2 weeks, but 6–8 weeks of treatment required for maximum effect | • Skin irritation in up to 20% (should not be used on face or groin)<br>• Risk of hypercalcemia and hypercalciuria when used at dose > 100 g/week |
| Retinoids | Tazorac (tazarotene 0.05%, 0.1% gel or cream) | • As effective as class 2 corticosteroids<br>• Rapid onset, with improvement in 1–2 weeks | • Skin irritation in up to 30%<br>• Class X drug – should not be used in pregnant or lactating women |
| Tar | Coal tar preparations (crude coal tar, tar shampoos, liquor carbonis detergens) | • Response in 2–4 weeks<br>• Less effective than corticosteroids, vitamin D3 analogs, and retinoids | • Offensive odor, messy, staining of clothing and skin<br>• Folliculitis, photosensitivity, potential risk of skin cancer |
| Salicylic acid | Formulations of 2%–10% in base. Available in combined formulations: Diprosalic® (salicylic acid 2–3%, betamethasone 0.05%), Coco-Scalp® (salicylic acid 2%, coal tar solution 12%, sulfur 4%) | • Particularly useful for palmoplantar psoriasis<br>• Does not usually result in clearance when used alone | Risk of salicylate toxicity when used on >20% BSA |
| Anthralin | Anthralin cream 1% | • Response in 2–4 weeks<br>• Less effective than corticosteroids, vitamin D3 analogs, and retinoids<br>• Can be used in patients who fail other topical therapies | *Severe* irritation (avoid contact with surrounding skin), purplish staining of clothing, skin, and other materials |

From Gottlieb [43] and Lebwohl [44], with permission

**Table 4.18** Systemic agents for psoriasis

| Drug | Dosage | Laboratory tests | Side effects |
|---|---|---|---|
| Methotrexate | 7.5–25 mg/week oral, subcutaneous, or intramuscular dose | • Pregnancy, liver function tests, CBC, renal function tests<br>• Liver biopsy when cumulative dose of 1.5 g reached<br>• Should be avoided if history of liver disease | Nausea, headache, phototoxic reactions, ulcerative stomatitis, hepatotoxicity, hepatic fibrosis, pulmonary fibrosis, myelosuppression, induction of lymphomas, teratogen (pregnancy should be avoided for 3 months in men and one ovulatory cycle in women after cessation of MTX) |
| Cyclosporine | 3–5 mg/kg/day oral, available in 25- or 100-mg gelatin capsules | Renal function tests, CBC, lipid panel, blood pressure monitoring, magnesium, potassium | Flares following withdrawal of medication, nephrotoxicity, hyperlipidemia, hypertension, gastrointestinal upset, flu-like symptoms, gingival hypertrophy, hypertrichosis; should not be used > 1 year duration |
| Acitretin | 25–50 mg every other day or daily | Pregnancy, liver function tests, lipid panel, CBC, renal function tests | Hepatotoxicity, hypertriglyceridemia, pseudotumor cerebri, alopecia, arthralgia, DISH syndrome, osteoporosis, premature epiphyseal closure, *teratogen* (for up to 3 years after cessation) |
| TNF-$\alpha$ inhibitors (infliximab, adalimumab, etanercept, ustekinumab) | Dosages and scheduling vary depending on disease severity | CBC, TB testing, renal function tests, hepatitis serologies in patients at risk | Serious infection (TB, invasive fungal infections, sepsis), increased incidence of lymphoma, pancytopenia, CHF, hypersensitivity reactions, neurological disorders, lupus-like syndrome |

From Gottlieb [43] and Lebwohl [44], with permission

**Table 4.19** Morphologic variants of sarcoidosis[a]

| Variant | Description | Characteristics |
|---|---|---|
| Lupus pernio | Indolent, violaceous, indurated papules, nodules, and plaques about the midface, lips, and ears | • Chronic fibrotic course with risk of nasal ulceration and septal perforation<br>• Associated with pulmonary infiltration, chronic uveitis, and lytic bone destruction (dactylitis of hands and feet) |
| Papular | • Red to violaceous papules, less than 1 cm in diameter, occurring anywhere on the body (including mucous membranes) OR<br>• Small, 2–6-mm eruptive micropapular lesions clustered on eyelids, lips, nape of neck, upper back, and hands | • Maculopapular lesions associated with less severe systemic manifestations and resolve over several years<br>• Diascopy of lesion reveals apple-jelly color<br>• Micropapular lesions may be assoc iated with acute hilar lymphadenopathy and ocular inflammation but has overall good prognosis |
| Annular plaques | Hypopigmented, atrophied plaque with central clearing and an infiltrated, active border involving face, scalp, back, and extensor surfaces | • Often presents bilaterally and resolves with scarring<br>• Angiolupoid designates annular sarcoid plaques with telangiectasias |
| Psoriasiform plaques | Crusted, scaly plaques on elbows and knees | • Polycyclic appearance and heals with scar |
| Subcutaneous (Darier-Roussy) | Round to oval, firm, mobile nodules with surface hypo- or hyperpigmentation involving the extremities | • Less severe systemic involvement, typically bilateral hilar lymphadenopathy<br>• May persist for several months |
| Ulcerative | Necrotic ulceration with a violaceous, rolled border and an atrophied base, most frequently involving pretibial area | • Nonhealing, treatment-resistant ulcers<br>• Commonly affects young women<br>• Early manifestation of systemic disease |
| Scar | Infiltration of old scars, resulting in reddish to violaceous coloration | • Occurs over days to weeks<br>• Reflects an exacerbation of the systemic disease |
| Alopecia | • Occurs over days to weeks<br>• Reflects an exacerbation of the systemic disease | • Most common in African American women<br>• Typically have systemic and other cutaneous involvement |

Data adapted from Fernandez-Faith and McDonnell [49] and Katta et al. [56]

[a]Other variants include verrucous, hypopigmented patches, ichthyosiform, erythrodermic, and mucosal

**Table 4.20** Sarcoid differential diagnosis based upon morphological variant

| | | |
|---|---|---|
| *Alopecia* | *Maculopapular* | *Plaque (annular)* |
| Cutaneous lupus erythematosus | Xanthelasma | Granuloma annulare |
| Lichen planopilaris | Lichen planus | Secondary syphilis |
| Pseudopelade | Rosacea | Leprosy |
| Alopecia areata | Trichoepithelioma | Annular elastolytic giant cell granuloma |
| Alopecia neoplastica | Syringoma | Tinea corporis |
| *Hypopigmentation* | Adenoma sebaceum | *Plaque (psoriasiform)* |
| Post-inflammatory hypopigmentation | Syphilis | Psoriasis |
| Vitiligo | Polymorphous light eruption | *Scar* |
| Pityriasis lichenoides chronica | Cutaneous lupus erythematosus | Tattoo pigment foreign body reaction |
| Syphilis | *Micropapular* | Keloid |
| Leishmaniasis | Lichen nitidus | *Subcutaneous (Darier-Roussy)* |
| Leprosy | Lichen planus | Tuberculosis |
| Pinta | Lichen scrofulosorum | Deep mycoses |
| Chemical-induced | *Plaque (general)* | Epidermoid cysts |
| *Ichthyosiform* | Discoid lupus erythematosus | Lipomatosis |
| Cutaneous lupus erythematosus | Necrobiosis lipoidica | Rheumatoid nodules |
| Dermatomyositis | Morphea | Cutaneous metastases |
| Malignancy (lymphoma, multiple myeloma, carcinoma) | Leprosy | Erythema induratum |
| Chronic malnutrition | Leishmaniasis | *Ulcerative* |
| Hypothyroidism | Lichen planus | Necrobiosis lipoidica |
| Leprosy | Cutaneous T-cell lymphoma | Ulcerative rheumatoid necrobiosis |
| Drug-induced | B-cell lymphoma | Necrobiotic xanthogranuloma |
| | Secondary syphilis | Pyoderma gangrenosum |
| | Gyrate erythema | |

From Fernandez-Faith and McDonnell [49], with permission

Skin involvement is divided into specific and nonspecific manifestations. Specific lesions (Table 4.19) show the classic noncaseating granulomas on histopathological examination, whereas nonspecific lesions do not [47]. However, the "specific" lesions of sarcoidosis can clinically mimic almost any type of skin disease, leading to a massive differential diagnosis for sarcoidosis pertaining to the particular morphology noted on clinical examination (Table 4.20). In brief, sarcoidosis can present as macular hypopigmentation, ichthyosis-like patches, deep nodules, annular, psoriasiform or verrucous plaques, scarring alopecia, micropapular lesions, and ulcerations (Figs. 4.5 and 4.6). In fact, sarcoidosis should be considered as a diagnostic possibility when confronted with almost *any* skin eruption in an African American patient. Violaceous-colored maculopapules and plaques are the most common type of specific lesion [49].

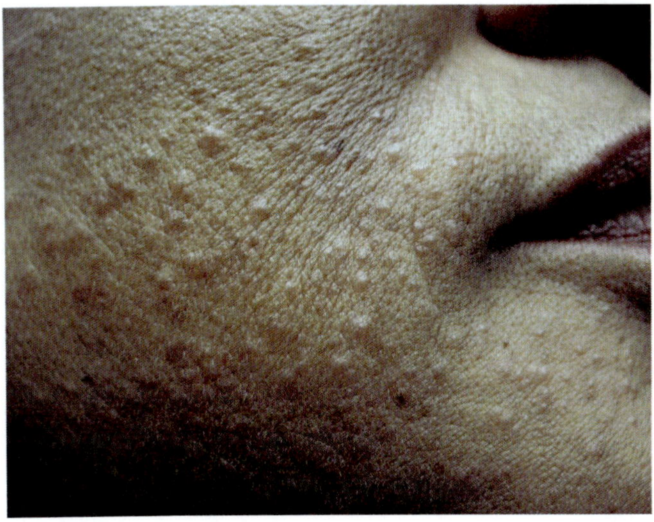

**Fig. 4.5** Profusion of tiny lesions characterize micropapular sarcoid

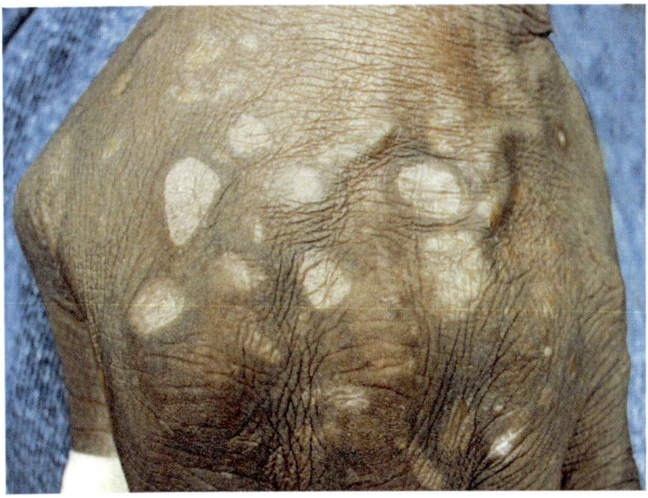

**Fig. 4.6** Hypopigmented macules may represent sarcoid in skin of color

Lupus pernio is the most characteristic sarcoid-specific lesion, consisting of indolent, violaceous, and indurated papules, plaques, and small nodules, primarily involving the nose, lips, and ears, as well as periorificial facial skin (Fig. 4.7). Lupus pernio is associated with granulomatous infiltration of the upper respiratory tract mucosa, leading to possible nasal septum perforation [47], and with dactylitis in black South Africans [50]. Sarcoidosis may also present as a painful, granulomatous, indurated

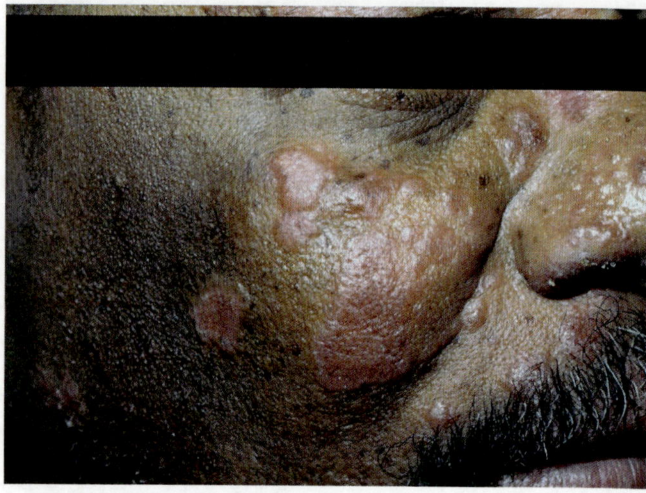

**Fig. 4.7** Typical lupus pernio type of sarcoid

infiltration of preexisting scars, known as scar sarcoidosis. Scar sarcoidosis can develop in areas of decorative, ritualistic, or therapeutic scarifications, most noted in cultural practices of West Africa [50] and India [51]. Scar sarcoidosis may also develop in areas of severe exogenous ochronosis due to excessive use of hydroquinone bleaching creams [50].

Erythema nodosum (EN) is a nonspecific but common sign of sarcoid in young, female patients. EN, though common in white patients with sarcoidosis (10–30%), is uncommon in black patients (<5%). Löfgren's syndrome is an acute, febrile illness with EN lesions, arthritis, arthralgias, and bilateral hilar lymphadenopathy; this condition generally portends a good prognosis with a high rate of spontaneous resolution in a few months to a year [49]. Similar to EN in sarcoidosis, Löfgren's syndrome occurs more frequently in whites than in other groups [52].

## *Epidemiology*

Northern European (Scandinavian, Irish), Caribbean, and African American populations have the highest reported incidence of sarcoidosis worldwide [46]. In the USA, the annual incidence is three to four times greater among African Americans than Caucasians; the highest incidence is found in African American women between the ages of 30 and 39 and is up to ten times greater than in Caucasians [46, 53]. Sarcoidosis is also common among Bantu populations of eastern and southern Africa and, surprisingly, uncommon among non-Bantu populations of western Africa, who share common ancestry with many African Americans. Sarcoidosis has a peak incidence in young adults between the ages of 20 and 40 years. Women are more commonly affected. It is generally accepted that black patients, regardless of country of origin, have a poorer prognosis when compared to their white or Asian counterparts.

## Etiology

In the pathogenesis of sarcoidosis, granuloma formation is possibly caused by a predominately TH1-mediated immune response to a poorly degradable exogenous antigen of low potency [54]. Several infectious etiologic agents, some more substantiated than others, have been implicated and include mycobacteria, *Propionibacterium acnes*, *Tropheryma whipplei*, spirochetes, fungi, and the DNA viruses (EBV, HSV, HHV-8) [54].

## Histopathology

Sarcoidosis-specific lesions will show noncaseating granulomas with a central zone of epithelioid and giant cells surrounded by a narrow border of lymphocytes and scattered plasma cells [49]. Foci of necrosis may be indicative of larger lesions and/or more widespread involvement [50, 55]. Schaumann bodies, laminated basophilic inclusions that represent degenerated lysosomes, and asteroid bodies, eosinophilic stellate inclusions that represent engulfed collagen, may be found within sarcoid giant cells but are not specific for sarcoidosis [49]. "Great imitator" not only applies to the clinical manifestations of sarcoidosis but also to the histopathological examination, since sarcoid granulomata may mimic other processes, particularly tuberculosis [49]; biopsy specimens should be subjected to Gram, periodic acid-Schiff, and Ziehl-Nielsen stains, as well as polarization studies [47].

## Laboratory

- *Hematologic* – anemia and leukopenia may be detected in 5–10%, eosinophilia in 20%, and elevated ESR in 50–70%.
- *Metabolic* – hypercalcemia and hypercalciuria may occur in 5–25% and lead to nephrocalcinosis and renal insufficiency.
- *Immunologic* – polyclonal hypergammaglobulinemia occurs in 50% and may be more common in blacks. Decreased T helper/suppressor cell ratio (less than 1:1) may also be noted.
- *Other* – serum angiotensin-converting enzyme (ACE) is elevated in up to 60% with a 40% false-negative rate and 10–15% false-positive rate. ACE level reflects the overall granuloma load and may be used to follow therapeutic response.

**Table 4.21** Sarcoid histopathology differential

| | |
|---|---|
| *Immunologic and foreign body* | |
| | Berylliosis |
| | Silicosis |
| | Zirconium granuloma |
| | Sea urchin granuloma |
| | Tattoo granuloma |
| *Infectious* | |
| | Tuberculosis |
| | Tuberculoid leprosy |
| | Atypical mycobacterium |
| | Deep fungal |
| | Cutaneous leishmaniasis |
| | Spirochetes |
| *Neoplasia* | |
| | Squamous cell carcinoma |
| | Breast carcinoma |
| | Bronchial carcinoma |
| | Lymphoma |
| *Other* | |
| | Actinic elastolytic granuloma |
| | Necrobiosis lipoidica |
| | Granulomatous rosacea |
| | Crohn's disease |

Adapted from Fernandez-Faith and McDonnell [49], with permission

## *Differential Diagnosis*

Diagnosis is dependent upon the clinical presentation, chest radiographic examination, and histopathological specimens [56]. The differential for both clinical and histopathological manifestations of sarcoidosis is extensive (Tables 4.20 and 4.21).

## *Treatment*

Therapy for cutaneous sarcoidosis is primarily based on clinical experience due to the current lack of evidence-based recommendations. Treatment is designed to suppress the various manifestations of the disease, but achievement of a cure is not possible at this date. In patients that have both cutaneous and extracutaneous manifestations, clinicians may utilize the response of skin lesions as a surrogate for overall therapeutic response. The most commonly employed treatment modalities are [45]:

- *Corticosteroids* – intralesional (triamcinolone acetonide 6–10 mg/ml repeated every 4 weeks), ultrapotent topical (clobetasol propionate 0.05% or halobetasol propionate 0.05% twice daily), and systemic (20–60 mg/day initially and tapered over 2 to 3 months to a minimal, maintenance dose)

- *Antimalarials* – (chloroquine 3.5 mg/kg/day, hydroxychloroquine 6.5 mg/kg/day). Require ophthalmologic examination every 6 months to a year
- *Methotrexate* – (10–30 mg/week divided on 2 consecutive days, given with oral folate 1 mg/day to prevent dose-dependent mucositis). Require routine CBC, renal function tests, liver function tests, and liver biopsy after cumulative dose > 1.5 g

Other less well-established therapies include, but are not limited to, pentoxifylline, tetracyclines, isotretinoin, thalidomide, infliximab and adalimumab, cyclosporine, chlorambucil, allopurinol, and melatonin [45].

## Scleroderma

Scleroderma is a chronic, autoimmune disorder characterized by cutaneous and systemic fibrosis, obliterative vasculopathy, and autoantibody proliferation [57–59]. Scleroderma is a multiorgan disease that requires a multidisciplinary approach – including rheumatology, pulmonology, and nephrology. Scleroderma is noted not only for a distinct presentation in skin of color but also for differing clinical course, autoantibody profile, and prognosis. Scleroderma is divided into localized scleroderma (morphea) and systemic sclerosis (SSc), as determined by the American College of Rheumatology guidelines (Table 4.22) [60]. The subtypes of localized scleroderma include plaque, generalized, bullous, linear, and deep [61]. Systemic sclerosis is divided into limited SSc (lSSc) and diffuse SSc (dSSc). The focus of this topic will be on the cutaneous manifestations of SSc, since there is a unique presentation in skin of color. A discussion of the many visceral manifestations of SSc is outside the scope of this chapter.

Limited SSc (formerly CREST syndrome) involves skin distal to the elbows and knees, whereas diffuse SSc involves the proximal extremities and trunk [62, 63]. Facial involvement, however, may occur with both [63, 64]. SSc usually begins with an inflammatory, nonpitting edema that gives way to progressive fibrosis, imparting the skin with a smooth, thickened, leathery, bound-down appearance [65, 66]. The fibrosis eventually stabilizes and lesions may undergo atrophy, giving the skin an improved appearance [37, 63, 67]. The time period over which the phases of SSc occur may be years to decades in limited SSc or may occur much more rapidly

**Table 4.22** ACR criteria for diagnosis of systemic sclerosis (scleroderma)[a]

| |
|---|
| *Major criterion* |
| Cutaneous sclerosis proximal to metacarpophalangeal or metatarsophalangeal joints |
| *Minor criterion* |
| Sclerodactyly |
| Digital pits, ulcers, or loss of fat pad |
| Bibasilar pulmonary fibrosis |

[a] Diagnosis requires major criterion or two minor criteria

**Table 4.23** Skin changes in SSc

| |
|---|
| Anhidrosis |
| Calcinosis |
| Digital pits/ulcers |
| Dry skin |
| Hair loss |
| Loss of distal phalanges |
| Masklike facies |
| Narrowing of nose |
| Pigment changes |
| Pruritus |
| Raynaud's phenomenon |
| Sclerodactyly |
| Telangiectasias |
| Tendon friction rubs |
| Thinning of lips (microstomia) |

Data adapted from Wolff et al.[37] and Steen [67]

in diffuse SSc [67]. Fibrosis begins on the fingers and progresses more proximally to involve the trunk; in contrast, the atrophy phase begins on the trunk and progresses distally [67]. Raynaud's phenomenon (blanching, cyanosis, and erythema of the distal fingers upon cold exposure or emotional stimulus) precedes the diagnosis of nearly all limited SSc cases and three-fourths of diffuse SSc cases [67]. There are several other cutaneous manifestations of scleroderma (Table 4.23).

SSc in skin of color is noted for focal, macular, perifollicular hypopigmentation, imparting a salt and pepper appearance to the involved skin, most commonly located on the hands, arms, and anterior trunk [66, 68, 69]. (Fig. 4.8a, b). Diffuse hyperpigmentation may also be present in SSc [67]. Changes in pigmentation may occur with a frequency of 82–93% in African Americans and are one of the most common cutaneous manifestations of SSc in this population [70, 71]. Facial telangiectasias may be more common in whites [70].

## *Epidemiology*

The prevalence of SSc in the USA is 240 cases per 1 million persons (240/million) and is significantly greater than the prevalence reported in Great Britain and Japan, 31/million and 38/million, respectively [63]. The incidence in the USA is approximately 19/million/year [72]. There is also a marked female predominance, with a female to male ratio ranging between 3:1 and 14:1 [63, 73, 74]. A Choctaw Native American group in southeastern Oklahoma has the highest prevalence of SSc, 660 cases/million, in the world [72]. Interestingly, SSc in this population is homogeneously noted for diffuse skin involvement, pulmonary fibrosis, and anti-topoisomerase I (Scl-70) antibodies [58]. African Americans are noted to have a greater risk for diffuse disease, younger age at onset, younger age at clinical presentation, pulmonary disease, and an overall worse prognosis than whites [64, 72, 75].

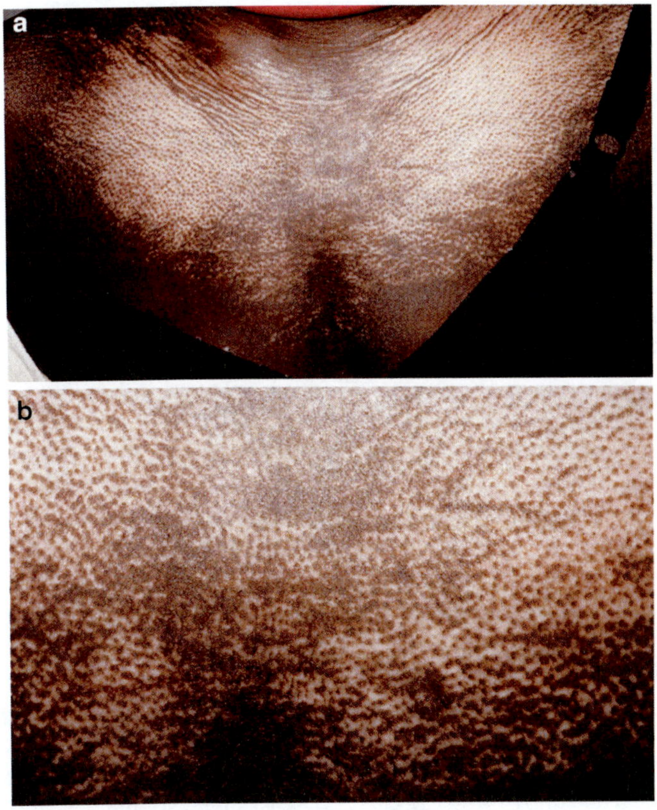

**Fig. 4.8** (**a**) Depigmentation of anterior chest in systemic sclerosis. (**b**) Close-up of the prior figure. Note the "salt and pepper" appearance due to follicular accentuation of dyschromia

Limited studies have also reported increased frequency of diffuse skin involvement in Hispanics compared to Caucasians [75].

## *Etiology*

Although the triggering event is unknown, vascular insult is an early event that precedes the ensuing fibrosis [57]. Pathogenetic mechanisms of SSc involve [57]:

- Early vascular injury with defective vasculogenesis
- Induction of profibrotic cytokines and growth factors (such as TGF-β and PDGF)
- Widespread activation of fibroblasts leading to dermal collagen accumulation with obliteration of dermal vasculature and appendages

The significance of autoantibodies in the pathogenesis of SSc is currently unknown [57].

## Laboratory

Autoantibodies can be seen in more than 95% of patients with SSc [59]. Anticentromere antibodies (ACA) are most specific for limited SSc and isolated pulmonary hypertension, whereas anti-topoisomerase I antibodies are associated with diffuse SSc, renal crisis, severe gastrointestinal and cardiac involvement, and debilitating interstitial fibrosis [59, 62]. ACA is more common in whites [62, 70], while African Americans more commonly have antibodies to topoisomerase I, fibrillarin, U1-RNP, and U3-RNP [62, 67, 75]. Antifibrillarin antibodies are nucleolar autoantibodies that are associated with a poorer prognosis [75]. Anti-U1-RNP has also been noted in African Americans with SLE [70] and may be seen in overlap syndromes [59]. Anti-U3-RNP is also associated with classic, diffuse SSc with multiorgan involvement; more than one half of persons with this antibody and SSc are African American [59]. Interestingly, anti-U3-RNP antibodies in SSc may also be more frequently associated with peripheral neuropathies and musculoskeletal involvement [59, 76]. The poor prognosis seen in blacks may be in part correlated to the serologic phenotype seen in this population [66]. However, African American ethnicity alone has been found to be an independent prognostic factor for more severe disease [77]. Therefore, African Americans with SSc should be screened regularly for visceral complications and treated aggressively early in the course of disease [59].

Other laboratory abnormalities may be present. Elevated creatine phosphokinase may be seen with inflammatory muscle involvement and elevated thyroid-stimulating hormone may indicate concurrent autoimmune thyroiditis or fibrosis of the thyroid gland [78]. Hypothyroidism may occur in 23% of whites but is much less frequent in blacks and Hispanics [70]. Elevated BUN/Cr suggests renal involvement, and urinalysis may show hematuria or proteinuria secondary to hypertension and glomerular damage [78].

## Histopathology

- Early lesions show a mild, mononuclear infiltrate surrounding dermal blood vessels, dermal appendages, and the dermal-subcutaneous junction [37].
- Late lesions are associated with thickening of the dermis and replacement of the subcutaneous fat with hyalinized collagen bundles [37]. Blood vessels show subintimal fibrosis with hyalinized thickening of vessel walls and may be compressed by surrounding dermal sclerosis [37, 68].

The pigmented lesions of SSc are associated with increased basal layer pigmentation, marked pigment incontinence, and increased dermal melanophages [68, 79].

**Table 4.24** Differential diagnosis of SSc

| |
|---|
| *Morphea variants* |
| Generalized morphea |
| Eosinophilic fasciitis (Shulman's syndrome) |
| Lichen sclerosus et atrophicus |
| *Pseudosclerodermas* |
| Scleromyxedema |
| Lichen myxedematosus |
| Scleredema adultorum of Buschke |
| *Drugs/toxin exposure* |
| Bleomycin |
| Polyvinyl chloride |
| Gadolinium (nephrogenic fibrosing dermopathy) |
| *Other* |
| Mixed connective tissue disease |
| Graft-vs.-host disease |
| Acrodermatitis chronica atrophicans (Lyme disease) |
| Porphyria cutanea tarda |
| Vitiligo (pigmentary changes) |
| DLE (pigmentary changes) |

Data adapted from Wolff et al. [37] and Sontheimer [65]

## *Differential Diagnosis*

Table 4.24 details the differential diagnosis for systemic sclerosis. Several conditions may manifest as sclerodermoid lesions. In addition, patients with SSc should avoid exposure to toxins known to cause sclerodermoid changes.

## *Treatment*

Unfortunately, there is a current lack of well-designed, therapeutic trials in the treatment for cutaneous sclerosis [65, 78]. Agents reported with varying efficacies include methotrexate, thalidomide, TNF-$\alpha$ inhibitors, INF-$\gamma$, D-penicillamine, and phototherapy [62]. Long-term systemic steroids are not useful in treating cutaneous sclerosis and may actually precipitate renal crisis and malignant hypertension [62, 65]. Raynaud's phenomenon has been treated with calcium channel blockers, topical prostaglandins, and topical nitroglycerin ointment, all of which may improve blood flow to the distal digits and prevent eventual ulceration [62]; cold exposure and cigarette smoking should be curtailed. Ulceration should be treated with antibiotic ointments and semiocclusive hydrocolloid dressings [65]. Symptoms of pruritus can be treated with bland emollients, antipruritic lotions (with menthol, phenol, camphor), and topical/systemic antihistamines [65].

## Seborrheic Dermatitis

Seborrheic dermatitis (SD) is a chronic, often recurrent inflammatory disorder that affects 1–3% of immunocompetent adults [80] and is characterized by erythematous plaques surmounted by thick, greasy scale. Infants are affected on the scalp (cradle cap), flexural surfaces, and diaper area with onset during the 3rd or 4th week after birth [81]; adults are affected symmetrically on the scalp, central face, eyebrows, nasolabial folds, external ear canals, postauricular creases, axillae, inframammary folds, and upper trunk [82]. Mild pruritus is common.

SD is common in blacks, typically presenting as hypopigmented, annular, scaly patches without appreciable underlying erythema [66]. In addition, annular patches extending from the hairline to the face and onto the upper back are much more common in blacks and are known as "seborrhea petaloides" (petaloid seborrhea) – confluent lesions with a flower-like appearance [66] (Fig. 4.9). The common presentation of annular SD lesions in blacks may be linked to an increased risk of fibroplasias [66].

The implicated organism in SD is *Malassezia* species. These lipophilic, saprophytic yeasts are commonly found in a distribution where sebaceous gland density is the greatest [81, 83]. Similar to pityriasis versicolor, yeast metabolites may inhibit melanocyte tyrosinase function and pigment production, accounting for the hypopigmentation that is particularly striking in pigmented skin.

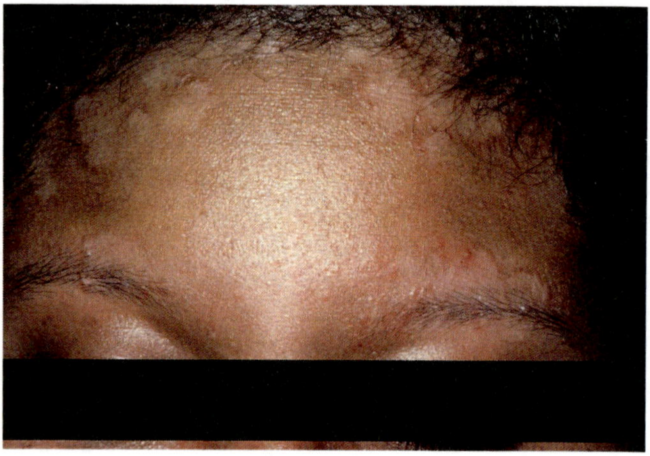

**Fig. 4.9** Petaloid seborrhea in black skin

## *Epidemiology*

SD is common (1–3%) in the general US population and may actually have a slightly increased incidence among African Americans (6.5%) [84] and West Africans (2.9–6%) [85]. SD occurs more commonly in males than females, possibly due to increased androgenic stimulation of sebaceous glands [82]. SD occurs most frequently in adolescents, young adults, and adults over 50 years of age [80]. SD in children typically disappears by 6–12 months of life, indicating a possible role of maternal hormonal stimulation [82]. SD has been reported to occur with a much higher incidence among HIV/AIDS patients, ranging from 30% to 83% [83]. The explosive onset of generalized, recalcitrant seborrhea may suggest underlying HIV/AIDS infection and requires immediate evaluation [81, 82]. SD shows seasonal variation, with improvement during the summer and exacerbation during winter [80, 82]. UVA and UVB light may inhibit the growth of *Malassezia* yeasts [82].

## *Etiology*

As discussed above, SD is currently thought to be caused by *Malassezia* yeasts, a normal constituent of human skin flora. Why certain individuals manifest SD, whereas others do not, remains a dermatologic conundrum. Current mechanisms implicated are inflammatory cytokines released by keratinocytes, increased lipase activity of *Malassezia* species causing the release of irritant fatty acids and arachidonic acid, abnormal host response to yeast colonization, and impaired host cell-mediated immunity facilitating yeast survival [86]. In addition, SD has been noted to be more common in neurologic disorders, such as parkinsonism, postcerebrovascular accidents, epilepsy, central nervous system trauma, depression, and spinal injuries [80, 81]; SD is also more frequent in patients with pityriasis versicolor and *Malassezia* folliculitis [87].

## *Differential Diagnosis*

Diagnosis is based upon clinical examination. Other papulosquamous disorders to consider include psoriasis, atopic dermatitis, pityriasis alba, pityriasis versicolor, dermatophytosis, and nutritional deficiency (riboflavin, pyridoxine, biotin, essential fatty acid) [81].

## *Treatment*

Therapeutic options overlap with those of pityriasis versicolor (Table 4.25).

**Table 4.25** Therapy for seborrheic dermatitis and pityriasis versicolor

| |
|---|
| *Topical regimen* |
| *Nonspecific* |
| – Selenium sulfide 2.5% for 7 days |
| – Propylene glycol in 50% water twice daily for 2 weeks |
| – Benzoyl peroxide 5–10% once daily for 4 weeks |
| – Sulfur-salicylic acid (2%:2%) nightly for 1 week |
| *Specific* |
| – Ketoconazole 2% cream, 2% shampoo, and 2% foaming gel once daily; duration varies; shampoo and foaming gel may be effective after a single use |
| – Fluconazole 2% for 5 days |
| – Terbinafine 1% solution, 1% cream, 1% gel, and 1% spray once to twice daily for 1–2 weeks |
| *Oral regimens* |
| – Ketoconazole in varying dosages and regimens (200 mg/d for 5 days to 4 weeks, 400 mg/d for 3 days, and 400 mg once/week for 2 weeks); may cause hepatotoxicity |
| – Itraconazole 200 mg/d for 5–7 days |
| – Fluconazole 300 mg once/week for 2 weeks |
| – Griseofulvin and terbinafine are *not* effective oral therapies against *Malassezia* species |
| *Prophylactic regimens* |
| – Ketoconazole 200–400 mg on the first 3 days of each month or 400 mg once per month |
| – Itraconazole 400 mg once per month for 6 months |

Data adapted from Gupta et al. [80, 98], Faergemann [87], and Sunenshine et al. [95]

## Syphilis

Syphilis, the sexually transmitted disease caused by the spirochete *Treponema pallidum*, initially presents as a solitary, painless, indurated ulceration (chancre) at the site of inoculation, typically some 3 weeks (range 9–90 days) after contact with an infected partner. This primary lesion resolves without scarring and, over the course of weeks to months, is followed by a secondary, papulosquamous eruption, involving the face, trunk, genitalia, palms, and soles. Constitutional symptoms with fever, fatigue, generalized lymphadenopathy, and arthralgias may also develop [88]. In addition, secondary syphilis can manifest as oral mucosal lesions, patchy "motheaten" alopecia, and moist, anogenital plaques, known as condylomata lata. In tertiary syphilis, gummas, psoriasiform plaques, and granulomatous nodules may appear on the skin. Granulomatous nodules may coalesce into nodular plaques with annular, serpiginous, or polycyclic borders [89]. Gummas are painless, heavily crusted, granulomatous nodules, a few millimeters to centimeters in diameter, that undergo secondary ulceration and heal with disfiguring scars [89].

Syphilis may follow an entirely typical evolution in skin of color; however, it may also demonstrate some unusual features. First, extragenital chancres are said to be rare in African American patients. Moreover, pustular and perifollicular papular rather than papulosquamous lesions may be more common during the secondary stage. Perhaps most notable, an annular syphilid, annular periorificial facial lesions,

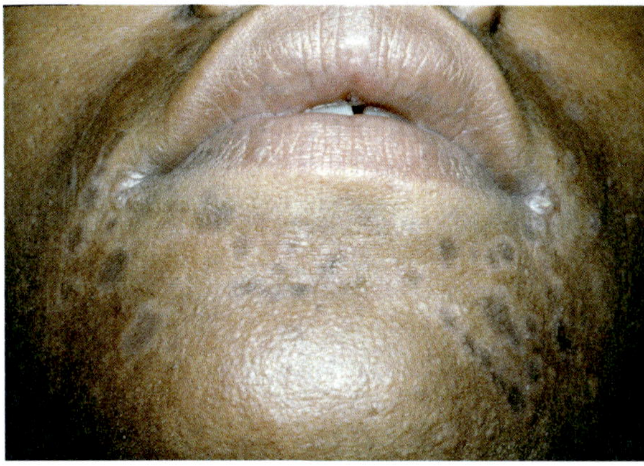

**Fig. 4.10** Annular syphilid presenting around the mouth

is more frequent in black patients (Fig. 4.10). Condylomata lata are reportedly more common in blacks with secondary syphilis, especially women. There have also been reports of extragenital condylomata lata in black patients, but whether this uncommon presentation is more common in blacks has yet to be substantiated [90]. Palmoplantar lesions of secondary syphilis in skin of color tend to resolve with a telltale post-inflammatory hyperpigmentation, which suggests the correct diagnosis. Gummas may be more common in blacks with untreated syphilis, while central nervous system involvement may be less frequent in late disease. A discussion of cardiovascular, neurological, and osseous manifestations of syphilis is beyond the scope of this text.

## *Epidemiology*

The incidence rate of primary and secondary syphilis in the United States reached a nadir in 2000, 2.1 per 100,000 persons [89, 91], and has been most recently reported at 3.8 per 100,000 persons [92]. Racial discrepancies between African Americans and whites in the incidence of reported syphilis cases peaked with an astounding ratio of 62:1 in 1992 [91] and have since declined to 7:1 in 2007 [92]. The incidence rates for primary and secondary syphilis for blacks, Hispanics, and whites, respectively, are 14, 4.2, and 2 (per 100,000 persons) [92]. The disproportionate incidence in blacks and Hispanics may be in part due to an inherent sampling bias of data collection from public health clinics where a higher proportion of blacks and Hispanics seek medical care [93]. There is also a disparity in the incidence of syphilis between men and women that is observed across various races, most likely due to men who have sex with men (MSM) and HIV coinfection [89]. More than 60% of new cases of syphilis occur in MSM [91]. Geographically, the highest rates are noted in the southern USA (5.1/100,000) and the lowest rates in the midwestern USA (1.9/100,000) [92].

**Table 4.26** Differential diagnosis of syphilis by stage

| |
|---|
| *Primary* |
| Behcet's syndrome |
| Bowen's disease |
| Chancroid |
| Fixed drug eruption |
| Genital herpes |
| Genital warts |
| Granuloma inguinale |
| Lymphogranuloma venereum |
| Mucosal lichen planus |
| *Secondary* |
| Atopic dermatitis |
| Dermatophytosis |
| Lichen planus |
| Pityriasis rosea |
| Psoriasis |
| Sarcoidosis |
| Seborrheic dermatitis |
| *Tertiary* |
| Cutaneous metastases |
| Deep mycoses |
| Primary cutaneous lymphoma |
| Tuberculosis |
| Ulcerated basal cell carcinoma |

Data adapted from Brown and Frank [88] and Lautenschlager [89]

## *Laboratory*

Dark field microscopy examination for direct visualization of treponemes is the gold standard and should be performed when feasible. However, screening for syphilis in the USA is often done by the nontreponemal tests, Venereal Disease Research Laboratory (VDRL) or rapid plasma reagin (RPR), and confirmed by the treponemal tests, fluorescent treponemal antibody absorption (FTA-ABS), *Treponema pallidum* particle agglutination assay (TPPA), or microhemagglutination assay (MHA-TP), due to false positives in the former [91]. Titer levels between RPR and VDRL are not equivalent, so the same nontreponemal assay should be used for diagnosis and for detection of serological response [88, 89, 94].Persons suspected of having syphilitic infection should be concurrently screened for other sexually transmitted infections, such as HIV, gonorrhea, chlamydia, and hepatitis B and C [88].

## *Differential Diagnosis*

Similar to sarcoidosis, syphilis is considered to be a great imitator of cutaneous diseases. A differential must be kept in mind for all of the varying stages of syphilis and for the varying presentations of syphilis during those stages (Table 4.26).

### *Treatment*

Standard treatment regimens are published by the public health authority in each country and should be followed. Penicillin G benzathine (Bicillin®-LA), 2.4 million units intramuscularly, remains the treatment of choice for syphilis of under 1 year duration; three injections of Penicillin G benzathine, one given each week for 3 consecutive weeks, are recommended for syphilis of over 1 year or of unknown duration. Patients who are allergic to penicillin should receive doxycycline 100 mg twice a day for 14 days for syphilis under 1 year duration and doxycycline 100 mg twice a day for 28 days for syphilis of greater than 1 year duration [94]. Pregnant women with syphilis and a penicillin allergy are an exception; they should be admitted to the intensive care unit and desensitized to penicillin for treatment [94]. Non-HIV-infected patients are expected to demonstrate a fourfold titer decrease by 6 months in early syphilis (< 1 year duration) and by 12 months in late syphilis (> 1 year duration) [88, 89, 94]. Serologic response is slower in patients coinfected with HIV, and titers typically decline over a longer period of time [94]. Failed serological response to therapy or continued symptoms warrants a lumbar puncture to evaluate for asymptomatic neurosyphilis [88, 91].

## Tinea (Pityriasis) Versicolor

Tinea (pityriasis) versicolor (PV) is a noncommunicable, recurring, cutaneous yeast infection caused by *Malassezia* species [95]. PV lesions present as white ("PV alba"), tan, pink, red ("PV rubra"), brown or black ("PV nigra"), round to oval macules that may coalesce to form large, geographic patches [80, 96, 97]. Scaling is often apparent, particularly if scraped with a sharp edge, *coup d'ongle* sign [95]. The lesions are typically distributed on the trunk and proximal arms but can also be present on the face and neck [96, 97]. Atypical distributions include the eyelids, axillae, groin, and genitalia [96]. In skin of color, lesions are not pink or red, but more commonly either tan/white or brown/black (Fig. 4.11). In people of African descent, particularly in children, hypopigmented facial lesions may be present. PV is generally asymptomatic, although pruritus may occur; the patient most often seeks medical attention due to cosmetic concerns.

### *Epidemiology*

Prevalence of PV varies greatly with the geographic location and climate, with rates from 30% to 50% in some tropical locations and from 1% to 4% in more temperate locations [87, 98]. PV is more common in people from Africa, the Caribbean, and Latin America. PV is most common in young adults and during the summer months in temperate climates; there is no gender predilection [96].

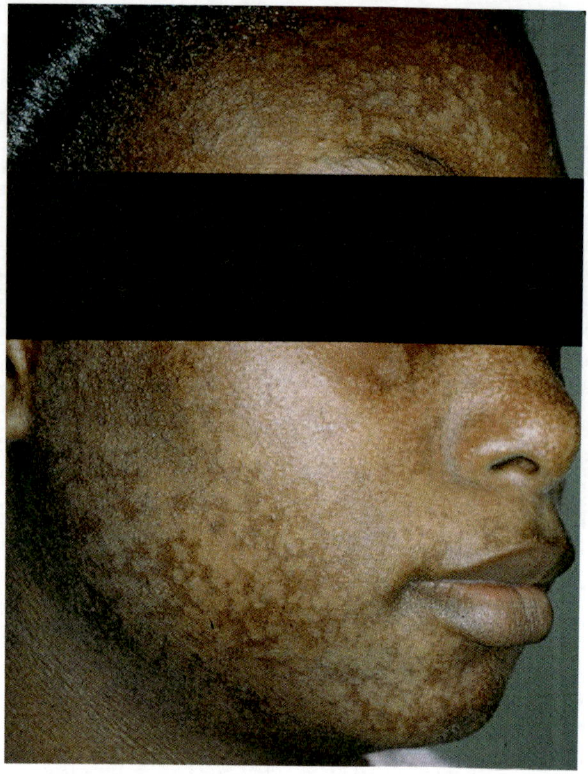

**Fig. 4.11** Tinea versicolor in black skin is often hypopigmented and may affect the face

## Etiology

Similar to seborrheic dermatitis, PV is due to infection of the stratum corneum with *Malassezia* yeasts, most commonly *M. globosa* and *M. sympodialis* [80, 96]. *Malassezia* species are saprophytic yeast that constitute normal human skin flora. For unknown endogenous and exogenous factors, the saprophytic, blastospore form may undergo transformation into a parasitic, mycelial form that allows the yeast to invade the stratum corneum, damage keratinocytes, and disintegrate keratin filaments [80, 96]. Endogenous host factors include malnutrition, oral contraceptives, oral anticoagulants, immunosuppression, corticosteroid therapy, hyperhidrosis, and genetic susceptibility [80, 97, 98]. Exogenous environmental factors include increased humidity, elevated temperatures, and occlusive clothing [96]; this accounts for the increased prevalence in subtropical and tropical locations and the predilection of PV for sites typically covered by clothing [95, 96]. *Malassezia* yeasts are lipophilic, which accounts for the increased incidence of PV in peripubertal and postpubertal populations, during times of increased sebum production [97, 98]. Similar to seborrheic dermatitis, the truncal distribution of PV also conforms to areas of

**Table 4.27** Differential diagnosis of PV

| |
|---|
| Confluent and reticulated papillomatosis |
| Erythrasma |
| Melasma |
| Pinta |
| Pityriasis alba |
| Pityriasis rosea |
| Pityriasis rotunda |
| Seborrheic dermatitis |
| Secondary syphilis |
| Tinea corporis |
| Vitiligo |

Data from Gupta et al. [80, 98] and Crespo-Erchiga and Florencio [96]

increased sebaceous gland density [87]. The mechanism of hypopigmentation has not been fully established, but damage to melanocytes, production of lipid-like substances (pityrialactone, pityriacitrine) that block ultraviolet light, and inhibition of melanocyte tyrosinase by azelaic acid or lipoxygenase have all been proposed [96, 98, 99]. Hyperpigmentation is thought to be due to hypertrophic, abnormal melanosomes, pronounced hyperemic, inflammatory response, or hyperkeratotic response to the proliferating fungus leading to a thickened stratum corneum [98, 99].

## *Laboratory*

A preparation of 10–15% potassium hydroxide (KOH) performed on scale from the edge of the lesion will show the classic spaghetti-and-meatballs appearance under direct microscopy, composed of pseudohyphae-and-blastospores, respectively. Wood's lamp examination may reveal bright yellow or gold fluorescence in up to one-third of cases, possibly due to indole compounds specific to *M. furfur* [80, 98].

## *Differential Diagnosis*

The diagnosis of PV relies on clinical recognition and is confirmed by KOH preparation. The differential diagnosis includes other disorders of skin dyspigmentation (Table 4.27). Vitiligo can be distinguished from PV due to its acral distribution (hands, feet, face), lack of overlying scale, and complete lack of pigmentation under Wood's lamp inspection [96]. Pityriasis alba typically affects the face and limbs and is nonfluorescent under Wood's lamp inspection, and patients often have a history of atopy [96].

### *Treatment*

Therapeutic options for PV [80, 95, 98] overlap with seborrheic dermatitis. Nonspecific agents physically or chemically remove infected stratum corneum, while specific agents have fungicidal or fungistatic properties [98, 100]. Systemic therapy is reserved for widespread, resistant, or recurrent lesions and for immunosuppressed patients [87]. Recurrence is common, occurring in 60% after 1 year of treatment and 80% after 2 years of treatment, and often necessitates prophylactic therapy [87]. For a comprehensive list of potential treatments, see Table 4.25.

## White Spot Parapsoriasis

White spot parapsoriasis is a poorly understood and poorly defined condition characterized by the development of a few to many, macular, 3–20-mm-diameter round to oval areas of nonpruritic hypopigmentation (Fig. 4.12). The face, upper trunk, and upper portions of the arms are most prominently affected. In some cases, the hypopigmented macules clearly follow the appearance of classic pityriasis lichenoides chronica [101, 102]. However, in other cases, the macular dyschromia appears without antecedent lesions and continues to expand in both size and domain for months to years [1, 103]. This entity is not associated with any systemic disorder; it does not develop into lymphoma despite a protracted course. As symptoms are rarely seen, the patient usually presents because of cosmetic distress.

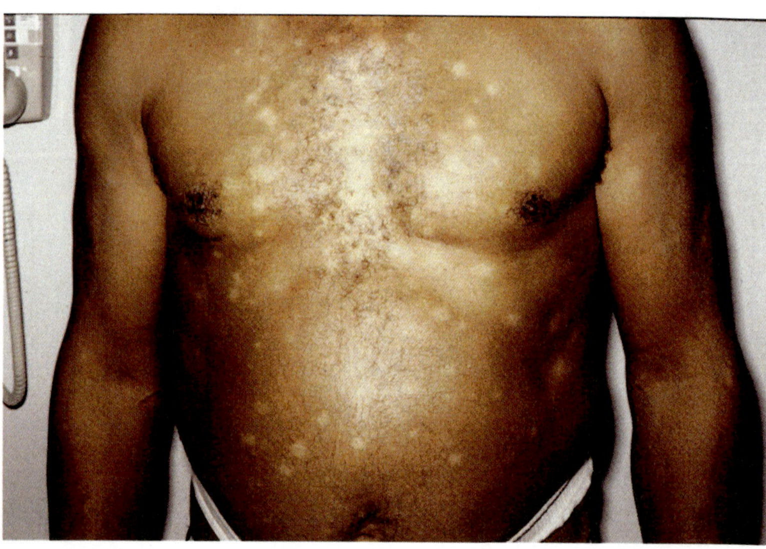

**Fig. 4.12** Progressive development of asymptomatic white macules with no precursor inflammatory lesions

## *Epidemiology*

Although white spot parapsoriasis (also known as white spot disease [104]) is not a new concept, this variant of parapsoriasis appears to either occur more commonly or be recognized more readily in the Southwest region of the United States. It is typically seen in skin of color: African American and Hispanic individuals to be precise. Many cases occur in the prepubertal pediatric population, but some also occur in middle-aged adults. It is the authors' experience that men are more often affected than women, but statistical validation for this belief is lacking.

## *Etiology/Pathophysiology*

The cause and pathogenesis are entirely unknown.

## *Laboratory*

All routine laboratory findings are normal.

## *Histopathology*

Histology of the hypopigmented lesions in white spot parapsoriasis is similar to that seen in a typical inflammatory pityriasis lichenoides chronica lesion: perivascular lymphohistiocytic infiltrate with exocytosis of cytologically normal lymphocytes into the epidermis [1, 101–104]. The latter demonstrates parakeratosis and focal spongiosis. Eosinophils are absent. In long-standing cases, the degree of inflammation diminishes, and reduced epidermal melanin deposition is the main pathological finding.

## *Differential Diagnosis*

The differential diagnosis is rather extensive and remarkably variable in nature. Among the many disorders which present in the same or in a similar clinical fashion are tinea versicolor, pityriasis alba, vitiligo, lichen sclerosus et atrophicus, guttate morphea, facial seborrhea, and the macular hypopigmented variants of mycosis fungoides and sarcoidosis. Tinea versicolor, pityriasis alba, and seborrhea tend to be scalier than white spot parapsoriasis. However, biopsy may be essential to rule out the remaining diagnostic considerations.

## *Treatment*

There is no uniformly effective therapy for white spot parapsoriasis. Topical corticosteroids are most often instituted, but rarely improve matters. Phototherapy, including the use of PUVA and UVB, may be useful in eradicating the more typical papules of PLC (when present) and in inducing repigmentation of the hypopigmented areas. Antibiotics and methotrexate are rarely effective in the treatment of white spot parapsoriasis. Disease course is generally prolonged, but spontaneous resolution has been observed in some fortunate patients.

# References

1. Rosen T, Orengo IF, Koff AB, Schell BJ. Clinical dermatology in black patients. Bari: Pigreco; 1995.
2. Wasserbauer N, Ballow M. Atopic dermatitis. Am J Med. 2009;122:121–5.
3. Nnoruka EN. Current epidemiology of atopic dermatitis in South-Eastern Nigeria. Int J Dermatol. 2004;43:739–44.
4. Dhar S, Kanwar AJ. Epidemiology and clinical pattern of atopic dermatitis in a North Indian pediatric population. Pediatr Dermatol. 1998;15:347–51.
5. Lee HJ, Cho SH, Ha SJ, et al. Minor cutaneous features of atopic dermatitis in South Korea. Int J Dermatol. 2000;39:337–42.
6. Allen HB, Jones NP, Bowen SE. Lichenoid and other clinical presentations of atopic dermatitis in an inner city practice. J Am Acad Dermatol. 2008;58:503–4.
7. Summey BT, Bowen SE, Allen HB. Lichen planus-like atopic dermatitis: expanding the differential diagnosis of spongiotic dermatitis. J Cutan Pathol. 2008;35:311–4.
8. Ben-Gashir MA, Hay RJ. Reliance on erythema scores may mask severe atopic dermatitis in black children compared with their white counterparts. Br J Dermatol. 2002;147:920–5.
9. Schachner L, Ling NS, Press S. A statistical analysis of a pediatric dermatology clinic. Pediatr Dermatol. 1983;1:157–64.
10. Lee CS, Lim HW. Cutaneous diseases in Asians. Dermatol Clin. 2003;21:669–77.
11. Bonness S, Bieber T. Molecular basis of atopic dermatitis. Curr Opin Allergy Clin Immunol. 2007;7:382–6.
12. Allam JP, Novak N. The pathophysiology of atopic eczema. Clin Exp Dermatol. 2006;31:89–93.
13. Peterson JD, Chan LS. A comprehensive management guide for atopic dermatitis. Dermatol Nurs. 2006;18:531–42.
14. Katta R. Lichen planus. Am Fam Physician. 2000;61:3319–24.
15. Ellgehausen P, Elsner P, Burg G. Drug-induced lichen planus. Clin Dermatol. 1998;16:325–32.
16. Nnoruka EN. Lichen planus in African children: a study of 13 patients. Pediatr Dermatol. 2007;24:495–8.
17. Marshman G. Lichen planus. Australas J Dermatol. 1998;39:1–11.

18. Boyd AS. New and emerging therapies for lichenoid dermatoses. Dermatol Clin. 2000;18:21–9.
19. Eisen D. The clinical features, malignant potential, and systemic associations of oral lichen planus: a study of 723 patients. J Am Acad Dermatol. 2002;46:207–14.
20. Alam F, Hamburger J. Oral mucosal lichen planus in children. Int J Paediatr Dent. 2001;11:209–14.
21. Sontheimer RD. Lichenoid tissue reaction/interface dermatitis: clinical and histological perspectives. J Invest Dermatol. 2009;129:1088–99.
22. Nagao Y, Sata M. Hepatitis C virus and lichen planus. J Gastroenterol Hepatol. 2004;19:1101–13.
23. Tan EM, Cohen AS, Fries JF, Masi AT, McShane DJ, Rothfield NF, et al. The 1982 revised criteria for the classification of systemic lupus erythematosus. Arthritis Rheum. 1982;25: 1271–7.
24. Hochberg MC. Updating the American College of Rheumatology revised criteria for the classification of systemic lupus erythematosus. Arthritis Rheum. 1997;40:1725.
25. McCauliffe DP. Cutaneous lupus erythematosus. Semin Cutan Med Surg. 2001;20:14–26.
26. Rothfield N, Sontheimer RD, Bernstein M. Lupus erythematosus: systemic and cutaneous manifestations. Clin Dermatol. 2006;24:348–62.
27. Martin S, Rosen T, Locker E. Metastatic squamous cell carcinoma of the lip. Occurrence in blacks with discoid lupus erythematosus. Arch Dermatol. 1979;115:1214.
28. Fabbri P, Cardinali C, Giomi B, et al. Cutaneous lupus erythematosus: diagnosis and management. Am J Clin Dermatol. 2003;4:449–65.
29. Tikly M, Burgin S, Mohanlal P, Bellingan A, George J. Autoantibodies in black South Africans with systemic lupus erythematosus: spectrum and clinical associations. Clin Rheumatol. 1996;15:261–5.
30. Nath SK, Namjou B, Kilpatrick J, et al. A candidate region on 11p13 for systemic lupus erythematosus: a linkage identified in African-American families. J Investig Dermatol Symp Proc. 2004;9:64–7.
31. González LM, Allen R, Janniger CK, Schwartz RA. Pityriasis rosea: an important papulosquamous disorder. Int J Dermatol. 2005;44:757–64.
32. Stulberg DL, Wolfrey J. Pityriasis rosea. Am Fam Physician. 2004;69:87–91.
33. Amer A, Fischer H, Li X. The natural history of pityriasis rosea in black American children: how correct is the "classic" description? Arch Pediatr Adolesc Med. 2007;161:503–6.
34. Chuh A, Chan H, Zawar V. Pityriasis rosea–evidence for and against an infectious aetiology. Epidemiol Infect. 2004;132:381–90.
35. Kempf W, Burg G. Pityriasis rosea–a virus-induced skin disease? An update. Arch Virol. 2000;145:1509–20.
36. Canpolat Kirac B, Adisen E, Bozdayi G, Yucel A, Fidan I, Aksakal N, et al. The role of human herpesvirus 6, human herpesvirus 7, Epstein-Barr virus and cytomegalovirus in the aetiology of pityriasis rosea. J Eur Acad Dermatol Venereol. 2009;23:16–21.
37. Wolff K, Johnson RA. Psoriasis. In: Sydor AM, Englis MR, editors. Fitzpatrick's color atlas and synopsis of clinical dermatology. 6th ed. New York: McGraw-Hill; 2009. p. 53–71.
38. Leder RO, Farber EM. The variable incidence of psoriasis in sub-Saharan Africa. Int J Dermatol. 1997;36:911–9.
39. Kormeili T, Lowe NJ, Yamauchi PS. Psoriasis: immunopathogenesis and evolving immunomodulators and systemic therapies; U.S. experiences. Br J Dermatol. 2004;151:3–15.
40. Gelfand JM, Stern RS, Nijsten T, Feldman SR, Thomas J, Kist J, et al. The prevalence of psoriasis in African Americans: results from a population-based study. J Am Acad Dermatol. 2005;52:23–6.
41. Nograles KE, Brasington RD, Bowcock AM. New insights into the pathogenesis and genetics of psoriatic arthritis. Nat Clin Pract Rheumatol. 2009;5:83–91.
42. Nickoloff BJ, Qin JZ, Nestle FO. Immunopathogenesis of psoriasis. Clin Rev Allergy Immunol. 2007;33:45–56.

43. Gottlieb AB. Therapeutic options in the treatment of psoriasis and atopic dermatitis. J Am Acad Dermatol. 2005;53:S3–16.
44. Lebwohl M. A clinician's paradigm in the treatment of psoriasis. J Am Acad Dermatol. 2005;53:S59–69.
45. Doherty CB, Rosen T. Evidence-based therapy for cutaneous sarcoidosis. Drugs. 2008;68:1361–83.
46. Tchernev G. Cutaneous sarcoidosis: the "great imitator": etiopathogenesis, morphology, differential diagnosis, and clinical management. Am J Clin Dermatol. 2006;7:375–82.
47. Katta R. Cutaneous sarcoidosis: a dermatologic masquerader. Am Fam Physician. 2002;65:1581–4.
48. Newman LS, Rose CS, Maier LA. Sarcoidosis. N Engl J Med. 1997;336:1224–34.
49. Fernandez-Faith E, McDonnell J. Cutaneous sarcoidosis: differential diagnosis. Clin Dermatol. 2007;25:276–87.
50. Jacyk WK. Cutaneous sarcoidosis in black South Africans. Int J Dermatol. 1999;38:841–5.
51. Chong WS, Tan HH, Tan SH. Cutaneous sarcoidosis in Asians: a report of 25 patients from Singapore. Clin Exp Dermatol. 2005;30:120–4.
52. Costabel U, Guzman J, Baughman RP. Systemic evaluation of a potential cutaneous sarcoidosis patient. Clin Dermatol. 2007;25:303–11.
53. Ahmed I, Harshad SR. Subcutaneous sarcoidosis: is it a specific subset of cutaneous sarcoidosis frequently associated with systemic disease? J Am Acad Dermatol. 2006;54:55–60.
54. Chen ES, Moller DR. Etiology of sarcoidosis. Clin Chest Med. 2008;29:365–77.
55. Marcoval J, Moreno A, Mañá J, Peyri J. Subcutaneous sarcoidosis. Dermatol Clin. 2008;26:553–6.
56. Katta R, Nelson B, Chen D, Roenigk H. Sarcoidosis of the scalp: a case series and review of the literature. J Am Acad Dermatol. 2000;42:690–2.
57. Gabrielli A, Avvedimento EV, Krieg T. Scleroderma. N Engl J Med. 2009;360:1989–2003.
58. Zhou X, Tan FK, Wang N, Xiong M, Maghidman S, Reveille JD, et al. Genome-wide association study for regions of systemic sclerosis susceptibility in a Choctaw Indian population with high disease prevalence. Arthritis Rheum. 2003;48:2585–92.
59. Steen VD. Autoantibodies in systemic sclerosis. Semin Arthritis Rheum. 2005;35:35–42.
60. Preliminary criteria for the classification of systemic sclerosis (scleroderma). Subcommittee for scleroderma criteria of the American Rheumatism Association Diagnostic and Therapeutic Criteria Committee. Arthritis Rheum. 1980;23:581–90
61. Peterson LS, Nelson AM, Su WP. Classification of morphea (localized scleroderma). Mayo Clin Proc. 1995;70:1068–76.
62. Costner MI, Grau RH. Update on connective tissue diseases in dermatology. Semin Cutan Med Surg. 2006;25:207–20.
63. Mayes MD. Classification and epidemiology of scleroderma. Semin Cutan Med Surg. 1998;17:22–6.
64. Nietert PJ, Mitchell HC, Bolster MB, Shaftman SR, Tilley BC, Silver RM. Racial variation in clinical and immunological manifestations of systemic sclerosis. J Rheumatol. 2006;33:263–8.
65. Sontheimer RD. Skin manifestations of systemic autoimmune connective tissue disease: diagnostics and therapeutics. Best Pract Res Clin Rheumatol. 2004;18:429–62.
66. Halder RM, Roberts CI, Nootheti PK. Cutaneous diseases in the black races. Dermatol Clin. 2003;21:679–87.
67. Steen VD. Clinical manifestations of systemic sclerosis. Semin Cutan Med Surg. 1998;17:48–54.
68. Ee HL, Tan SH. Reticulate hyperpigmented scleroderma: a new pigmentary manifestation. Clin Exp Dermatol. 2005;30:131–3.
69. Adelowo OO, Oguntona S. Scleroderma (systemic sclerosis) among Nigerians. Clin Rheumatol. 2009;28:1121–5.
70. Reveille JD, Fischbach M, McNearney T, Friedman AW, Aguilar MB, Lisse J. Systemic sclerosis in 3 US ethnic groups: a comparison of clinical, sociodemographic, serologic, and immunogenetic determinants. Semin Arthritis Rheum. 2001;30:332–46.

71. Kuwana M, Kaburaki J, Arnett FC, Howard RF, Medsger Jr TA, Wright TM. Influence of ethnic background on clinical and serologic features in patients with systemic sclerosis and anti-DNA topoisomerase I antibody. Arthritis Rheum. 1999;42:465–74.
72. Mayes MD, Lacey Jr JV, Beebe-Dimmer J, Gillespie BW, Cooper B, Laing TJ, et al. Prevalence, incidence, survival, and disease characteristics of systemic sclerosis in a large US population. Arthritis Rheum. 2003;48:2246–55.
73. Steen VD, Oddis CV, Conte CG, Janoski J, Casterline GZ, Medsger Jr TA. Incidence of systemic sclerosis in Allegheny County, Pennsylvania. A twenty-year study of hospital-diagnosed cases, 1963–1982. Arthritis Rheum. 1997;40:441–5.
74. Tamaki T, Mori S, Takehara K. Epidemiological study of patients with systemic sclerosis in Tokyo. Arch Dermatol Res. 1991;283:366–71.
75. Reveille JD. Ethnicity and race and systemic sclerosis: how it affects susceptibility, severity, antibody genetics, and clinical manifestations. Curr Rheumatol Rep. 2003;5:160–7.
76. Aggarwal R, Lucas M, Fertig N, Oddis CV, Medsger Jr TA. Anti-U3 RNP autoantibodies in systemic sclerosis. Arthritis Rheum. 2009;60:1112–8.
77. Greidinger EL, Flaherty KT, White B, Rosen A, Wigley FM, Wise RA. African-American race and antibodies to topoisomerase I are associated with increased severity of scleroderma lung disease. Chest. 1998;114:801–7.
78. White B. Clinical approach to scleroderma. Semin Cutan Med Surg. 1998;17:213–8.
79. Pope JE, Shum DT, Gottschalk R, Stevens A, McManus R. Increased pigmentation in scleroderma. J Rheumatol. 1996;23:1912–6.
80. Gupta AK, Batra R, Bluhm R, Boekhout T, Dawson Jr TL. Skin diseases associated with *Malassezia* species. J Am Acad Dermatol. 2004;51:785–98.
81. Schwartz RA, Janusz CA, Janniger CK. Seborrheic dermatitis: an overview. Am Fam Physician. 2006;74:125–30.
82. Johnson BA, Nunley JR. Treatment of seborrheic dermatitis. Am Fam Physician. 2000;61(2703–2710):2713–4.
83. Gupta AK, Nicol KA. Seborrheic dermatitis of the scalp: etiology and treatment. J Drugs Dermatol. 2004;3:155–8.
84. Halder RM, Nootheti PK. Ethnic skin disorders overview. J Am Acad Dermatol. 2003;48:S143–8.
85. Ogunbiyi AO, Daramola OO, Alese OO. Prevalence of skin diseases in Ibadan, Nigeria. Int J Dermatol. 2004;43:31–6.
86. Gupta AK, Madzia SE, Batra R. Etiology and management of Seborrheic dermatitis. Dermatology. 2004;208:89–93.
87. Faergemann J. Management of seborrheic dermatitis and pityriasis versicolor. Am J Clin Dermatol. 2000;1:75–80.
88. Brown DL, Frank JE. Diagnosis and management of syphilis. Am Fam Physician. 2003;68:283–90.
89. Lautenschlager S. Cutaneous manifestations of syphilis: recognition and management. Am J Clin Dermatol. 2006;7:291–304.
90. Rosen T, Hwong H. Pedal interdigital condylomata lata: a rare sign of secondary syphilis. Sex Transm Dis. 2001;28:184–6.
91. Kent ME, Romanelli F. Reexamining syphilis: an update on epidemiology, clinical manifestations, and management. Ann Pharmacother. 2008;42:226–36.
92. Centers for Disease Control and Prevention. Sexually transmitted disease surveillance, 2007. Atlanta: U.S. Department of Health and Human Services; 2008.
93. Singh AE, Romanowski B. Syphilis: review with emphasis on clinical, epidemiologic, and some biologic features. Clin Microbiol Rev. 1999;12:187–209.
94. Zetola NM, Klausner JD. Syphilis and HIV infection: an update. Clin Infect Dis. 2007;44:1222–8.
95. Sunenshine PJ, Schwartz RA, Janniger CK. Tinea versicolor. Int J Dermatol. 1998;37:648–55.
96. Crespo-Erchiga V, Florencio VD. *Malassezia* yeasts and pityriasis versicolor. Curr Opin Infect Dis. 2006;19:139–47.

97. Mollet I, Ongenae K, Naeyaert JM. Origin, clinical presentation, and diagnosis of hypomelanotic skin disorders. Dermatol Clin. 2007;25:363–71.
98. Gupta AK, Batra R, Bluhm R, Faergemann J. Pityriasis versicolor. Dermatol Clin. 2003;21:413–29.
99. Aljabre SH, Alzayir AA, Abdulghani M, Osman OO. Pigmentary changes of tinea versicolor in dark-skinned patients. Int J Dermatol. 2001;40:273–5.
100. Elewski BE, Abramovits W, Kempers S, Schlessinger J, Rosen T, Gupta AK, Abraham S, Rowell R. A novel foam formulation of ketoconazole 2% for the treatment of seborrheic dermatitis on multiple body regions. J Drugs Dermatol. 2007;6:1001–8.
101. Warin AP. Hypochromic variant of pityriasis lichenoides chronic. Clin Exp Dermatol. 1978;3:85–7.
102. Clayton R, Warin A. Pityriasis lichenoides chronic presenting as hypopigmentation. Br J Dermatol. 1979;100:297–302.
103. Guillet G, Helenon R, Gauthier Y, Surleve-Bazeille JE, Plantin P, Sassolas BP. Progressive macular hypomelanosis of the trunk: primary acquired hypopigmentation. J Cutan Pathol. 1988;15:286–9.
104. MacKee GM, Wise W. White spot disease. J Cutan Dis. 1914;32:629–60.

# Chapter 5
# Nonscarring Alopecias

**Victoria H. Barbosa**

For most people, hair is an important part of how one looks and how one feels about him- or herself. In fact, it can be an important part of one's identity overall. Some people take their hair for granted until they start to lose it. Alopecia can be an emotionally devastating condition for patients regardless of its severity. Decrease in quality of life has been documented for many different forms of alopecia [1, 2]. Most dermatologists know this intuitively from their own experience in treating these patients who may be unhappy about or even distraught by their condition. The diagnosis of a nonscarring alopecia allows us to offer hope to these patients. The preservation of the hair follicle that is characteristic of these conditions means that there is the possibility of, and in some instances an excellent chance of regrowth.

## Grooming-Induced Alopecias

While there is a wide degree of individual variation, the physical characteristics of hair vary based upon a person's racial background. For instance, Asian hair tends to be straightest and round in cross section. The hair of people of African descent tends to be tightly curled and elliptical in cross section. Caucasian hair falls in between the two. African hair has a lower tensile strength in its virgin state than the hair of people of other ethnicities. This means that it is more fragile and prone to breakage [3, 4]. In addition, many of the hairstyle styling techniques including temporary straightening, permanent straightening, and coloring the hair further increase its fragility. It has been documented that African hair grows slower than Caucasian or

V.H. Barbosa, M.D, M.PH, M.BA. (✉)
Millenium Park Dermatology, 30 N Michigan Avenue Suite 1429, Chicago 60602, IL, USA
e-mail: vbarbosa@millenniumparkdermatology.com

A.F. Alexis and V.H. Barbosa (eds.), *Skin of Color: A Practical Guide to Dermatologic Diagnosis and Treatment*, DOI 10.1007/978-0-387-84929-4_5,

Asian hair [5]. So, hair in people of African descent breaks off more easily and grows back more slowly than the hair of people of other ethnicities. The importance of hair to African Americans and the care that is taken to maintain it is reflected in the amount of money that is spent to maintain the hair. African Americans make up 13% of the United States population but make up one third of the purchases of hair care products [6].

## *Primer on Hairstyling*

Understanding the hair care habits and styling practices of people with very curly hair, and people of African descent in particular, is essential for any dermatologist who treats them. A patient's confidence in the physician will be greater if the patient sees that the physician is knowledgeable. A dermatologist must also be able to recognize grooming-induced disorders and recommend treatment plans that the patients will follow.

The most important distinction that people of African descent make in terms of their hair is whether or not their hair is "natural." This is an imprecise designation because it means different things to different people. For some, natural hair is simply hair that does not have a relaxer to straighten in. For others it means no chemicals at all, including hair color. And for still others it means no relaxer, color, or heat use. So, while it is important for a dermatologist to be familiar with the terminology of whether or not the hair is natural, a thorough history must specifically ascertain use of relaxers, texturizers, color, and heat.

Hair relaxers are used by most African American women at some point in their lives. These products are used to rearrange disulfide bonds to permanently straighten the hair. They are very alkaline, usually with a pH range from 12 to 14 depending on the product. Relaxers are divided into two categories, commonly referred to as *lye* and *no lye*. Lye relaxers contain sodium hydroxide as the active ingredient. *No lye* relaxers most commonly contain guanidine hydroxide. Because this substance is not stable, these relaxers come in a kit containing calcium hydroxide and guanidine carbonate. Potassium hydroxide and lithium hydroxide are also used in some products, particularly in texturizers. It should be noted that some patients refer to relaxers as *perms*. These should not be confused with the permanent wave products that are used by people with straight hair, also referred to as *perms*. Permanent wave solutions contain thiols as the active ingredient. Thiols like ammonium thioglycolate are also used in some African American hair care products. These products are generally referred to as *waves* or *curls*.

Texturizers are used to relax the curl pattern without leaving the hair completely straight. In taking a history, one should ask specifically about their use. Because they do not leave the hair completely straight, some people do not consider it a chemical. Ironically, texturizers contain the same alkaline ingredients that relaxers do. It is important to note that texturizers may be used by men as well as women, while relaxers are mainly used by women.

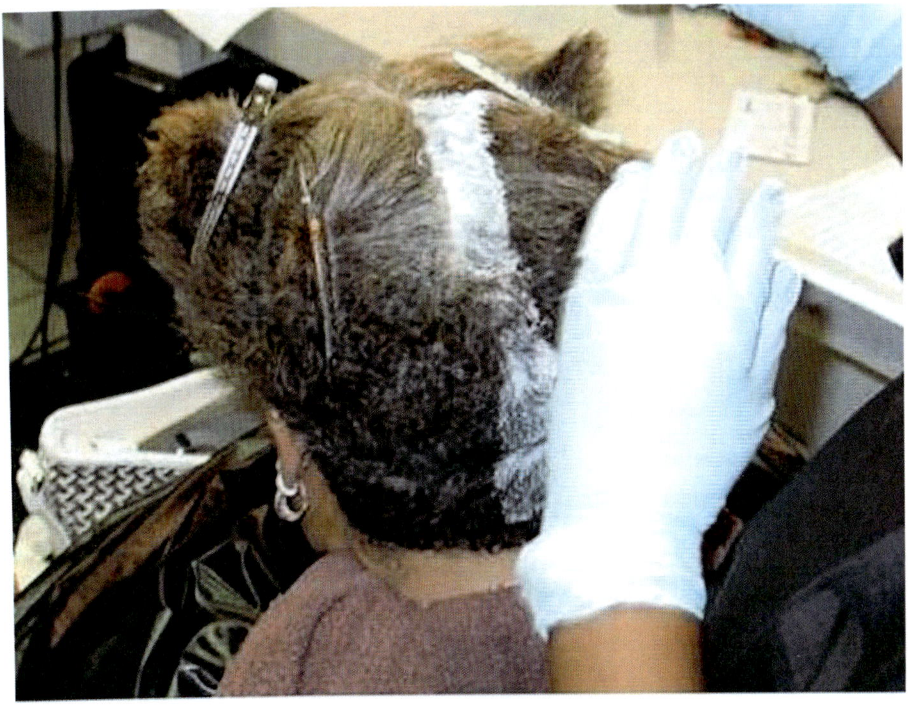

**Fig. 5.1** Proper relaxer application entails applying the product to the new growth only

Proper use of the relaxer includes applying the product to the new growth only (Fig. 5.1). The product should be left on the hair for a duration consistent with package instructions, which generally ranges from 15 to 20 min. The product should be rinsed earlier if burning occurs. Hair color can be used with relaxer but not necessarily on the same day. It depends on the hair color. Semipermanent color and temporary color, also referred to as a rinse, can be used on the same day as relaxer. However, permanent hair color must be spaced out by at least 2 weeks.

Individuals tend to have strong preferences about whether they prefer their hair with or without relaxer. In most cases, there is not a clear answer as to which is better. Natural hair has higher tensile strength than relaxed hair, so it is stronger. However, the natural kinks and twists make it more difficult to comb, and relaxed hair requires a lower force with which to comb it. The higher force needed to comb natural hair can result in breakage. The effects of relaxer on the scalp are not well understood.

Aside from whether the hair is natural or relaxed, people might opt to wear the hair in a number of different styles. Heat is frequently used to temporarily straighten natural hair or to style relaxed hair. Heated appliances include curling irons, flat irons, hot combs, blow dryers, and cap dryers. These appliances can reach temperatures in excess of 400° Fahrenheit. Direct heat on the hair can weaken the hair, particularly if it was not adequately dry before applying the direct heat (Fig. 5.2).

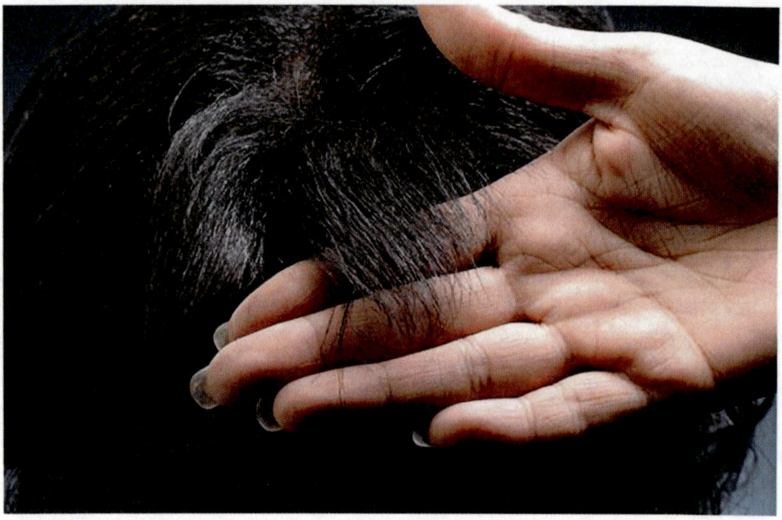

**Fig. 5.2** Breakage from curling iron

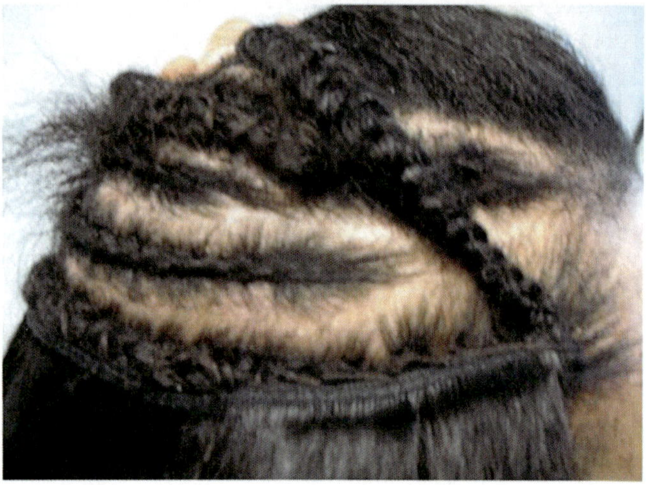

**Fig. 5.3** A hair weave on a thin strip of fabric is sewn onto cornrows with a needle and thread

Braided styles, in which three sections of hair are intertwined, or twists, in which one section of hair is coiled or two sections of hair are intertwined, can be performed on straight or curly hair. Loose strands of human or synthetic hair may be added to a person's own hair to provide additional length and volume. Weaves are similar to extensions in that additional hair is added to one's own hair. Rather than the strands of hair being loose, they are attached to a thin strip of fabric. The fabric can either be sewn onto a patient's cornrows using a needle and thread (Fig. 5.3) or

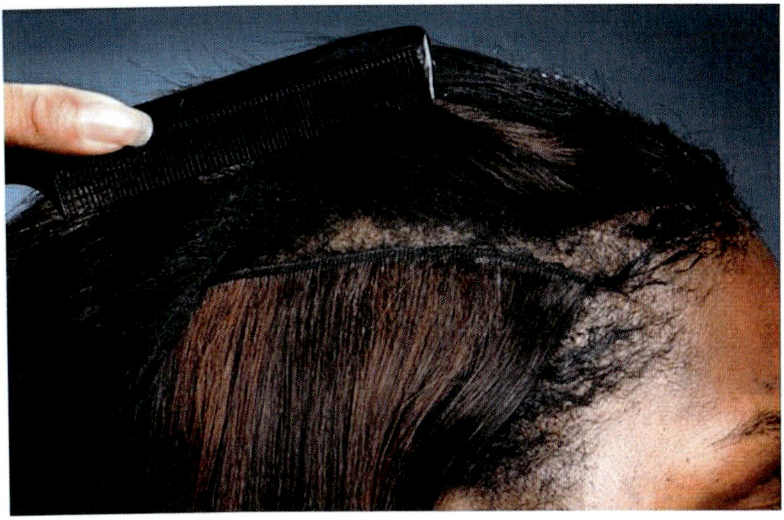

**Fig. 5.4** Hair weave strips are glued directly onto the scalp

the strips can be glued directly onto the scalp (Fig. 5.4). Braids and twists with extensions are normally worn for 8–12 weeks, while weaves are normally worn for 6–8 weeks. The hair and scalp are shampooed during this time.

People with very curly hair usually wash their hair once a week or every other week. People without a relaxer who wear their hair curly might shampoo more frequently, and people with very fragile hair might shampoo less frequently. Because sebum weigh down curly hair as fast as it does straight hair, the cosmetic need for shampoo frequency is decreased compared to people of other ethnicities. In addition, wet hair is more prone to breakage than dry hair is, and the use of heated styling appliances is another source of damage to the hair fiber. So, shampoo and styling represent opportunities for hair breakage and hence are weighed differently against the need for scalp cleansing than in people with straighter, stronger hair. Moisturizing shampoos are frequently used and are followed by at least one and often several conditioners. Deep conditioners which are left on for 10 min under a heated dryer or warm towel can be an important set in protecting the hair fibers. Leave-in conditioners are also frequently used at the time of shampoo and in between shampoos.

## Relaxer-Induced Alopecia

Most women who have used relaxers have experienced breakage at one time or another. This frequently occurs as a result of improper use of the product. Relaxer should only be applied to the new growth and not for more time that is indicated in package instructions. More is definitely not better. Fortunately, hair breakage from relaxer damage grows back, but patients may experience ongoing breakage until all the damaged hair has broken off. Use of hair conditioners can support patients through this time. It should be noted that some patients develop a severe irritant dermatitis from misuse of relaxers, which can also result in localized or diffuse alopecia. Severe irritant dermatitis can result in blisters and/or erosions. There have been care reports of scarring alopecia following relaxer application, but this is not a common occurrence [7, 8]. Some studies have demonstrated that relaxer use is prevalent among patients with central centrifugal cicatricial alopecia, a condition that predominantly affects African American women [9, 10]. However, relaxer use is prevalent among all African American women. More research is needed to understand the association between the two. The author does encourage patients who have been diagnosed with CCCA or any other scarring alopecia to discontinue, or at least significantly decrease, relaxer use.

Suggestions for minimizing damage from relaxers:

- Use a mild relaxer instead of *regular* or *super* strength.
- Decrease application time.
- Only apply product to new growth rather than to the entire hair shaft.
- Space out relaxer application to at least every 8 weeks.
- Space out relaxer and permanent hair color application at least 2 weeks apart.
- Be sure to remove all relaxer from the hair and scalp with a neutralizing shampoo.
- Use conditioners liberally.

## Traction Alopecia

Traction alopecia is caused by repeated pulling on the hair from hairstyling or hair care. Common culprits include braided styles such as individual braids, cornrows, and weaves, as well as ponytails and repeated use of rollers to set the hair. The classic pattern of traction alopecia is thinning at the anterior hairline from tight ponytails or braided styles, although thinning at the posterior hairline is also seen (Fig. 5.5). With an increase in the popularity of individual braids and weaves, traction can also be appreciated in a more diffuse pattern from braids pulling on hair throughout the scalp. When identified early, the styling can be modified and hair will regrow. However, over time, traction alopecia can lead to scarring and become irreversible. Hence, it is important for the physician to encourage modification of hairstyles. Data on treatment is limited. Minoxidil was effective in a case series [11]. Some physicians will try potent topical steroids or intralesional kenalog for a few weeks up to 6 months to attempt to stimulate regrowth.

Suggestions for minimizing traction alopecia include:

- Rotate the pattern of braided and twisted hairstyles.
- Avoid tight braiding, opting instead to refresh the hairstyle more frequently.
- Avoid use of rubber bands and elastic ponytail holders.
- Avoid sleeping in rollers; opt instead to wrap or pin curl the hair at night.
- Wear a satin bonnet or use a satin pillowcase at bedtime.

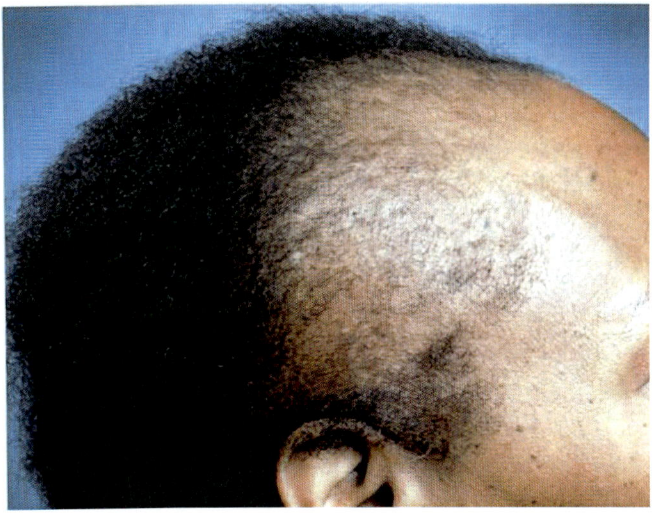

**Fig. 5.5** Classic pattern of traction alopecia

## Androgenetic Alopecia

Androgenetic alopecia is a hereditary form of hair loss that becomes noticeable for most patients in their 30s and 40s. As with most forms of hair loss, the cause of androgenetic alopecia (AGA) is not fully understood, though recent studies have demonstrated susceptibility loci on chromosomes 20p11 and 3q26 [12, 13]. Testosterone is converted to DHT by 5-alpha reductase, and the DHT causes follicles to miniaturize so that they ultimately stop producing terminal hairs, producing vellus hairs instead. There is no variation in prevalence by ethnicity.

AGA is often called "patterned alopecia" because distinct patterns of hair loss occur, and those patterns are different for men and for women. Men experience a thinning at the temples and at the crown, with eventual loss of the anterior hairline. Advanced cases demonstrate retention only of some parietal and occipital hair or may progress to complete baldness. Male pattern alopecia is graded using the Norwood-Hamilton classification. Women tend to have thinning at the crown with less temporal involvement than men. Women also tend to retain the anterior hairline. This female pattern is depicted in the Ludwig classification which depicts three grades of severity. Diagnosis is a clinical one, with hair pull test and trichoscopy serving as useful tools to distinguish this from other forms of hair loss.

Depending on the history and physical examination, a CBC and iron studies, thyroid function tests, total and free testosterone, and DHEA-S and vitamin D are laboratory tests that can be considered.

Treatment options for men with androgenetic alopecia include topical minoxidil 5% foam or solution. The type II 5-alpha reductase inhibitor finasteride at 1 mg per day is also very effective. Dutasteride 0.5 mg po daily has demonstrated effectiveness in treating male AGA, although this is an off-label use for this type I and type II 5-a reductase inhibitor [14]. Once the patient's disease is stable, he may be a candidate for hair transplantation. Treatment options for women are a bit different. Minoxidil 2% is indicated for use in women, but many physicians use 5% minoxidil off-label in this patient population. They should be warned about the increased risk of hypertrichosis at this higher dose. While finasteride is not appropriate for use in women who are able to conceive, spironolactone can provide a reasonable treatment alternative. Transplantation is also a reasonable alternative for women whose disease has stabilized.

## Telogen Effluvium

Telogen effluvium is a common condition in which patients complain of hair shedding. This disorder is caused by a physical or emotional stress causing a sudden or gradual increase in the percentage of follicles in telogen phase. Normally, anywhere from 5% to 15% of the follicles are in the resting phase, which lasts about 3 months. Conversely, 85–95% of hair follicles are usually in the anagen phase in which hair is actively growing. In telogen effluvium (TE), the percentage of follicles in telogen phase increases to 25% or more. As new anagen hairs grow, they push out the telogen hairs. So approximately 3 months after the stressor, a patient begins to notice an increase in shedding [15].

Epidemiological data is sparse, but TE is believed to be a common condition with no racial or ethnic differences in prevalence. It may be more common in women because pregnancy and delivery are two inciting events. Other common causes include physical stressors such as trauma, surgery, febrile illness, and change in diet. Underlying medical conditions including thyroid disease, malignancy, renal disease, and hepatic disease have also been implicated. Medications that cause TE include beta blockers, anticoagulants, and retinoids. Sometimes the inciting event is obvious, other times not. So, a thorough history is important.

Physical examination is notable for diffuse hair thinning without any discrete patches of alopecia. In early phase or with mild disease, this may be difficult to appreciate. Patients will often bring old photos to serve as a base of comparison for the physician. The scalp appears unremarkable, without erythema or scale. A hair pull test can be diagnostic and is best performed if the hair has not been shampooed for 24–48 h before the office visit. A hair pull reveals 10% of hairs or more with white clubs in TE.

A biopsy is usually not needed but is the most definitive way to diagnose telogen effluvium. The telogen follicles are most easily seen on horizontal section. Twenty-five percent or more of the follicles are in the telogen phase. Laboratory evaluation should be guided by the history. While data is lacking, many physicians will check a complete blood count, iron, ferritin, total iron binding capacity in menstruating women, and vitamin D. In addition, thyroid function, renal function, liver function, etc., should be checked as dictated by the history.

A periodic 24-h hair count can be a useful tool for the physician as well as a source of reassurance for patients. After avoiding shampooing for one day, the patient collects all of the hair that he or she sheds in a 24-h period of time and counts it. More than 100 hairs collected is indicative of a disorder. This process also allows for quantification of the magnitude of the problem and serves as a base of comparison for future hair counts.

Reassurance is the most important aspect of care for TE. Most patients exhibit features of acute disease, which begins suddenly and usually resolves within 6 months. Some patients exhibit a chronic pattern, with an onset that is often more insidious and a course which persists longer than 6 months, often a year to 2 years and sometimes longer. Some physicians will add minoxidil for treatment of acute or chronic TE. In addition, some will use spironolactone for the treatment of chronic disease.

## Anagen Effluvium

Anagen effluvium (AE) occurs as a result of a direct insult to the hair follicle. Chemotherapeutic agents are a common cause of AE. It is also been reported in pemphigus vulgaris because the follicle is a target for the pemphigus autoantibodies and in alopecia areata when significant inflammation damages the follicle.

The alopecia usually begins 1–2 weeks after the toxic agent has been administered but becomes more noticeable after 1–2 months. Alopecia may be diffused or patterned [16]. The scalp appears normal, without alopecia, scale, or loss of follicular ostia. A hair pull demonstrates anagen hairs which are fully pigmented, in contrast to the white clubs on the end of telogen hairs.

Hair usually regrows after an anagen effluvium, although there are reports of permanent hair loss after chemotherapy [17]. Loss of hair cannot be prevented, but scalp cooling can be used to try to minimize hair loss, and minoxidil shortens the duration of the condition [18].

## Alopecia Areata

Alopecia areata is believed to be a T cell-mediated autoimmune disease. It is the most common autoimmune disease in the United States, affecting 5.3 million people. It is seen in people off all races, ages, and both genders without a predilection for any racial group [19].

Alopecia areata is distinguished by its discrete round patches of hair loss (Fig. 5.6). The scalp is the most frequent site of involvement, but eyebrows, eyelashes, beard region, and any area on the body can be involved. In each area of alopecia, hairs that taper toward the follicle may be seen. These are commonly referred to as exclamation point hairs and are often most noticeable at the margin on the patch. In alopecia totalis, the entire scalp is involved, and in alopecia universalis,

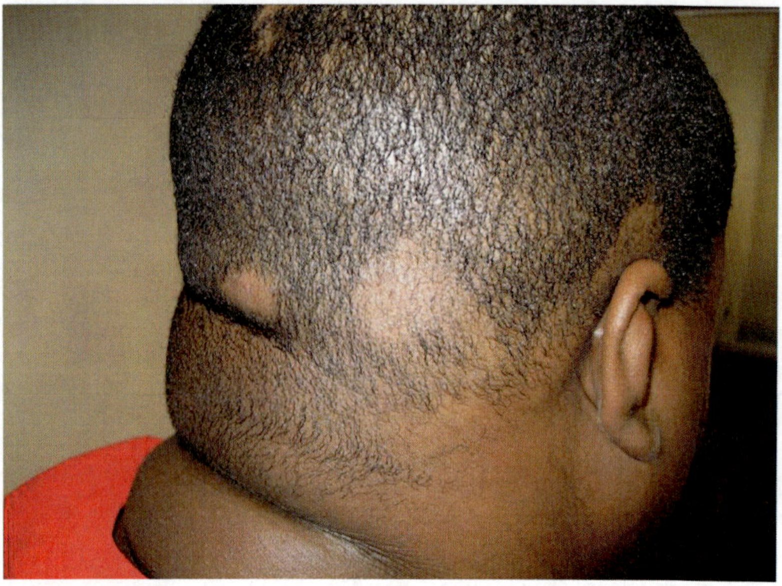

**Fig. 5.6** Discrete round patches of hair loss in alopecia areata

all of the body hair is lost. In diffuse alopecia areata, there are no distinct patches, but rather hair is lost throughout the scalp. For most patients, the patches are asymptomatic, but some may experience burning or itching.

Treatment of alopecia areata is guided by the location of involvement, the extent of involvement, and the age of the patient. The mainstay of treatment is intralesional triamcinolone, at strengths ranging from 2.5 mg/cm$^3$ to 20 mg/cm$^3$. Five mg/cm$^3$ is a reasonable starting point for scalp lesions, with 2.5 mg/cm$^3$ being a more appropriate starting point for facial lesions. For people with extensive scalp involvement or for people who are too young to tolerate needles, topical steroids can be substituted for injections. A recent report demonstrates similar efficacy between clobetasol propionate cream 0.05% and pimecrolimus 1%, so this may be used as well [20]. Minoxidil at 2% or 5% may be added to try to stimulate regrowth. Second-line topical treatments include irritation therapy with anthralin and sensitization with squaric acid dibutylester or diphencyprone. Diffuse areas can be treated with ultraviolet light therapy. Systemic agents may be used in rapidly progressive disease and in extensive disease. Options with demonstrated efficacy include prednisone and cyclosporine. There is a recent report of treating eyelash alopecia with bimatoprost [21].

## Trichotillomania

Trichotillomania is a form of traumatic alopecia where the patient pulls out his or her own hair. Pulling can occur anywhere on the body, with the scalp, eyebrows, and eyelashes being common locations. Patients cannot control the urge to pull their hair.

They often experience a sense of tension prior to the pulling which is replaced by a sense of relief or gratification afterward. It is, in fact, a psychological disorder rather than a dermatological one. However, most of the patients who seek treatment present to the dermatologist first, so dermatologists must be adept at distinguishing it from other forms of nonscarring alopecia.

Trichotillomania (TTM) is classified as an impulse control disorder in the DSM IV-TR [22]. However, there is ongoing discussion in the psychiatric community about the proper categorization of this condition and even the most appropriate name. It is commonly grouped with onychophagia (nail biting) and dermatillomania (skin picking) as body-focused repetitive behaviors. These questions will continue to be debated as our understanding of TTM progresses, and changes may be noted in the DSM V. It may be categorized as part of the obsessive compulsive spectrum [23].

The prevalence data on TTM is very limited overall, and no racial or ethnic differences are believed to exist. A recent study of 791 college students demonstrated a TTM prevalence of 3.91% [24]. This study population was 89.5% Caucasian, and nonwhites were slightly more likely to screen positive for an impulse control disorder in general, but this finding was not specific to TTM. A study of 200 African American college students demonstrated a TTM prevalence of 6.3% [25]. Women are affected more commonly than men. More studies are needed to better understand the epidemiology of this condition.

Diagnosis is made primarily by history and physical examination. The patient may or may not be aware of their behavior, but parents, sibling, and or teachers may have observed it. On physical examination, patchy hair loss is noticed on the scalp, eyebrows, eyelashes, or other body areas. Broken off hairs of different lengths are observed. Hair pull reveals predominantly anagen hairs, and KOH rules out tinea capitis. Biopsy is not usually necessary.

Treatment options for trichotillomania include cognitive behavior therapy and pharmacological intervention. Medications that have traditionally been used to treat TTM include selective serotonin reuptake inhibitors and tricyclic antidepressants, both categories of drugs have demonstrated some effectiveness but with varying results. Small recent studies have shown promise with other classes of medication, including aripiprazole and dronabinol [26, 27]. Treatment should progress in conjunction with a psychiatrist and/or a licensed clinical psychologist.

## Alopecia Syphilitica

Sir William Osler called syphilis "the great imitator." This is as true for alopecia syphilitica as it is for other manifestations of the disease. The hair loss may be patchy or "moth eaten" in appearance, mimicking alopecia areata or trichotillomania. Or, it may be diffuse and be difficult to distinguish from telogen effluvium. Alopecia syphilitica occurs in approximately 4% of people with secondary syphilis and may affect the beard, eyebrows, and body hair as well as the scalp [28].

Syphilis is still a significant problem in the United States. According to the Centers for Disease Control and Prevention, the overall prevalence of syphilis continues to rise, though levels have stabilized in women and in neonates. Men who have sex with men as a group have the most significant increase in disease. While they represented just 4% of people with primary or secondary syphilis in the year 2000, they comprised 62% of cases by 2009. People of color are affected disproportionately by syphilis. African Americans accounted for 52% of all cases of primary and secondary syphilis in 2009. The rates for Black, Hispanic, and Whites in that year were 19.2, 4.5, and 2.1 per 100,000, respectively. These differences are likely accounted for by disparities in healthcare and presence of comorbid conditions [29].

Alopecia syphilitica can easily be misdiagnosed based on physical examination alone. The physician must keep this condition in mind because laboratory evaluation is key to diagnosis. First, a nontreponemal screening test, either VDRL or an RPR, should be performed. Because of the high rate of false positives, a positive screening test should be verified with one of the treponemal tests, such as an FTA-ABS, MHA-TP, TPHA, TPPA, or EIA for IgG and IgM.

Biopsy is not usually necessarily if the threshold for laboratory investigation is low. If a sample of scalp is obtained, findings might include an increased number of telogen hairs, lymphocytic infiltration around the follicles, fibrous tracts and/or blood vessels, plasma cells, follicular plugging, and/or a sparse, follicle-oriented melanin clumping [30, 31]. A recent case reported detection of the T. pallidum spirochete in the hair follicle [32]. Penicillin remains the treatment of choice for syphilis, and the hair grows back after appropriate treatment.

## Summary

It is important for dermatologists to pay close attention to patients' complaints of alopecia. It may appear that one's level of concern is out of proportion to the amount of hair loss that the physician observes. However, we know that the patient's experience with hair loss affects their sense of well-being and quality of life. Having the knowledge, tools, and patience to distinguish the type of the alopecia, be it scarring or nonscarring alopecia, and further between types of nonscarring alopecia will ultimately serve the patients well. Proper diagnosis will dictate the doctor's message to the patient about likelihood of regrowth, which is what they most want to hear. It will also impact the physician's management. Careful history and examination, bearing localized and systemic causes of alopecia in mind, will allow for a thorough work-up that minimizes unnecessary testing and aids in proper diagnosis. In this way, patients can be reassured about transient conditions, and appropriate treatment can begin for more progressive conditions.

## References

1. Reid EE, Haley AC, Borovicka JH, Rademaker A, West DP, Colavincenzo M, Wickless H. Clinical severity does not reliably predict quality of life in women with alopecia areata, telogen effluvium, or androgenic alopecia. J Am Acad Dermatol. 2011;66(3):e97–102.

2. Dubois M, Baumstarck-Barrau K, Gaudy-Marqueste C, Richard MA, Loundou A, Auquier P, Grob JJ. Quality of life in alopecia areata: a study of 60 cases. J Invest Dermatol. 2010;130(12):2830–3.
3. Porter CE, Diridollou S, Holloway BV. Holloway. Int J Dermatol. 2005;44 Suppl 1:4–5.
4. Porter CE, Dixon F, Khine CC, Pistorio B, Bryant H, de la Mettrie R. The behavior of hair from different countries. J Cosmet Sci. 2009;60(2):97–109.
5. Loussouarn G. African hair growth parameters. Br J Dermatol. 2001;145(2):294–7.
6. Grubow L, Morris E. The imperative relevance of ethnic hair care. GCI Magazine. 2010.
7. Khumalo NP, Pillay K, Ngwanya RM. Acute 'relaxer'-associated scarring alopecia: a report of five cases. Br J Dermatol. 2007;156(6):1394–7.
8. Miller JJ. Relaxer-induced alopecia. Am J Contact Dermat. 2001;12(4):238–9.
9. Shah SK, Alexis AF. Central centrifugal cicatricial alopecia: retrospective chart review. J Cutan Med Surg. 2010;14(5):212–22.
10. Gathers RC, Jankowski M, Eide M, Lim HW. Hair grooming practices and central centrifugal cicatricial alopecia. J Am Acad Dermatol. 2009;60(4):574–8.
11. Khumalo NP, Ngwanya RM. Traction alopecia: 2% topical minoxidil shows promise. Report of two cases. J Eur Acad Dermatol Venereol. 2007;21(3):433–4.
12. Hillmer AM, Brockschmidt FF, Hanneken S, Eigelshoven S, Steffens M, Flaquer A, Herms S, Becker T, Kortüm AK, Nyholt DR, Zhao ZZ, Montgomery GW, Martin NG, Mühleisen TW, Alblas MA, Moebus S, Jöckel KH, Bröcker-Preuss M, Erbel R, Reinartz R, Betz RC, Cichon S, Propping P, Baur MP, Wienker TF, Kruse R, Nöthen MM. Susceptibility variants for male-pattern baldness on chromosome 20p11. Nat Genet. 2008;40(11):1279–81.
13. Hillmer AM, Flaquer A, Hanneken S, et al. Genome-wide scan and fine-mapping linkage study of androgenetic alopecia reveals a locus on chromosome 3q26. Am J Hum Genet. 2008;82(3):737–43.
14. Eun HC, Kwon OS, Yeon JH, Shin HS, Kim BY, Ro BI, Cho HK, Sim WY, Lew BL, Lee WS, Park HY, Hong SP, Ji JH. Efficacy, safety, and tolerability of dutasteride 0.5 mg once daily in male patients with male pattern hair loss: a randomized, double-blind, placebo-controlled, phase III study. J Am Acad Dermatol. 2010;63(2):252–8.
15. Elizabeth CW Hughes, MD; Chief Editor: Dirk M Elston, MD. Telogen effluvium . http://emedicine.medscape.com/article/1071566-overview#a0104
16. Yun SJ, Kim SJ. Hair loss pattern due to chemotherapy-induced anagen effluvium: a cross-sectional observation. Dermatology. 2007;215(1):36–40.
17. Palamaras I, Misciali C, Vincenzi C, Robles WS, Tosti A. Permanent chemotherapy-induced alopecia: a review. J Am Acad Dermatol. 2011;64(3):604–6. Review.
18. Trüeb RM. Chemotherapy-induced alopecia. Semin Cutan Med Surg. 2009;28(1):11–4. Review.
19. Petukhova L, Cabral RM, Mackay-Wiggan J, Clynes R, Christiano AM. The genetics of alopecia areata: what's new and how will it help our patients? Dermatol Ther. 2011;24(3):326–36.
20. Ucak H, Kandi B, Cicek D, Halisdemir N, Dertlıoğlu SB. The comparison of treatment with clobetasol propionate 0.05% and topical pimecrolimus 1% treatment in the treatment of alopecia areata. J Dermatol Treat. 2011. Epub ahead of print
21. Vila TO, Camacho Martinez FM. Bimatoprost in the treatment of eyelash universalis alopecia areata. Int J Trichol. 2010;2(2):86–8.
22. American Psychiatric Association. DSM-IV: Diagnostic & Statistical Manual of Mental Disorders. 4th ed. Washington, DC: American Psychiatric Association; 2000. p. 674–7.
23. Phillips, KA. Report of the DSM-V Anxiety, obsessive-compulsive spectrum, posttraumatic, and dissociative disorders work group. Apr 2009 available at http://www.psych.org/MainMenu/Research/DSMIV/DSMV/DSMRevisionActivities/DSM-V-Work-Group-Reports/Anxiety-Obsessive-Compulsive-Spectrum-Posttraumatic-and-Dissociative-Disorders-Work-Group-Report.aspx
24. Odlaug BL, Grant JE. Impulse-control disorders in a college sample: results from the self-administered Minnesota Impulse Disorders Interview (MIDI). Prim Care Companion J Clin Psychiatry. 2010;12(2). pii: PCC.09m00842

25. Mausueto CS, Thomas AM, Brice AL. Hair pulling and its affective correlates in an African American university sample. J Anxiety Disord. 2007;21(4):590–9.
26. White MP, Koran LM. Open-label trial of aripiprazole in the treatment of trichotillomania. J Clin Psychopharmacol. 2011;31(4):503–6.
27. Grant JE, Odlaug BL, Chamberlain SR, Kim SW. Dronabinol, a cannabinoid agonist, reduces hair pulling in trichotillomania: a pilot study. Psychopharmacology (Berl). 2011;218(3): 439–502.
28. Bi MY, Cohen PR, Robinson FW, Gray JM. Alopecia syphilitica-report of a patient with secondary syphilis presenting as moth-eaten alopecia and a review of its common mimickers. Dermatol Online J. 2009;15(10):6.
29. CDC Trends in Sexually Transmitted Diseases in the United States: 2009 National Data for Gonorrhea, Chlamydia and Syphilis available at http://www.cdc.gov/std/stats09/trends2009.pdf
30. Jordaan HF, Louw M. The moth-eaten alopecia of secondary syphilis. A histopathological study of 12 patients. Am J Dermatopathol. 1995;17(2):158–62.
31. Lee JY, Hsu ML. Alopecia syphilitica, a simulator of alopecia areata: histopathology and differential diagnosis. J Cutan Pathol. 1991;18(2):87–92.
32. Nam-Cha SH, Guhl G, Fernández-Peña P, Fraga J. Alopecia syphilitica with detection of *Treponema pallidum* in the hair follicle. J Cutan Pathol. 2007;34 Suppl 1:37–40.

# Chapter 6
# Cicatricial Alopecias

**Yolanda M. Lenzy and Amy J. McMichael**

Scarring forms of hair loss, or cicatricial alopecias, are a particularly challenging group of diseases to diagnose and treat. Diagnosis can be difficult clinically and confusing pathologically. There is no widely tested therapeutic progression of treatment, and there are many published medical and surgical treatments that have been discussed. When addressing the cicatricial alopecias, a systematic approach is necessary to sort through the nuances of diagnosis and to begin diagnosis specific treatment.

This chapter will provide a practical approach to the diagnosis and management of the most common types of primary cicatricial alopecias. In primary scarring alopecias, the target of the inflammation is the hair follicle. In secondary scarring alopecias, the hair follicle is an *innocent bystander* in the disease process and is destroyed in a nonspecific manner. Examples of secondary scarring alopecias include deep burns, radiation dermatitis, cutaneous malignancies, cutaneous sarcoidosis, morphea, necrobiosis lipoidica, and certain chronic infections such as cutaneous tuberculosis [1, 2]. Secondary forms of scarring hair loss are quite common and must be considered in the differential diagnosis of late-stage primary scarring hair loss when inflammatory clues are no longer available to help with diagnosis. The diagnostic hallmark of all forms of cicatricial alopecia (primary and secondary) is visible loss of follicular ostia. In this chapter, we will focus on helpful clinical clues that help distinguish the various primary scarring alopecias and allow distinction from potentially similar non-scarring alopecias. Treatments will be discussed based on the inflammatory level of typical pathologic examination of each entity.

Y.M. Lenzy, M.D., M.P.H
Department of Dermatology, Boston University School of Medicine, Boston, MA 02118, USA

A.J. McMichael, M.D. (✉)
Department of Dermatology, Medical Center Boulevard, Wake Forest University School of Medicine, Winston-Salem, NC 27157, USA
e-mail: amcmicha@wakehealth.edu

A.F. Alexis and V.H. Barbosa (eds.), *Skin of Color: A Practical Guide to Dermatologic Diagnosis and Treatment*, DOI 10.1007/978-0-387-84929-4_6,

**Table 6.1** NAHRS classification of cicatricial alopecia

| |
|---|
| *Lymphocytic mediated* |
| Central centrifugal cicatricial alopecia |
| Chronic cutaneous lupus erythematosus |
| Classic lichen planopilaris |
| Frontal fibrosing alopecia |
| Graham-Little syndrome |
| Pseudopelade (Brocq) |
| Keratosis follicularis spinulosa decalvans |
| *Neutrophil mediated* |
| Dissecting cellulitis/folliculitis (perifolliculitis capitis abscedens et suffodiens) |
| Folliculitis decalvans |
| Tufted folliculitis |
| *Mixed* |
| Folliculitis keloidalis |

Several classification systems have been described for primary cicatricial alopecias [3, 4]. The North American Hair Research Society (NAHRS) has classified the primary cicatricial alopecias by histopathologic findings into four categories – lymphocytic, neutrophilic, mixed, and nonspecific [3] (Table 6.1). The overlap in both clinical and histological features sometimes blurs the distinction between disorders. We will discuss the five most commonly seen types of scarring alopecias: central centrifugal cicatricial alopecia, lichen planopilaris, discoid lupus erythematosus, dissecting cellulitis of the scalp, and folliculitis decalvans.

## Lymphocytic Cicatricial Alopecias

### *Central Centrifugal Cicatricial Alopecia*

#### Previous Names

- Hot comb alopecia
- Follicular degeneration syndrome
- Pseudopelade of the central scalp

#### Key Features

- Chronic, progressive cicatricial alopecia centered on the crown or vertex that gradually expands symmetrically with the most active disease at the periphery (Fig. 6.1)
- Most commonly seen in women of African descent
- Role of hair care practices probable but unclear

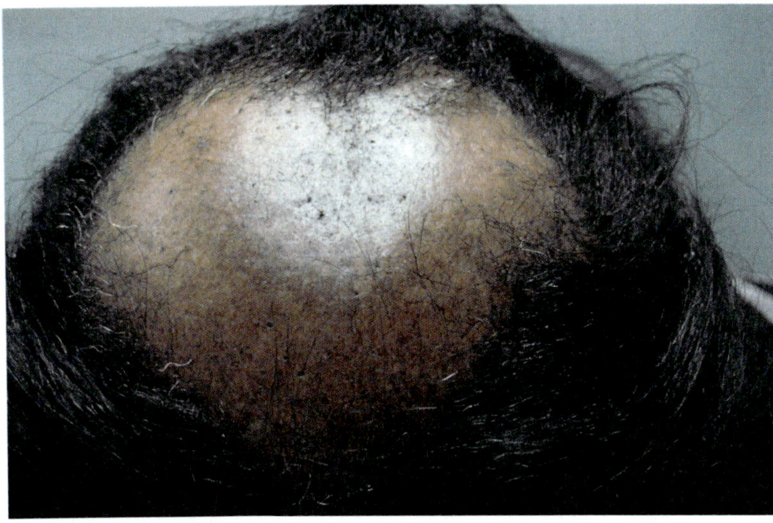

**Fig. 6.1** CCCA with classic changes of scarring on vertex scalp

## Epidemiology

Central centrifugal cicatricial alopecia (CCCA) is most commonly seen in women of African descent but has been described in men [5] and rarely occurs in women of other ethnic groups. Among African Americans, CCCA is likely responsible for more cases of scarring alopecia than all other forms combined [6], but there is no incidence or prevalence data available for this entity. Onset of the condition often occurs between the third and fifth decades. Because a considerable amount of hair is often lost before the patient notices thinning, the actual onset of hair loss may actually begin years before the patient takes notice.

## Etiology

Many factors have been proposed to contribute to the pathogenesis of CCCA including genetic predisposition, use of hot combs and pomades [7], chemical relaxers [8–11], sewn-in and glued-in hair weaves, and cornrows/braids with extension hair [12]. Interestingly, Gathers recently reported poor correlation between the use of relaxers, hot combs, and genetic predisposition and CCCA in a study of 51 CCCA patients and 50 controls [12].

## Clinical Features

In many cases of CCCA, there are no symptoms at all. In some cases, patients complain of pruritus, tenderness, burning, pain, or tingling, sometimes described as a

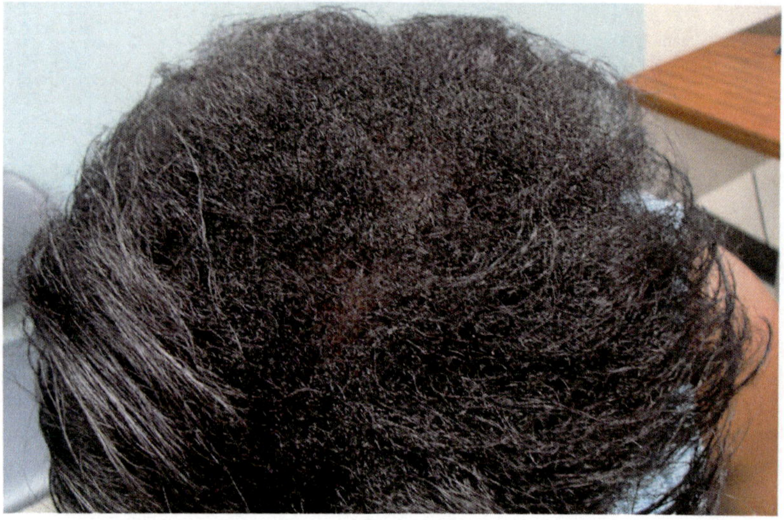

**Fig. 6.2** Breakage in the vertex area with no hair loss

"pins and needles" sensation. Patients with CCCA may also experience scaling, pustules, and crusting. If pustules, scaling, or pain is observed, it is important to rule out infection with a KOH or fungal or bacterial cultures [13]. The disease begins and remains most severe on the crown or vertex of the scalp, gradually expanding in a centrifugal fashion. Close view of the scalp will often reveal mottled hyper-/hypopigmentation along with the typical loss of follicular ostia.

CCCA shows a spectrum of severity from slowly progressive (over decades) and relatively noninflammatory to rapidly progressive (over years) and highly inflammatory disease [14]. Patients with the highly inflammatory variant have been described to have folliculitis decalvans (see the "Folliculitis Decalvans" section below). Two other problems, hair breakage and traction alopecia, may be present in some women with CCCA, but it is not clear how they are related to the scarring process of CCCA (Fig. 6.2). End-stage traction alopecia similarly presents with loss of follicular orifices, and its relationship to CCCA has been speculated [15]. Male pattern hair loss (MPHL) and female pattern hair loss (FPHL), although classified as non-scarring, have the potential for transitioning to a scarring type of hair loss [16]. This causes difficulty in the clinical distinction of FPHL and MPHL from CCCA, often necessitating a biopsy.

## Treatment

There have been no clinical trials for the treatment of patients with CCCA, so little data exists on the most effective treatment regimen for CCCA. Therefore, management of CCCA is both approached symptomatically and aimed to halt the centrifugal

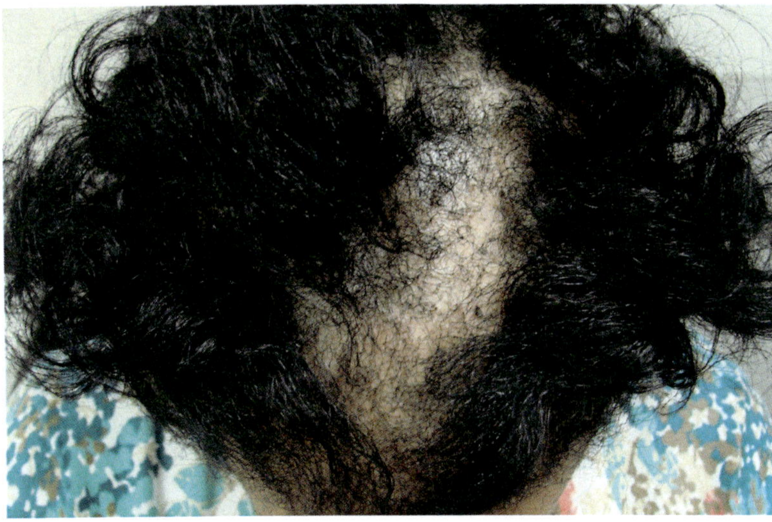

**Fig. 6.3** Miniaturized hairs in the vertex scalp of patient with CCCA

progression of the disease. To relieve inflammation and decrease pruritus, intralesional steroids, topical steroids, increasing the frequency of hair washing, and anti-dandruff shampoos are commonly used as treatments. A trial of a series of 6–8 monthly intralesional Kenalog injections (5–10 mg/cc) with concomitant use of potent topical steroids (e.g., clobetasol or fluocinonide) to the peripheral alopecic zone is often helpful. For highly inflammatory cases, a long-acting oral tetracycline (e.g., doxycycline or minocycline) or an antimalarial (e.g., hydroxychloroquine) can be effective in controlling inflammation [17, 18]. After a sufficient course of anti-inflammatory therapy, typically after 6 intralesional injections, minoxidil 2% or 5% solution or foam can be helpful as an adjuvant therapy to prolong anagen cycling for viable hairs and promote regrowth of hairs that are miniaturized in the area (Fig. 6.3) [19]. In addition, a recommendation of gentle hair care practices should also be made, and potentially damaging hair care practices should be discouraged, including reducing the frequency of chemical relaxer use or discontinuing them and limiting the use of heat and traction, hardening gels, and sprays to the scalp.

For end-stage and/or stable disease, hair transplantation is a viable option in select patients with sufficient donor area and a negative history of keloids. Experts in hair transplantation for cicatricial alopecia recommend that patients are managed medically for at least 6–9 months prior to the procedure [20]. A test graft session with a 3–4-month waiting period is recommended to evaluate the viability of the transplanted hairs [20]. Extensive keloid formation has been reported following hair transplantation in the literature [21]. Callender and colleagues, however, have found the occurrence of disfiguring keloids to be nearly nonexistent in their experience [20].

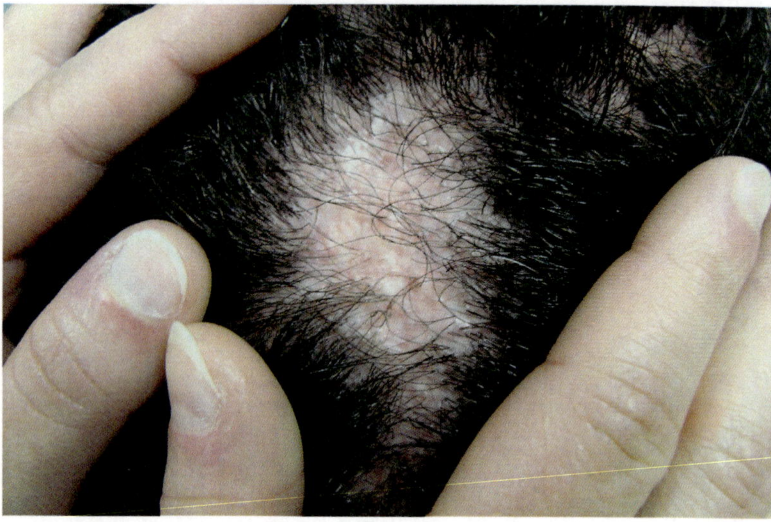

**Fig. 6.4** LPP clinically showing perifollicular erythema with mild scale

## *Lichen Planopilaris*

### Subgroups

- Classic lichen planopilaris (LPP)
- Frontal fibrosing alopecia (FFA)
- Fibrosing alopecia in a pattern distribution (FAPD)
- Graham-Little syndrome

### Key Features

- Inflammatory cicatricial alopecia with highly variable patterns of hair loss.
- Most commonly, there are scattered foci of hair loss with associated perifollicular erythema and perifollicular scale (Fig. 6.4).
- Most common cause of Brocq's alopecia (end-stage scarring alopecia).

### Epidemiology and Clinical Features

Four main subgroups are currently described: (1) classic LPP, (2) FFA, (3) FAPD, and (4) Graham-Little syndrome. Classic LPP is typically seen in women with a mean age of 50 years [22] though many men also have this diagnosis, and Caucasians are more commonly affected than individuals of color. Fifty percent of patients with LPP lack evidence of lichen planus at sites other than the scalp [23]. Patients with

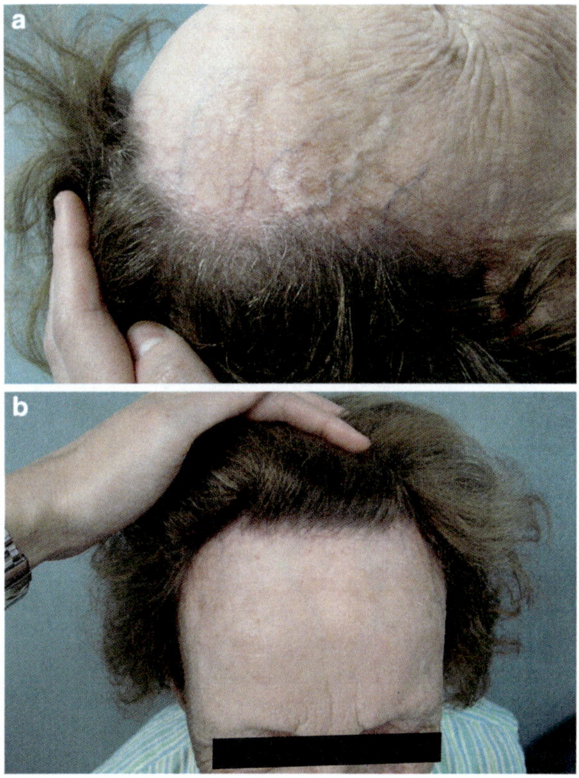


**Fig. 6.5** (**a**) FFA on frontal hairline and (**b**) FFA with eyebrow involvement

LPP are often quite symptomatic with itching, burning, and tenderness or pain of the scalp [24]. Examination reveals patchy alopecia or a more diffuse involvement of the scalp with characteristic perifollicular erythema and perifollicular scale at the margins of the areas of alopecia [25]. A positive pull test of anagen hairs is commonly present at the margin, indicating disease activity.

FFA predominately affects postmenopausal women (mean age, 67 years) but the pathogenesis seems to be unrelated to hormone replacement status [25]. FFA is characterized by a band-like frontotemporal alopecia which progresses to involve the temporal-parietal scalp and the eyebrows (Fig. 6.5a, b). The skin pallor in the band of alopecia anterior to the frontal hairline is a helpful clinical clue in recognizing this subtype [24]. The scarring in the band-like area can manifest as atrophy as well, so this should be assessed prior to any intralesional or topical treatment.

FAPD is a more recently described variant of LPP that presents as an accelerated hair loss in the central scalp of women and men with underlying pattern hair loss [26]. Patients with FAPD present similarly to classic LPP with perifollicular erythema, follicular hyperkeratosis, and loss of follicular orifices, but the involvement is centered upon the central scalp (Fig. 6.6). The net result is a reduction in the number of terminal hair follicles either by the underlying miniaturization process of pattern hair loss or by replacement of follicles by fibrous tracts [16].

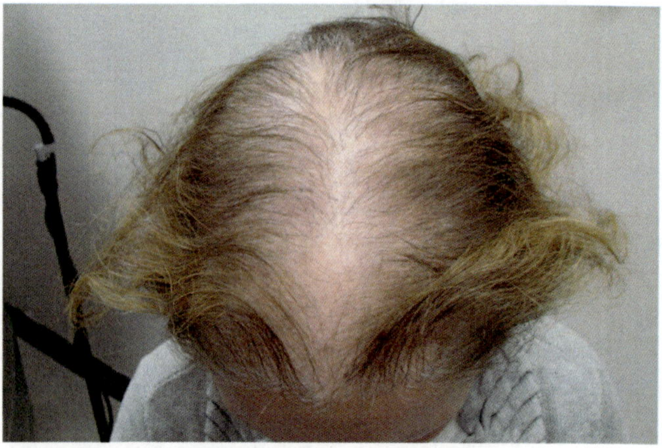

**Fig. 6.6** Fibrosing alopecia in a pattern distribution

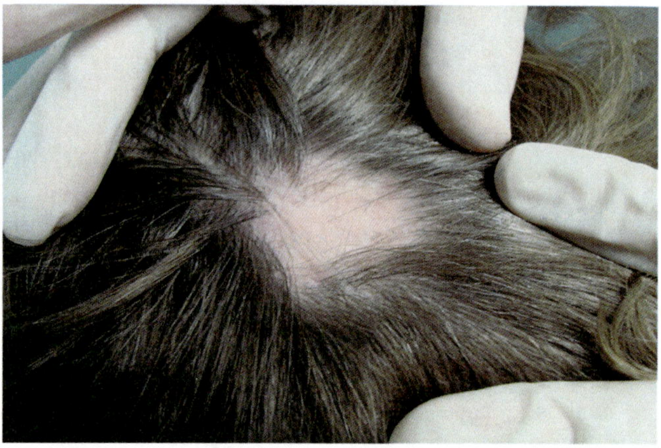

**Fig. 6.7** Pseudopelade, localized with scarring and no scale or erythema

Graham-Little syndrome is a rare variant characterized by lesions of classic LPP on the scalp, along with non-scarring alopecia of the axillary and pubic hair and keratosis pilaris on the trunk and extremities [27].

Pseudopelade of Brocq is now thought to be a form of LPP without the aforementioned signs of inflammation [28, 29] (Fig. 6.7). This pattern has been described as "footprints in the snow" [30]. The areas may show erythema and slight atrophy in the well-demarcated circular plaques on the scalp. Often, the main differential with this form of scarring alopecia is alopecia areata. A biopsy can easily show the scarring pattern of pseudopelade.

**Table 6.2** Therapeutic ladder for LPP

| | |
|---|---|
| *Topical (agents may be used in combination)* | |
| | Intralesional triamcinolone |
| | Superpotent topical steroids |
| *Systemic* | |
| | Hydroxychloroquine |
| | Methotrexate |
| | Cyclosporine |
| | Mycophenolate mofetil |

## Pathogenesis

New research points to the role of the peroxisome proliferator-activated receptor-$\gamma$ (PPAR-$\gamma$) in the pathogenesis of LPP. Karnik and colleagues found that PPAR-$\gamma$ is required for maintenance of a functional epithelial stem cell compartment in murine hair follicles and that the targeted deletion of PPAR-$\gamma$ generates skin pathology that resembles LPP and that LPP patients show gene expression changes that indicate a defect in lipid metabolism and peroxisome biogenesis [31]. This new knowledge may have treatment implications with the use of PPAR-$\gamma$ agonists (e.g., thiazolidinediones) [32].

## Treatment

The goal of current treatment is to alleviate symptoms and signs and to arrest the disease process. A helpful approach involves the use of a therapeutic ladder to guide therapy based upon the extent of involvement and clinical disease activity (Table 6.2).

*Topical/Intralesional Therapy*. The first-line treatment for moderately active LPP lesions is intralesional triamcinolone acetonide at a suggested concentration of 10 mg/cc every 4–6 weeks optionally in combination with topical class I or class II corticosteroids [33, 34]. The vehicle chosen for the scalp varies, depending on the needs and hairstyles of the patient, with ointment, oil, or foam [35] often preferred by many blacks and topical solutions or foams preferred by white patients.

*Hydroxychloroquine*. For rapidly progressive or extensive disease, hydroxychloroquine, an antilymphocytic antimalarial, is often the first-line systemic agent given its safety and low side-effect profile. The usual starting dose is 200 mg twice daily and is usually continued for 6–12 months [18]. A baseline ophthalmologic exam, a complete blood count, and liver function tests are recommended prior to the start of therapy and repeated every 6 months once the patient is stable on the medication. The ophthalmologic exam is repeated yearly. Hydroxychloroquine is well tolerated, but occasional patients complain of gastrointestinal intolerance to the drug [18].

*Methotrexate (MTX)*. For patients with persistent symptoms and hair loss after a 3–6-month trial of hydroxychloroquine, a second-line systemic agent is considered.

Currently, we use methotrexate, an antilymphocytic immunosuppressant that competitively binds dihydrofolate reductase and inhibits DNA synthesis in immunocompetent cells [36]. In vitro studies demonstrate that MTX's effect on the proliferation of lymphoid cells is 1,000 times greater than its effect on keratinocytes [11]. There have been no clinical trials of MTX in LPP or lichen planus (LP), but there are case series reporting MTX to be an effective and tolerable treatment for erosive and generalized form of LP [37, 38]. A test dose of 5 mg is given and a CBC and liver function tests are drawn 7 days later to monitor for leucopenia and thrombocytopenia. The dose is then increased to 15 mg weekly. Monitoring for drug toxicity involves drawing a complete blood count and liver function tests every 1–2 weeks during the first 2–4 weeks and after dose escalation, then every 3–4 months long term. Liver biopsy in chronic MTX usage, after every 1.5–2.0 g total dose for low-risk patients, is generally recommended [36].

*Cyclosporine.* Cyclosporine can be used as a third-line drug for patients whose clinical activity is severe and persistent after taking hydroxychloroquine and methotrexate, primarily as a short-term or "bridge" therapy. Cyclosporine (CsA) is a calcineurin inhibitor which also acts by suppressing T cell activation and downregulating proinflammatory cytokines responsible for macrophage activation. Beneficial effects of short-term CsA therapy (2–5 months) at dosages of 3–5 mg/kg/day in patients with LPP have been reported [39]. Pretreatment evaluation includes documentation of blood pressure x2, serum creatinine x2, urinalysis, CBC, BUN, and LFTs. Blood pressure and kidney and liver function are monitored every 2 weeks for 1 month and then monthly. Adverse effects include nephrotoxicity which is usually reversible, hypertension, liver toxicity, flu-like symptoms, and hypertrichosis [18].

*Mycophenolate Mofetil.* Mycophenolate mofetil is an immunomodulating drug that inhibits activated T lymphocytes. The effectiveness and safety profile of mycophenolate mofetil have made it a preferred drug for many autoimmune and inflammatory disorders including bullous pemphigoid [40], pemphigus vulgaris [41], and lichen planus of the skin and oral mucosa [42]. Mycophenolate mofetil can be used in patients for whom the above therapies fail. The recommended starting dose is 0.5 g twice daily for the first month, escalated to 1 g twice daily for 5–6 months as tolerated [18]. Baseline and monthly CBC and liver function tests should be followed.

## Other Therapies

Additional therapies with reported effectiveness in LPP and its variants include finasteride (2.5 mg/day) [43] and thalidomide [44]. Minoxidil 2% or 5% may be started during the maintenance phase, and surgical modalities such as hair transplantation or scalp reduction are options in clinically inactive cases [20]. While studies are lacking, some clinicians have begun to use pioglitazone to treat LPP in light of the preliminary research findings regarding patients' defect in lipid metabolism and peroxisome biogenesis.

## *Chronic Cutaneous Lupus Erythematosus*

### Synonym

- Discoid lupus erythematosus

### Key Features

- Annular or "discoid" lesions with erythema, scale, and pigmentary changes most pronounced on the scalp, ears, and face.
- Increased occurrence among women and African Americans.
- Majority of patients do not have systemic lupus erythematosus.

### Epidemiology

Discoid lupus erythematosus (DLE) is a form of chronic lupus erythematosus that commonly affects the scalp and results in cicatricial alopecia. Women are more commonly affected than men and the disease is more common in adults (with onset typically at the age of 20–40 years) than in children [33]. DLE has been reported to be increased among African American women [45, 46]. Approximately 25% of children and 5–10% of adults with DLE develop systemic lupus erythematosus [45]. Therefore, a thorough history and physical exam with ANA, CBC, and urinalysis should be carried out in every patient diagnosed with DLE [47]. The incidence of concurrent alopecia areata is higher in patients with DLE [48] as compared to the normal population.

### Clinical Features

Erythema, scale, and pigmentary changes are more pronounced in DLE than in other forms of scarring alopecia [49]. Annular lesions with central hypopigmentation and peripheral hyperpigmentation are commonly seen in dark-skinned individuals (Fig. 6.8). Follicular plugging is a common clinical feature. Active lesions can be tender and pruritic, and patients may report worsening after UV exposure [33]. These lesions can be seen on the scalp or any other part of the body, especially in sun-exposed areas.

### Treatment

The lymphocytic alopecia therapeutic ladder (Table 6.2) is recommended for DLE.

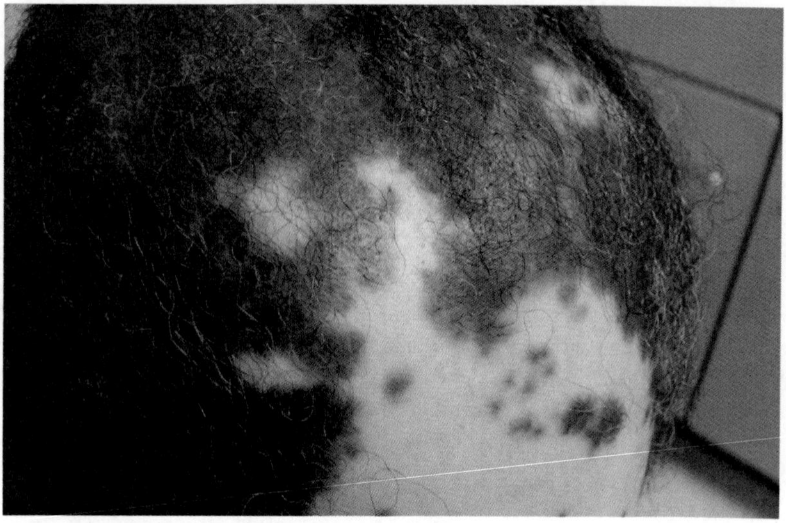

**Fig. 6.8** DLE showing typical hypo- and hyperpigmentation

# Neutrophilic Cicatricial Alopecias

## *Dissecting Cellulitis of the Scalp*

### Synonyms

- Perifolliculitis capitis abscedens et suffodiens
- Dissecting folliculitis
- Hoffman's disease

### Key Features

- A component of the *follicular occlusion tetrad*
- Follicular pustules, nodules, plaques, and sinus tracts
- Deep inflammation (deep dermis and subcutaneous fat)

### Epidemiology

Dissecting cellulitis of the scalp (DCS) may present as part of the *follicular occlusion tetrad* that includes hidradenitis suppurativa, acne conglobata, and pilonidal sinus and is seen most commonly in black men in the 2nd to 4th decade of life, but it has been reported in whites [50] and in women.

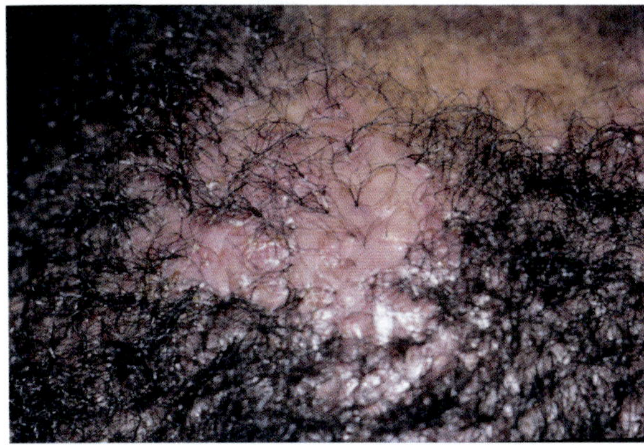

**Fig. 6.9** Dissecting cellulitis with hypertrophic scarring and tufting of hair follicles

**Table 6.3** Therapeutic ladder for DCS

| |
|---|
| *Medical* |
| Oral antibiotics |
| Isotretinoin |
| Combination of antibiotic and isotretinoin |
| TNF blockers |
| *Surgical* |
| Incision and drainage |
| Surgical excision (if inactive) |
| *Destructive* |
| Laser hair epilation |

## Clinical Features

Patients present with recurrent eruptions of follicular pustules and nodules concentrated on the crown, vertex, and occiput. These inflammatory lesions rapidly evolve into boggy plaques with sinus tract formation (Fig. 6.9). Pain can be pronounced and patients often complain of foul-smelling discharge. DCS can wax and wane in severity for years, then eventually results in scarring alopecia. Although follicular hyperkeratosis rather than infection is thought to play a primary role in pathogenesis, bacterial superinfection can occur [14]. As follicular rupture ensues, neutrophils, macrophages, and lymphocytes produce tumor necrosis factor (TNF) and other proinflammatory cytokines [51].

## Treatment

There are no FDA-approved treatments for DCS. Various case reports indicate efficacy of a range of therapies which can be divided into medical, surgical, and destructive (Table 6.3). Medical therapies reported for DCS include oral antibiotics (tetracyclines, dapsone, rifampicin), isotretinoin [50, 52], vitamin supplements (namely zinc) [53], and most recently TNF blockers, leading to resolution of the inflammatory lesion and hair regrowth [51, 54]. Combination medical therapies have reported success in recalcitrant patients failing monotherapy including isotretinoin and dapsone [55] and rifampicin and isotretinoin [56]. Incision and drainage is often a common first step in treating the fluctuant nodules and abscesses. Wide excision with primary closure or split-thickness skin grafting has been reported as successful surgical treatment when the disease is no longer active [53]. A growing literature of various destructive modalities has been reported for DCS in recent years. In the 1960s, standard treatment consisted of X-ray therapy, which is no longer performed due to increased occurrence of skin cancers. For recalcitrant cases, destruction of the hair follicle with various lasers ($C0_2$ [57], 800-nm pulse diode [58], long-pulse non-Q-switched ruby [59], and the 1,064-nm Nd:YAG [60]) have been reported with good effect.

## *Folliculitis Decalvans*

### Key Features

- Painful, perifollicular papules and pustules
- *S. aureus* usually isolated from pustules
- Superficial inflammation (superficial dermis)

### Epidemiology and Clinical Features

Folliculitis decalvans (FD) affects men and women from young adulthood to middle age. The term "folliculitis decalvans" has been applied in different ways by different authors but is usually applied to highly inflammatory forms of cicatricial alopecia where painful, perifollicular papules and pustules dominate the clinical picture. Tufted hair follicles or multiple hairs emerging from a single follicle are often seen in cases of folliculitis decalvans. Tufted follicles are a late-state feature that can be seen with a variety of inflammatory alopecias including DLE, LPP, DCS, and acne keloidalis nuchae [61]. Histologically, folliculitis decalvans manifests as a dense perifollicular inflammation of the upper follicles, while DCS involves the deeper follicles. Folliculitis decalvans occurs in otherwise healthy persons who do not have infections at other sites or demonstrable systemic or local immune abnormalities [62].

There is debate over the classification and etiology of FD, involving whether it is a subset of CCCA with pustule formation [14] or whether it represents a distinct entity caused by a specific infection: *Staphylococcus aureus* [62]. Sperling and colleagues contend that the pustules of folliculitis decalvans are a manifestation of either bacterial superinfection or an intense immune response to degenerating follicular components and classified folliculitis decalvans as a subset of CCCA [14]. Prospective, double-blinded studies are needed to quell the debate [63].

### Treatment

Bacterial cultures and sensitivities from intact pustules are the first step in management of folliculitis decalvans. *S. aureus* is usually isolated, and occasionally other microbes are cultured [62]. Treatment is geared to the predominant pathogen cultured. Oral rifampicin 300 mg twice daily and oral clindamycin 300 mg twice daily for 10 weeks have been shown to lead to significant improvement [18]. For patients who do not tolerate clindamycin, oral ciprofloxacin, cephalexin, or doxycycline can be substituted [18]. Zinc and fusidic acid has reported effectiveness in a limited number of patients [64]. Topical mupirocin daily for 1 week then once monthly is recommended if the patient is a staphylococcus carrier [18].

## Conclusion

Cicatricial alopecias are a diverse group of cutaneous disorders of different clinical presentations, etiology, and pathogenesis. The treatment of cicatricial alopecias is challenging and patient expectations must be clear. Patient participation in support groups through the Cicatricial Alopecia Research Foundation (CARF, www.carfintl.org) can be helpful. Study of the disorders on the molecular level as well as population-based trials will likely provide much needed insight into pathophysiology of the cicatricial alopecias and better inform prevention and treatment efforts.

## References

1. Sperling L, et al. Alopecias. In: Bolognia J, Jorizzo JL, Rapini RP, editors. Dermatology. St. Louis, MO: Elsevier; 2008. p. 996.
2. Finner AM, Otberg N, Shapiro J. Secondary cicatricial and other permanent alopecias. Dermatol Ther. 2008;21(4):279–94.
3. Olsen EA, Bergfeld WF, Cotsarelis G, et al. Summary of North American hair research society (NAHRS)-sponsored Workshop on Cicatricial Alopecia, Duke University Medical Center, February 10 and 11, 2001. J Am Acad Dermatol. 2003;48(1):103–10.
4. Sperling LC. Scarring alopecia and the dermatopathologist. J Cutan Pathol. 2001;28(7):333–42.
5. Sperling LC, Skelton 3rd HG, Smith KJ, Sau P, Friedman K. Follicular degeneration syndrome in men. Arch Dermatol. 1994;130(6):763–9.
6. Sperling LC, Sau P. The follicular degeneration syndrome in black patients. "Hot comb alopecia" revisited and revised. Arch Dermatol. 1992;128(1):68–74.
7. LoPresti P, Papa CM, Kligman AM. Hot comb alopecia. Arch Dermatol. 1968;98(3):234–8.
8. McMichael AJ. Ethnic hair update: past and present. J Am Acad Dermatol. 2003;48 (6 Suppl):S127–33.
9. Nnoruka EN. Hair loss: is there a relationship with hair care practices in Nigeria? Int J Dermatol. 2005;44 Suppl 1:13–7.
10. McMichael AJ. Hair and scalp disorders in ethnic populations. Dermatol Clin. 2003;21(4):629–44.

11. Bulengo-Ransby SM, Bergfeld WF. Chemical and traumatic alopecia from thioglycolate in a black woman: a case report with unusual clinical and histologic findings. Cutis. 1992;49(2): 99–103.
12. Gathers RC, Jankowski M, Eide M, Lim HW. Hair grooming practices and central centrifugal cicatricial alopecia. J Am Acad Dermatol. 2009;60(4):574–8.
13. Martin ES, Elewski BE. Tinea capitis in adult women masquerading as bacterial pyoderma. J Am Acad Dermatol. 2003;49(2 Suppl Case Reports):S177–9.
14. Sperling LC, Solomon AR, Whiting DA. A new look at scarring alopecia. Arch Dermatol. 2000;136(2):235–42.
15. Ackerman AB, Walton NW, Jones RE, Charissi C. "Hot comb alopecia"/ "Follicular degeneration syndrome" in African American women is traction alopecia. Dermatopath: Practical Conceptual. 2000;6:6–21.
16. Olsen EA. Female pattern hair loss and its relationship to permanent/cicatricial alopecia: a new perspective. j investig dermatol Symp proc. 2005;10(3):217–21.
17. Scott DA. Disorders of the hair and scalp in blacks. Dermatol Clin. 1988;6(3):387–95.
18. Price VH. The medical treatment of cicatricial alopecia. Semin Cutan Med Surg. 2006;25(1):56–9.
19. Taylor S. Practical tips for managing hair disorders in African-American females. Pract Dermatol. 2006;3(7):25–7.
20. Callender VD, McMichael AJ, Cohen GF. Medical and surgical therapies for alopecias in black women. Dermatol Ther. 2004;17(2):164–76.
21. Brown MD, Johnson T, Swanson NA. Extensive keloids following hair transplantation. J Dermatol Surg Oncol. 1990;16(9):867–9.
22. Chieregato C, Zini A, Barba A, Magnanini M, Rosina P. Lichen planopilaris: report of 30 cases and review of the literature. Int J Dermatol. 2003;42(5):342–5.
23. Mehregan DA, Van Hale HM, Muller SA. Lichen planopilaris: clinical and pathologic study of forty-five patients. J Am Acad Dermatol. 1992;27(6 Pt 1):935–42.
24. Mirmirani P. Cicatricial Alopecia. In: healthcare I, editor. Hair and scalp diseases: medical, surgical and cosmetic treatments. New York: Informa Healthcare; 2008. p. 137–48.
25. Kossard S, Lee MS, Wilkinson B. Postmenopausal frontal fibrosing alopecia: a frontal variant of lichen planopilaris. J Am Acad Dermatol. 1997;36(1):59–66.
26. Zinkernagel MS, Trueb RM. Fibrosing alopecia in a pattern distribution: patterned lichen planopilaris or androgenetic alopecia with a lichenoid tissue reaction pattern? Arch Dermatol. 2000;136(2):205–11.
27. Bianchi L, Paro Vidolin A, Piemonte P, Carboni I, Chimenti S. Graham Little-Piccardi-Lassueur syndrome: effective treatment with cyclosporin A. Clin Exp Dermatol. 2001; 26(6).
28. Amato L, Mei S, Massi D, Gallerani I, Fabbri P. Cicatricial alopecia; a dermatopathologic and immunopathologic study of 33 patients (pseudopelade of Brocq is not a specific clinicopathologic entity). Int J Dermatol. 2002;41(1):8–15.
29. Silvers DN, Katz BE, Young AW. Pseudopelade of Brocq is lichen planopilaris: report of four cases that support this nosology. Cutis. 1993;51(2):99–105.
30. Ronchese F. Pseudopelade. Arch dermat. 1960;82:336–43.
31. Karnik P, Tekeste Z, McCormick TS, et al. Hair follicle stem cell-specific PPARgamma deletion causes scarring alopecia. J Invest Dermatol. 2009;129(5):1243–57.
32. Harries MJ, Paus R. Scarring alopecia and the PPAR-gamma connection. J Invest Dermatol. 2009;129(5):1066–70.
33. Otberg N, Wu WY, McElwee KJ, Shapiro J. Diagnosis and management of primary cicatricial alopecia: part I. Skinmed. 2008;7(1):19–26.
34. Cevasco NC, Bergfeld WF, Remzi BK, de Knott HR. A case-series of 29 patients with lichen planopilaris: the Cleveland clinic foundation experience on evaluation, diagnosis, and treatment. J Am Acad Dermatol. 2007;57(1):47–53.
35. George YA RS, Gottlieb J, et al. Betamethasone valerate 0.12 % in foam vehicle scalp dermatitis in African Americans. Cosmet Dermatol. 2002;15:23–7.

36. Callen JP K-SC, Wolverton SE. Methotrexate. In: Comprehensive dermatologic drug therapy. Seconth ed. Philadelphia: Saunders; 2007.
37. Turan H, Baskan EB, Tunali S, Yazici S, Saricaoglu H. Methotrexate for the treatment of generalized lichen planus. J Am Acad Dermatol. 2009;60(1):164–6.
38. Nylander Lundqvist E, Wahlin YB, Hofer PA. Methotrexate supplemented with steroid ointments for the treatment of severe erosive lichen ruber. Acta Derm Venereol. 2002;82(1):63–4.
39. Mirmirani P, Willey A, Price VH. Short course of oral cyclosporine in lichen planopilaris. J Am Acad Dermatol. 2003;49(4):667–71.
40. Bohm M, Beissert S, Schwarz T, Metze D, Luger T. Bullous pemphigoid treated with mycophenolate mofetil. Lancet. 1997;349(9051):541.
41. Enk AH, Knop J. Treatment of pemphigus vulgaris with mycophenolate mofetil. Lancet. 1997;350(9076):494.
42. Frieling U, Bonsmann G, Schwarz T, Luger TA, Beissert S. Treatment of severe lichen planus with mycophenolate mofetil. J Am Acad Dermatol. 2003;49(6):1063–6.
43. Tosti A, Piraccini BM, Iorizzo M, Misciali C. Frontal fibrosing alopecia in postmenopausal women. J Am Acad Dermatol. 2005;52(1):55–60.
44. George SJ, Hsu S. Lichen planopilaris treated with thalidomide. J Am Acad Dermatol. 2001;45(6):965–6.
45. Callen JP. Chronic cutaneous lupus erythematosus. Clinical, laboratory, therapeutic, and prognostic examination of 62 patients. Arch Dermatol. 1982;118(6):412–6.
46. McCarty DJ, Manzi S, Medsger Jr TA, Ramsey-Goldman R, LaPorte RE, Kwoh CK. Incidence of systemic lupus erythematosus. Race and gender differences. Arthritis Rheum. 1995;38(9):1260–70.
47. Tebbe B, Mansmann U, Wollina U, et al. Markers in cutaneous lupus erythematosus indicating systemic involvement. A multicenter study on 296 patients. Acta Derm Venereol. 1997;77(4): 305–8.
48. Werth VP, White WL, Sanchez MR, Franks AG. Incidence of alopecia areata in lupus erythematosus. Arch Dermatol. 1992;128(3):368–71.
49. Headington JT. Cicatricial alopecia. Dermatol Clin. 1996;14(4):773–82.
50. Koca R, Altinyazar HC, Ozen OI, Tekin NS. Dissecting cellulitis in a white male: response to isotretinoin. Int J Dermatol. 2002;41(8):509–13.
51. Sukhatme SV, Lenzy YM, Gottlieb AB. Refractory dissecting cellulitis of the scalp treated with adalimumab. J Drugs Dermatol. 2008;7(10):981–3.
52. Scerri L, Williams HC, Allen BR. Dissecting cellulitis of the scalp: response to isotretinoin. Br J Dermatol. 1996;134(6):1105–8.
53. Williams CN, Cohen M, Ronan SG, Lewandowski CA. Dissecting cellulitis of the scalp. Plast Reconstr Surg. 1986;77(3):378–82.
54. Brandt HR, Malheiros AP, Teixeira MG, Machado MC. Perifolliculitis capitis abscedens et suffodiens successfully controlled with infliximab. Br J Dermatol. 2008;159(2):506–7.
55. Bolz S, Jappe U, Hartschuh W. Successful treatment of perifolliculitis capitis abscedens et suffodiens with combined isotretinoin and dapsone. J Dtsch Dermatol Ges. 2008;6(1):44–7.
56. Georgala S, Korfitis C, Ioannidou D, Alestas T, Kylafis G, Georgala C. Dissecting cellulitis of the scalp treated with rifampicin and isotretinoin: case reports. Cutis. 2008;82(3):195–8.
57. Glass LF, Berman B, Laub D. Treatment of perifolliculitis capitis abscedens et suffodiens with the carbon dioxide laser. J Dermatol Surg Oncol. 1989;15(6):673–6.
58. Boyd AS, Binhlam JQ. Use of an 800-nm pulsed-diode laser in the treatment of recalcitrant dissecting cellulitis of the scalp. Arch Dermatol. 2002;138(10):1291–3.
59. Chui CT, Berger TG, Price VH, Zachary CB. Recalcitrant scarring follicular disorders treated by laser-assisted hair removal: a preliminary report. Dermatol Surg. 1999;25(1):34–7.
60. Krasner BD, Hamzavi FH, Murakawa GJ, Hamzavi IH. Dissecting cellulitis treated with the long-pulsed Nd:YAG laser. Dermatol Surg. 2006;32(8):1039–44.
61. Wu WY, Otberg N, McElwee KJ, Shapiro J. Diagnosis and management of primary cicatricial alopecia: part II. Skinmed. 2008;7(2):78–83.
62. Powell JJ, Dawber RP, Gatter K. Folliculitis decalvans including tufted folliculitis: clinical, histological and therapeutic findings. Br J Dermatol. 1999;140(2):328–33.

63. Powell J, Dawber RP. Folliculitis decalvans and tufted folliculitis are specific infective diseases that may lead to scarring, but are not a subset of central centrifugal scarring alopecia. Arch Dermatol. 2001;137(3):373–4.
64. Abeck D, Korting HC, Braun-Falco O. Folliculitis decalvans. Long-lasting response to combined therapy with fusidic acid and zinc. Acta Derm Venereol. 1992;72(2):143–5.

# Chapter 7
# Pseudofolliculitis Barbae and Acne Keloidalis Nuchae

**Marcelyn K. Coley, A. Paul Kelly, and Andrew F. Alexis**

## Pseudofolliculitis Barbae

Pseudofolliculitis barbae (PFB) is an inflammatory disorder characterized by papules and pustules in the beard area. It represents a foreign-body inflammatory response to ingrown hairs.

### *Epidemiology*

The prevalence of PFB is reported to be between 45% and 83% in black men [1, 2]. However, the condition also affects men from other racial groups as well as women.

M.K. Coley, M.D.
Department of Dermatology, SUNY Downstate Medical Center,
450 Clarkson Avenue, 11203 Brooklyn, NY, USA
e-mail: mkcoley@gmail.com

A.P. Kelly, M.D.
Division of Dermatology, Charles Drew University of Medicine and Science,
Former King/Drew Medical Center, The David Geffen School of Medicine,
2983 Burdeck Drive, 94602 Oakland, CA, USA
e-mail: aA.Paulkelly@yahoo.com

A.F. Alexis, M.PH., M.D. (✉)
Skin of Color Center, Department of Dermatology, St. Luke's Roosevelt Hospital
and Columbia University College of Physicians and Surgeons
New York, NY, USA
e-mail: alexisderm@yahoo.com

A.F. Alexis and V.H. Barbosa (eds.), *Skin of Color: A Practical Guide to Dermatologic Diagnosis and Treatment*, DOI 10.1007/978-0-387-84929-4_7,

## *Pathogenesis and Etiology*

PFB is related to the coarse and tightly curled nature of the hair shaft characteristically found in individuals of African descent, which predisposes newly cut hair to curl back and penetrate the skin inciting an inflammatory reaction. Shaving is a major predisposing factor producing the sharp edge on the hair shaft, which punctures and reenters the skin triggering a chronic foreign-body inflammatory response to the hair shaft in the epidermis and/or dermis. Other forms of hair removal have also been implicated such as plucking and waxing. A recent study identified a single nucleotide polymorphism in the companion layer-specific keratin K6hf (k75) that may contribute a partial risk for development of the condition [3]. The mutation likely leads to a structurally weakened companion layer of the follicle which, in the context of close shaving of a curly hair shaft, contributes to an increased risk of ingrown hairs.

## *Diagnosis*

PFB is clinically characterized by erythematous or hyperpigmented follicular and perifollicular papules or pustules. Generally, the submaxillary (Fig. 7.1), chin, submental, and anterior neck regions are involved (Fig. 7.2), whereas the mustache and sideburn areas are usually spared. A similar clinical presentation can be seen in other areas where hair removal is practiced including the axillae, pubic region, and legs. PFB tends to follow a chronic course as long as shaving continues. Potential sequelae include postinflammatory hyperpigmentation (PIH) (Fig. 7.3) and keloidal or hypertrophic scarring (Fig. 7.4).

## *Laboratory Investigations*

A clinical diagnosis is usually made. However, when pustules are present, bacterial culture and sensitivity should be performed followed by treatment with the appropriate antibiotics as needed for secondary infection. Hormonal abnormalities such as those caused by polycystic ovarian syndrome or androgen-producing tumors should be considered when a hirsute female patient presents with PFB. Screening studies include serum free and total testosterone, dehydroepiandrosterone (DHEAS), and luteinizing hormone and follicle-stimulating hormone (LH/FSH) [4].

## *Differential Diagnoses*

Other diagnoses to consider include true bacterial folliculitis, acne vulgaris, and tinea barbae. Bacterial folliculitis will have positive bacterial cultures, whereas only those secondarily infected papules of PFB will. Acne also occurs on non-hair-bearing areas of the face and may present with comedones, in contrast to PFB. Tinea barbae typically affects one side of the face and is typically scaly and annular (Table 7.1).

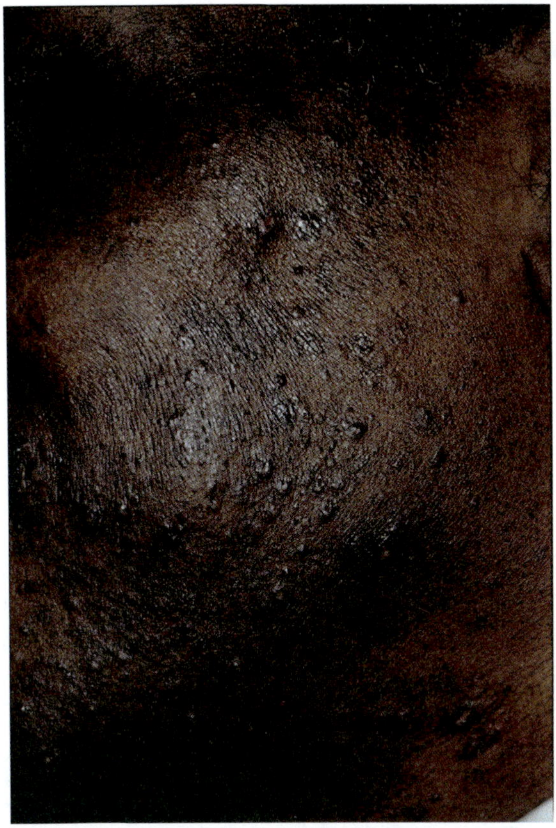

**Fig. 7.1** PFB. Moderate: multiple papules on the left cheek

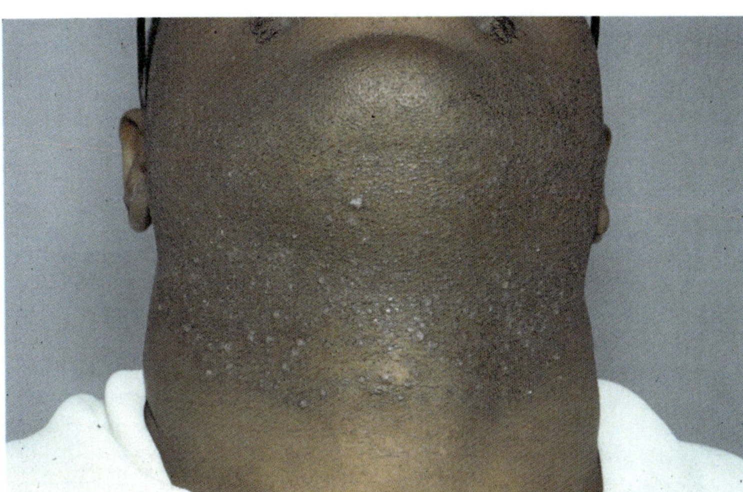

**Fig. 7.2** PFB. Papules and pustules of the anterior neck and submandibular area

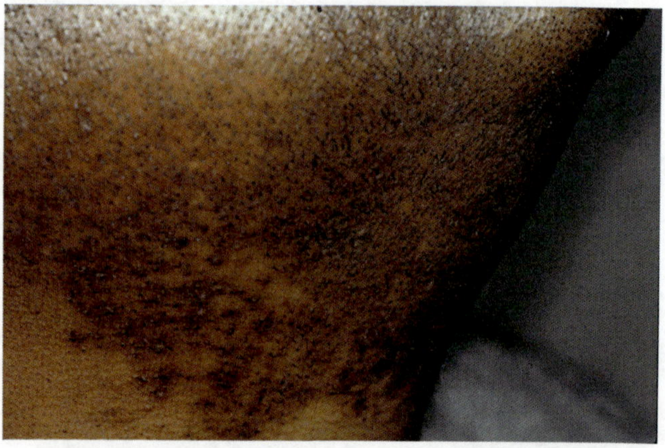

**Fig. 7.3** PFB. Hyperpigmentation secondary to PIH on the right cheek and anterior neck

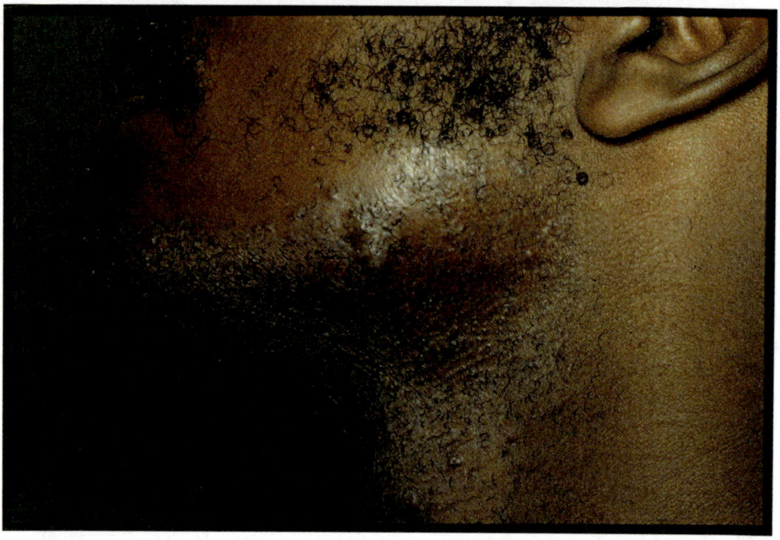

**Fig. 7.4** PFB. A small keloid on the left mandibular area. Papules and pustules on the left anterior neck and submandibular area

**Table 7.1** Differential diagnoses for PFB

| Condition | Distinguishing features |
|---|---|
| Bacterial folliculitis | Primary bacterial infection |
| Traumatic folliculitis | No evidence of infection or ingrowth of hair; resolves 1–2 days after discontinuation of shaving |
| Acne vulgaris | Comedones present; distribution beyond beard |
| Tinea barbae | Unilateral; typically male formers |
| Keloids/hypertrophic scars | Usually history of trauma |
| Sarcoidosis | Dermal papules |

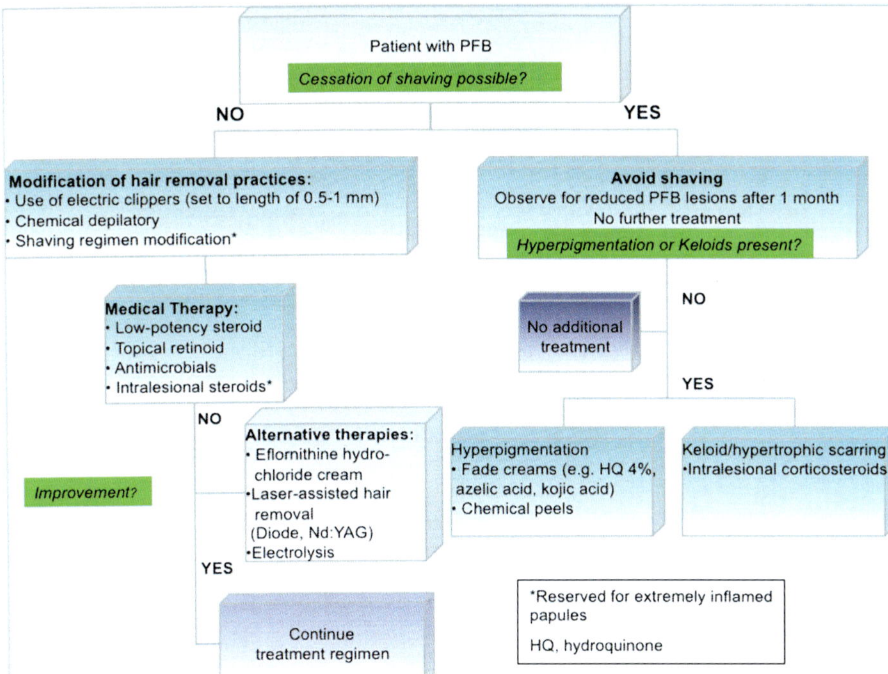


**Fig. 7.5** Approach to the patient with PFB

## *Treatment*

### First-Line Therapy

An important part of management is educating patients on the etiologic factors of PFB and discussing shaving practices. Cessation of shaving and allowing beard growth results in resolution of papules in most cases [5]. However, for many patients this is not a favorable option due to either occupational requirements or personal preferences. Therefore, various therapeutic approaches are often necessary including modification of shaving or hair removal practices, prescribing topical therapies, or performing in-office procedures (Fig. 7.5).

### Hair Removal Practices

Several shaving techniques are recommended for men with PFB. Prior to shaving, embedded hairs should be gently released. Single-blade razors are generally recommended over multiblade razors because of the increased potential for transfollicular reentry when closer-shaving multiblade razors are used. However, a recent open-label company-sponsored study found that daily shaving with a five-blade razor

**Shaving Recommendations to Reduce "razor bumps"**

1. Prior to shaving, wash face with warm water and a mild cleanser (e.g. Cetpahil® cleanser). A washcloth or Buf-Puf® can be used to gently release ingrown hairs.
2. Lather the beard with a soothing cream (e.g. Aveeno Therapeutic Shave Gel or Neutrogena Skin Clearing Shave Cream)
3. Shaving using a single-edged razor with foil guard (e.g. The Bump Fighter®). The following shaving tips should be kept in mind:
   - Do not pull the skin taut while shaving
   - Shave with the grain (the direction of hair growth)
   - Shave any given area only once
   - Use soft strokes – do not apply excessive pressure
   - Shave at least every 3 days (less frequent shaving allows enough time for growing hair to curl back into the skin)
4. After shaving, a magnifying mirror can be used to identify ingrown hairs. They can be released by gently inserting a toothpick or sterile needle under the loop of hair and pulling outward.

Additional creams/lotions may be prescribed. Please follow the instructions with a checkmark below.

❑ After shaving:
Apply ________________________ to the affected area

❑ Every night:
Apply ________________________ to the affected area

**Fig. 7.6** Sample patient education material to for PFB (razor bumps)

(Gillete Fusion Power™, Proctor & Gamble, Cincinnati, OH) did not exacerbate PFB [6]. Further studies are needed to confirm the best shaving practices for men with PFB (Fig. 7.6). Electric shavers commonly are recommended to patients because they can be set to cut the hair to the desired length. The suggested lengths are 0.5–1 mm [7]. But this may be unpopular for men who prefer a closer shave.

Chemical depilatories may be used as an alternate way to remove hair. Barium sulfide and calcium thioglycolate weaken disulfide bonds in keratin, allowing the hair to be easily wiped off the face. These formulations exist in a cream, paste, or powder form. The product is applied to moistened skin and allowed to sit for 5 or 10 min (barium sulfate and calcium thioglycolate, respectively). The substance is then gently scraped off using a blunt instrument such as a wooden spatula. The resultant blunt hair tip makes extrafollicular and transfollicular penetration less likely [8]. Caution must be used as these substances are known for their potential to cause contact irritant dermatitis with prolonged exposure. For this reason, the package instructions should be closely adhered to. A test spot is advocated prior to proceeding with treatment to the entire hair-bearing area.

## Medical Treatment

Medical therapy generally targets inflammation and secondary infection. Topical retinoids, antibiotics, and low-potency corticosteroids are useful. Nightly topical retinoids (e.g., adapalene, tazarotene, or tretinoin) help to minimize hyperkeratinization that can form with repeated nicking of the epithelium [8]. Retinoids also help to improve PIH. Low-potency steroids (i.e., desonide, hydrocortisone) are often used in place of aftershave products to help reduce inflammation. Antimicrobials inhibit the colonization of bacteria that may lead to secondary infection. Benzoyl peroxide washes are commonly recommended prior to shaving. Topical antibiotics are also useful for their anti-inflammatory properties [9]. One study found that a benzoyl peroxide 5%/clindamycin 1% gel was significantly more effective in reducing PFB lesions than vehicle [9]. In cases of severely inflamed papules or hypertrophic or keloidal scarring, monthly injections of intralesional corticosteroids (e.g., triamcinolone acetonide, 5–40 mg/ml) may be useful. Associated hyperpigmentation can be treated with bleaching agents, such as hydroquinone 4%, azelaic acid 15% (or 20%), or kojic acid twice daily.

A recent addition to medical therapy is the use of eflornithine hydrochloride cream, 13.9% (Vaniqa, SkinMedica, Carlsbad, CA), an FDA-approved treatment for unwanted facial hair in women. It has however been prescribed off label for use in men. It works by slowing the hair growth rate through inhibition of ornithine decarboxylase, an enzyme involved in hair cell division. The cream is applied twice daily to the affected area. Results can be expected after approximately 2 months of use. It is, however, necessary to continue with some form of concurrent hair removal, as this is not a depilatory.

## Epilation

Although not commonly recommended, electrolysis remains the only permanent form of hair removal and can lead to cure if there is complete destruction of the hair follicle. This, however, may be difficult in patients of color as the follicle is curved and often distorted making it challenging to precisely target the hair bulb. Electrolysis may potentially exacerbate PFB if only partial destruction of the follicle occurs [10].

With the advent of laser devices that can safely be used on darker skin types, laser-assisted hair reduction is a significant advance in the treatment of PFB. The diode 800–810 nm [3, 11–13] and the long-pulsed 1,064-nm Nd:YAG [11, 14–16] are the lasers of choice for laser-assisted hair removal in patients with Fitzpatrick skin types IV–VI. Weaver et al. found that the Nd:YAG 1,064-nm laser at fluences of 24–40 J/cm [2] and pulse duration of 30–40 ms with continuous contact cooling was safe and effective in the treatment of PFB in skin types V–VI [15]. Side effects may include erythema, itching, and transient hyper- or hypopigmentation. Schulze et al. recently found that weekly treatments with lower than traditional fluences at 12 J/cm [2] were also effective and resulted in a significant reduction in PFB lesions [16].

Special precautions must be taken in order to minimize the risk of adverse effects when performing laser hair removal in skin of color patients. Hydroquinone 4% can be used for 1–2 weeks prior to treatment to help prevent PIH, although in this author's (AFA) experience this is not necessary when the long-pulsed 1,064-nm laser is used with the appropriate settings for a given patient. Longer pulse durations, conservative fluences, and aggressive epidermal cooling are recommended for skin of color patients in order to minimize the risk of thermal injury and associated dyschromia. Pretreatment cooling can be achieved by applying a refrigerated gel on the skin prior to treatment. Intraoperative cooling is achieved either through a chilled sapphire tip or copper-plated hand piece (i.e., contact cooling) or a cryogen spray that cools the skin prior to delivery of the laser pulse [17]. The latter, however, carries a risk of dyschromia in darker skin if the cryogen spray is used too aggressively. Posttreatment cooling with ice packs (10–15 min) is also recommended to help reduce thermal injury. Photoprotection with sunscreen along with sun avoidance before, during, and after the treatment period is also strongly advised. Generally, treatments are safely spaced 4 weeks or more apart.

#### Alternative Therapies

Chemical peels can be used as an adjunctive therapy, primarily addressing hyperkeratinization and hyperpigmentation [4] that occurs secondary to repeated shaving and in response to the inflammation, respectively. Chemical peels with superficial peeling agents, such as salicylic acid and glycolic acid, have been shown to be safe and effective in darker skin types [18–20]. Additionally, reduced numbers of PFB lesions have been observed with consistent use [19–21]. One proposed regimen is 30% salicylic acid peels done at 4-week intervals and maintained with glycolic acid 15% cream or gel applied twice daily to the area, between peels [20]. This is continued until the expected clinical goal is achieved.

## Acne Keloidalis Nuchae

Acne keloidalis nuchae (AKN) is a chronic inflammatory follicular disorder of the occipital scalp and posterior neck that primarily affects men of African descent. It was first described by Kaposi in 1869 and has since been referred to by various names including dermatitis papillaris capillitii and folliculitis keloidalis. Especially in severe cases, AKN is associated with considerable psychological effects and impaired quality of life.

### *Epidemiology*

AKN is most commonly seen in black men but can also occur in Hispanics, Asians [22], and whites 23–25 as well as women. The reported prevalence is up to 13.7%

among black men [26–28]. It typically occurs in postpubertal men through the age of 50 [29]. AKN rarely occurs in women [30, 31], with a male to female ratio of at least 20:1 [29].

## *Pathogenesis*

The etiology of AKN is poorly understood. Several mechanisms of disease have been proposed. It appears that AKN has the propensity to occur at some time after having a low haircut or after shaving, suggesting that trauma may play a role. Like the mechanism proposed for pseudofolliculitis, it is thought that the tightly coiled nature of the hair of individuals affected with the disease has some bearing on the development of the condition. However, this hypothesis has been challenged by a recent study by Sperling et al. [5]. It is important to note that AKN is neither a keloid nor is it related to acne vulgaris.

In one study, no association between the occurrence of AKN and family history of AKN was observed nor was a personal or family history of keloids found to be associated [27]. However, 15% of patients with AKN seen at a teaching hospital in Nigeria reported a family history of AKN [32]. No specific genetic factors have been identified, although there has been one case report of familial acne keloidalis involving a father and all three of his sons [33]. George et al. suggested that seborrheic constitution, early reproductive years, and increased fasting blood testosterone concentration were associated with AKN [32], with two-third of subjects having coexisting seborrheic dermatitis and one-third coexisting PFB. It is postulated that the increased mast cell density and dilatation of dermal capillaries may predispose to the concentration of lesions in the occipital region [32].

Other proposed etiologic factors in the development of AKN include chronic irritation from shirt collars, chronic low-grade folliculitis, and autoimmune processes [29]. One case series suggests that AKN is a transepithelial elimination disorder similar to perforating folliculitis [34]. Sperling et al. proposed that AKN is a mixed primary scarring alopecia [35] due to the various overlapping histological features that it shares with other primary cicatricial alopecias.

## *Diagnosis*

Clinically, characteristic firm flesh-colored fibrotic papules can be found on the posterior scalp and neck (Fig. 7.7). In more severe cases, lesions may extend up to the vertex scalp. Pustules or crusted papules are often present. In later stages, lesions tend to coalesce, forming keloid-like plaques. Tufted hairs may also be apparent, with as many as 20 hairs coming out of a single opening on the scalp (Fig. 7.8). Subjects often complain of soreness or itching in affected areas.

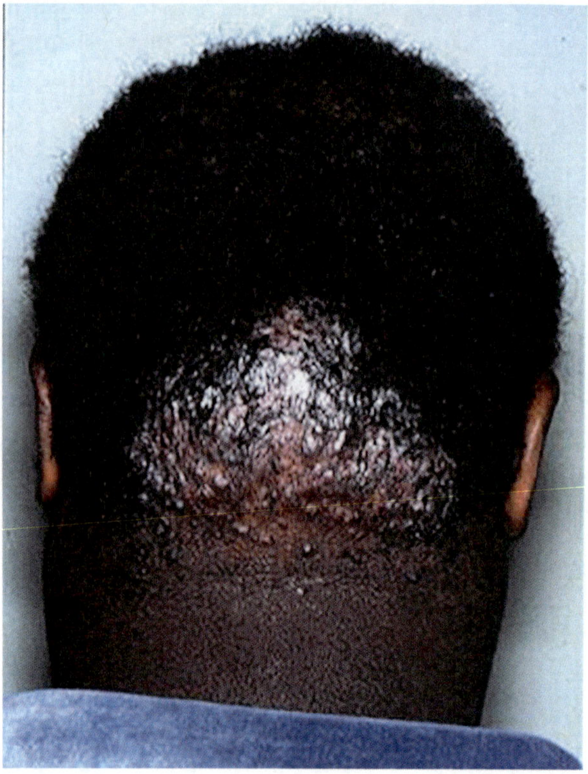

**Fig. 7.7** AKN. Papules coalescing into a plaque with scarring alopecia on posterior scalp

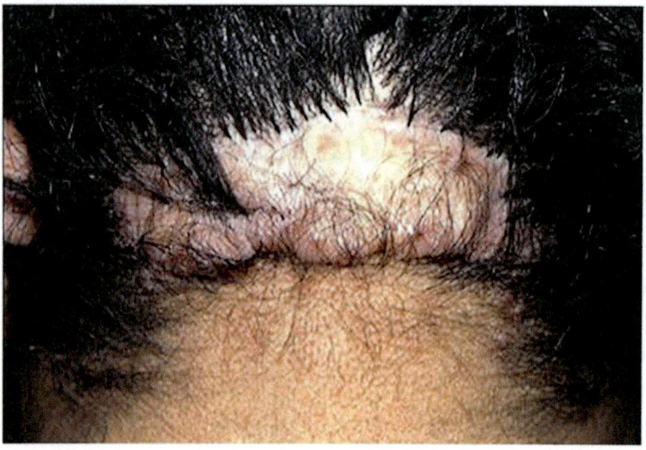

**Fig. 7.8** AKN. Tufted hairs of the left upper border

**Table 7.2** Differential diagnoses for AKN

| Condition | Distinguishing features |
|---|---|
| Folliculitis/perifolliculitis | Primary bacterial infection |
| Pseudofolliculitis barbae | Distribution beyond scalp/posterior neck unlikely |
| Keloid 2′ to trauma | Usually develops sometime after incidence of trauma or inflammation |
| Acne mechanica | Associated with use of head gear (e.g., helmet) |
| Folliculitis decalvans | Primarily parietal and vertex scalp, erythema, and pustules/crusting |
| Dissecting cellulitis | Painful nodules and abscesses |

## *Histopathology*

Studies are generally not needed to make the diagnosis. However, on histopathology, evidence of follicular and perifollicular inflammation is present [36]. Composition changes occur as the lesions progress. For example, in early lesions, infiltrates are primarily neutrophilic and lymphocytic, but in later lesions, plasma cells and sometimes mast cells predominate [36]. The inflammation begins in the upper third portion of the hair follicle. There is a paucity of sebaceous glands. Later on, disrupted hair follicles are surrounded by granulomatous inflammation. Dermal fibrosis seen in some patients resembles the thick, hyalinized, eosinophilic collagen fibers of keloids [36]. Herzberg et al. [36] proposed a sequence of inflammatory events as follows: acute inflammation, which results in a weakened follicular wall. This allows the release of the naked hair shafts into the dermis, which triggers a foreign-body reaction causing further acute and chronic granulomatous inflammation manifested as a papule. Fibroblasts undergo activation, producing collagen and thus scar tissue in the region. This causes further distortion and occlusion of the follicle resulting in hair retention in the inferior follicle and further granulomatous inflammation and scarring, with ultimate formation of apparent scarring and plaque formation [36]. Inflammation and scarring through the mechanisms described may also contribute to the development of tufted hair folliculitis seen late in the disease process [37].

## *Differential Diagnosis*

Although sharing a portion of its name, AKN and acne vulgaris are not the related. The scalp is not a common place to develop acne. Early cases may be confused with bacterial folliculitis or pseudofolliculitis, though pseudofolliculitis rarely occurs on the posterior scalp or neck. Keloid scarring secondary to trauma should be considered, especially when presenting in more advanced stages. Other rare differential diagnoses to consider include dissecting cellulitis of the scalp (perifolliculitis capitis abscedens et suffodiens), folliculitis decalvans, and sarcoidosis (Table 7.2).

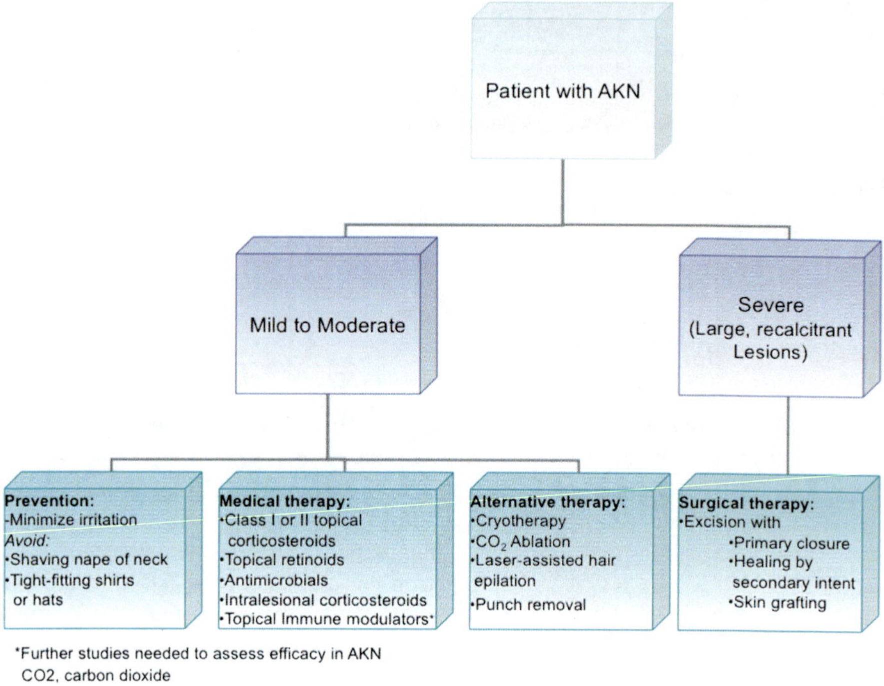


**Fig. 7.9** Approach to the patient with AKN

## *Treatment*

### First Line

The best approach to this condition is one of prevention and attenuation of disease progression, as later stages are more difficult to treat. Minimizing irritation to the areas involved is important. Therefore, counseling patients on avoidance of tight shirt collars, tightly fitting hats, or the like should be emphasized. Although only anecdotal evidence suggests an association between short haircuts and AKN, minimization of trauma from razors or electric hair clippers is generally recommended by most authorities (Fig. 7.9).

Twice-daily application of high-potency (class I or II) topical corticosteroids is a first-line therapy for mild to moderate AKN. The choice of vehicle should be based on efficacy as well as patient preference. In this author's (AFA) experience, gels and foams are the preferred vehicles for topical therapies in AKN. A recent clinical study examined the use of clobetasol 0.05% foam in men with AKN (applied twice daily, alternating 2 weeks on and 2 weeks off therapy) [9]. Subjects responded well, noting decreased lesions. The cosmetic acceptability of the foam vehicle by patients was also noted. Topical retinoids are often used in combination with corticosteroids to help flatten lesions. When lesions become secondarily infected, topical or oral antibiotics are indicated. Appropriate antibiotics should be selected based on bacterial cultures. A recent small open-label study showed success with the use of topical imiquimod and pimecrolimus, applied twice daily for 8 weeks [38].

Intralesional corticosteroid (triamcinolone acetonide 10–40 mg/ml) injections are effective for larger lesions and should also be considered for cases resistant to topical monotherapy. Corticosteroid injections are generally repeated on a monthly basis until desired results are obtained.

## Surgical

Advanced cases of AKN may require surgical intervention. Usually, these are larger areas of involvement that have failed combination medical therapies. The affected area can be surgically excised with subsequent primary closure [39], closure by secondary healing [22, 40], or skin grafting [41]. Larger lesions may require multi-staged excisions [39] or tissue expansion [42, 43]. Of the closure options, skin grafting is the least favored because of the potential for depressed atrophic scars [37]. Cosmetic results are best when AKN lesions are excised with a horizontal elliptical excision adjacent to the posterior hairline, as opposed to more circular excisions for those above the posterior hairline [40]. This will result in easier wound closure with the least amount of tension. Additionally, this may help to minimize splaying of the wound. If the neck must be extended in order to obtain primary closure of the wound (i.e., to allow greater approximation of the skin), then postoperative movement of the neck may need to be restricted (e.g., with a soft collar) for a period of time to prevent splaying. Even when these precautions are taken, splaying may still occur, especially for larger defects, with a final stretched scar potentially extending up to the size of the initial excision or to that of secondary-intention wounds. Of note, it is important to convey to patients that healing by secondary intention may take 6–12 weeks to close [22, 39, 40] and requires careful wound care.

To prevent recurrences and establish the best environment for optimal wound closures, it is important that excisions be carried down to a depth inferior to the base of the hair follicles [39]. In cases of recurrences, patients may be treated with twice-daily applications of high-potency topical and monthly intralesional corticosteroids [39]. Care must be taken not to introduce steroids too early, as wound healing and contraction may be negatively impacted [37, 40].

## Alternative Therapies

Other approaches include minimally invasive therapies such as cryotherapy [29], carbon dioxide ($CO_2$) laser ablation with healing by secondary intent [44], and laser-assisted hair epilation of trapped hairs with the long-pulse diode laser. [45] Early studies suggest that the long-pulse Nd:YAG laser may also be effective in AKN [37]. Individual fibrotic papules may be removed using a hair transplant punch followed by primary or secondary closure.

# References


1. Alexander AM, Delph WI. Pseudofolliculitis barbae in the military. A medical, administrative and social problem. J Natl Med Assoc. 1974;66:459–64. 79.
2. McMichael AJ. Hair and scalp disorders in ethnic populations. Dermatol Clin. 2003;21: 629–44.
3. Winter H, Schissel D, Parry DAD, et al. An unusual Ala12Thr polymorphism in the 1A [alpha]-Helical segment of the companion layer-specific keratin K6hf: evidence for a risk factor in the etiology of the common hair disorder pseudofolliculitis barbae. J Invest Dermatol. 2004;122:652–7.
4. Quarles FN HB, Johnson BA, et al. Pseudofolliculitis barbae. Dermatol Ther. 2007;20: 133–6.
5. Strauss JS, Kligman AM. Pseudofolliculitis of the beard. AMA Arch Derm. 1956;74:533–42.
6. Gillette. Advances in shaving technology: a review of the optimal shaving regimen for men highlighting technical advances associated with the fusion five-blade razor and its myth-busting effect on pseudofolliculitis Barbae. Proctor & Gamble :1–24 http://www.pgdermatology.com/downloads/documents/Gillette_WhitePaper.pdf. Last accessed 30 May 2012.
7. Halder RM, Roberts CI, Nootheti PK, et al. Dermatologic disease in blacks. In: Halder RM, editor. Dermatology and dermatological therapy of pigmented skins. Boca Raton: Taylor & Francis Group; 2006. p. 331–55.
8. Perry PK, Cook-Bolden F, Rahman Z, et al. Defining pseudofolliculitis barbae in 2001: a review of the literature and current trends. J Am Acad Dermatol. 2002;46:S113–9.
9. Cook-Bolden FE, Barba A, Halder R, et al. Twice-daily applications of benzoyl peroxide 5%/ clindamycin 1% gel versus vehicle in the treatment of pseudofolliculitis barbae. Cutis. 2004;73:18–24.
10. Kelly AP. Pseudofolliculitis barbae. In: Kelly AP, Taylor SC, editors. Dermatology for skin of color. China: McGraw-Hill; 2009. p. 211–6.
11. Battle EF, Hobbs LM. Laser-assisted hair removal for darker skin types. Dermatol Ther. 2004;17:177–83.
12. Greppi I. Diode laser hair removal of the black patient. Lasers Surg Med. 2001;28:150–5.
13. Smith EP, Winstanley D, Ross EV. Modified superlong pulse 810 nm diode laser in the treatment of pseudofolliculitis barbae in skin types V and VI. Dermatol Surg. 2005;31:297–301.
14. Ross EV, Cooke LM, Overstreet KA, et al. Treatment of pseudofolliculitis barbae in very dark skin with a long pulse Nd:YAG laser. J Natl Med Assoc. 2002;94:888–93.
15. Weaver III SM, Sagaral EC. Treatment of pseudofolliculitis barbae using the long-pulse Nd:YAG Laser on skin types V and VI. Dermatol Surg. 2003;29:1187–91.
16. Schulze R, Meehan KJ, Lopez A, et al. Low-fluence 1,064-nm laser hair reduction for pseudofolliculitis barbae in skin types IV, V, and VI. Dermatol Surg. 2009;35:98–107.
17. Kundu RV. Hair removal in ethnic skin. In: Alam M, Bhatia AC, Kundu RV, editors. Cosmetic dermatology for skin of color. Columbuso: McGraw Hill; 2009. p. 70–7.
18. Grimes PE. The safety and efficacy of salicylic acid chemical peels in darker racial-ethnic groups. Dermatol Surg. 1999;25:18–22.
19. Grimes PE. Agents for ethnic skin peeling. Dermatol Ther. 2000;13:159–64.
20. Roberts WE. Chemical peeling in ethnic/dark skin. Dermatol Ther. 2004;17:196–205.
21. Perricone NV. Treatment of pseudofolliculitis barbae with topical glycolic acid: a report of two studies. Cutis. 1993;52:232–5.
22. Bajaj V, Langtry JAA. Surgical excision of acne keloidalis nuchae with secondary intention healing. Clin Exp Dermatol. 2008;33:53–5.
23. Azurdia RM, Graham RM, Weismann K, et al. Acne keloidalis in Caucasian patients on cyclosporin following organ transplantation. Br J Dermatol. 2000;143:465–6.
24. Goh MSY, Magee J, Chong AH. Keratosis follicularis spinulosa decalvans and acne keloidalis nuchae. Australas J Dermatol. 2005;46:257–60.

25. Grunwald MH, Ben-Dor D, Livni E, et al. Acne keloidalis-like lesions on the scalp associated with antiepileptic drugs. Int J Dermatol. 1990;29:559–61.
26. Child F, Fuller L, Higgins E, et al. A study of the spectrum of skin disease occurring in a black population in south-east London. Br J Dermatol. 1999;141:512–7.
27. Knable JAL, Hanke CW, Gonin R. Prevalence of acne keloidalis nuchae in football players. J Am Acad Dermatol. 1997;37:570–4.
28. Salami T, Omeife H, Samuel S. Prevalence of acne keloidalis nuchae in Nigerians. Int J Dermatol. 2007;46:482–4.
29. McMichael A, Sanchez DG, Kelly P. Folliculitis and the follicular occlusion tetrad. In: Bolognia JL, Jorizzo JL, Rapini RP, editors. Dermatology, vol. 1. Secondth ed. Spain: Mosby Elsevier; 2008. p. 517–30.
30. Dinehart SM, Tanner L, Mallory SB, et al. Acne keloidalis in women. Cutis. 1989;44:250–2.
31. Ogunbiyi A, George A. Acne keloidalis in females: case report and review of literature. J Natl Med Assoc. 2005;97:736–8.
32. George AO, Akanji AO, Nduka EU, et al. Clinical, biochemical and morphologic features of acne keloidalis in a black population. Int J Dermatol. 1993;32:714–6.
33. D'Souza P, Iyer V, Ramam M. Familial acne keloidalis. Acta Derm Venereol. 1998;78:382.
34. Goette DK, Berger TG. Acne keloidalis nuchae: a transepithelial elimination disorder. Int J Dermatol. 1987;26:442–4.
35. Sperling LC, Homoky C, Pratt L, et al. Acne keloidalis is a form of primary scarring alopecia. Arch Dermatol. 2000;136:479–84.
36. Herzberg AJ, Dinehart SM, Kerns BJMT, et al. Acne keloidalis transverse microscopy, immunohistochemistry, and electron microscopy. Am J Dermatopathol. 1990;12:109–21.
37. Kelly AP. Acne keloidalis. In: Kelly AP, Taylor SC, editors. Dermatology for skin of color. China: McGraw-Hill; 2009. p. 205–10.
38. Barr J, Friedman A, Balwin H. Use of imiquimod and pimecrolimus cream in the treatment of acne keloidalis nuchae. J Am Acad Dermatol. 2005;52:P64.
39. Gloster Jr HM. The surgical management of extensive cases of acne keloidalis nuchae. Arch Dermatol. 2000;136:1376–9.
40. Glenn MJ, Bennett RG, Kelly AP. Acne keloidalis nuchae: treatment with excision and second-intention healing. J Am Acad Dermatol. 1995;33:243–6.
41. Cosman B, Wolff M. Acne keloidalis. Plast Reconstr Surg. 1972;50:25–30.
42. Marasco PV, Marks MW, Argenta LC. Surgical management of acne keloidalis. Eur J Plast Surg. 1993;16:70–2.
43. Pestalardo C, Cordero AJ, Ansorena J, et al. Acne keloidalis nuchae: tissue expansion treatment. Dermatol Surg. 1995;21:723–4.
44. Kantor GR, Ratz JL, Wheeland RG. Treatment of acne keloidalis nuchae with carbon dioxide laser. J Am Acad Dermatol. 1986;14:263–7.
45. Shah GK. Efficacy of diode laser for treating acne keloidalis nuchae. Indian J Dermatol Venereol Leprol. 2005;71:31–4.

# Chapter 8
# Disorders of Hyperpigmentation

**So Yeon Paek and Amit G. Pandya**

Acquired disorders of hyperpigmentation affect individuals of all skin types. However, pigmentary lesions may be more visible in skin of color and are often resistant to treatment. Dyschromias, in addition to acne, eczema, alopecia, and seborrheic dermatitis, are among the most common diagnoses in black patients seen by dermatologists [1, 2]. Etiology, diagnosis, treatment, and recommendations for melasma, postinflammatory hyperpigmentation, nevus of Ota/Ito, and periorbital hypermelanosis are reviewed.

## Melasma

Melasma (chloasma, *mask of pregnancy*) is an acquired hyperpigmentation of sun-exposed areas of the face, including the forehead, nose, cheeks, and upper lip, which predominantly affects women with Fitzpatrick skin types III–VI. The prevalence of melasma has been reported as 4% in Malaysia, 0.98% in Indonesia [3], 3.8% in Korea [4], 15.8% in Iran [5], and 8.8% among premenopausal women in the Dallas-Fort Worth area of Texas [6].

S.Y. Paek, M.D. (✉)
3031 W. Grand Blvd, 8th floor, Detroit, MI 48202, USA

Henry Ford Hospital, Detroit, MI, USA
e-mail: doctor.paek@gmail.com

A.G. Pandya, M.D.
Department of Dermatology, University of Texas Southwestern Medical Center,
5323 Harry Hines Blvd, Dallas, TX 75390-9190, USA
e-mail: amit.pandya@utsouthwestern.edu

A.F. Alexis and V.H. Barbosa (eds.), *Skin of Color: A Practical Guide to Dermatologic Diagnosis and Treatment*, DOI 10.1007/978-0-387-84929-4_8,

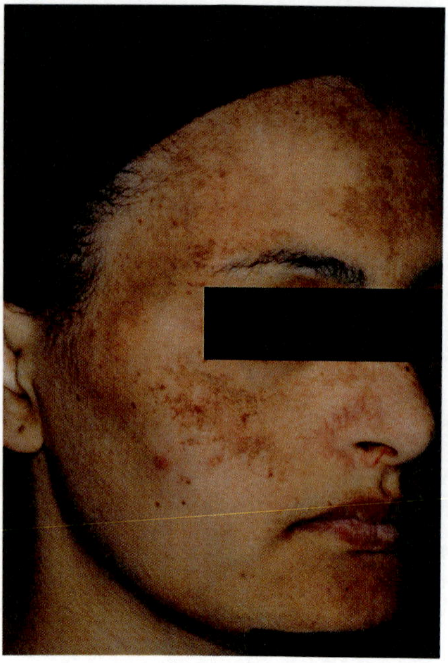

**Fig. 8.1** Melasma of cheeks, nose, and forehead

## *Etiology*

The exact cause of melasma remains to be determined, but current theories implicate genetic influences, hormones, and UV exposure as major factors in the pathogenesis of the disease. The high incidence of melasma observed within families suggests a genetic predisposition to the disease. Published studies in different populations have reported a positive family history of this disorder, including 54.7% of patients with melasma in Iran [5], 10.2% in Singapore [7], and 70.4% of Latinos in Puerto Rico [8]. Given the association of melasma with pregnancy and oral contraceptive use [9], several investigators explored the relationship of hormone expression in melasma and found upregulation of estrogen receptor expression in lesional skin [10]. Melanocytes of healthy skin demonstrated increased cell proliferation when incubated with estradiol, estriol, and progesterone due to the presence of nuclear and cytosol estrogen receptors [11]. A study of local hormone expression in lesional biopsies of women with melasma also revealed overexpression of $\alpha$-MSH with unchanged melanocortin-1 receptor expression after UV exposure [12], inferring the additional role of ultraviolet radiation in the disease.

## *Clinical Diagnosis and Histopathology*

The clinical diagnosis of melasma can be made by recognizing one of three patterns of hyperpigmented patches with well-circumscribed but irregular borders (Fig. 8.1).

The most common pattern is centrofacial, characterized by lesions on the forehead, nose, cheeks, chin, and upper lip, followed by malar and mandibular patterns [13]. Differential diagnoses for melasma include drug-induced or postinflammatory hyperpigmentation, facial acanthosis nigricans, actinic lichen planus, friction melanosis, solar lentigines, Hori's nevus, and nevus of Ota/Ito.

Melasma is also classified into three histologic patterns: epidermal (70%), dermal (10–15%), and mixed (20%), as determined by Wood's light and biopsy examination [14]. Epidermal melasma is light brown in color and more responsive to treatment, while dermal melasma is often blue-gray and resistant to treatment by depigmenting agents. Biopsies of lesional skin have demonstrated basal and suprabasal melanin deposition and dendritic melanocytes with pigment [15]. Dermal melasma contains less epidermal pigmentation than the epidermal pattern. Recent studies have demonstrated dermal perivascular melanophages in patients with all three histologic types of melasma, bringing into question the utility of Wood's light exam to predict the level of pigmentation and potential response to therapy [16].

## *Treatment*

A variety of treatment modalities have been used in the management of melasma, including topical agents, chemical peels, and laser and light therapies. Principles of therapy involve utilizing agents that disrupt melanogenesis through tyrosinase inhibition or melanin removal and preventing future damage with sun protection. Treatment success can be measured using melasma area and severity index (MASI) scoring, narrow-band reflectance spectroscopy or colorimetry, and quality-of-life scales. The 10-item, validated MELASQOL (melasma quality-of-life scale) measures social life, emotional well-being, and recreation/leisure and was found to be superior to SKINDEX-16 and DLQI (dermatology life quality index) in assessing the impact of melasma [17]. Interestingly, quality-of-life measures were not correlated with severity of disease, confirming the difficulty of determining psychological impact based on physical findings alone. Since its development, the MELASQOL has been adapted and validated for patients speaking Spanish [18] and Portuguese [19].

### Topical Agents

*Sunscreens.* In 1962, Pathak et al. found that UVA (290–320 nm) and UVB (320–400 nm) radiation induce melanin formation [20]. Subsequent studies revealed that long-wave visible light (400–760 nm), in addition to UV light, induces pigmentation in patients with Fitzpatrick skin types IV–VI [21]. Mahmoud et al. compared the effects of ultraviolet (UV) radiation and visible light on the skin and found that visible light induces darker pigmentation with delayed lightening in dark skin [22]. Since sunscreens do not protect very well against visible light, avoidance of UV exposure should be emphasized until visible light-blocking agents can be developed. A prospective study of 200 Moroccan women treated with broad-spectrum sunscreen against UVA and UVB light every 2 h daily at less than 3 months of pregnancy resulted in only 2.7% of participants developing melasma, even though over 50% were expected to develop melasma during pregnancy based on a previous study in that location [23, 24] (level of evidence II-iii). To protect against UVA and UVB exposure, patients should apply an oil-free, broad-spectrum sunscreen with SPF of at least 15 [25]. Although SPF 15 is the minimum based on the literature, the American Academy of Dermatology (AAD) now recommends year-round use of a sunscreen with SPF of at least 30, regardless of skin type. Protective hats and clothing, sun avoidance, and agents such as titanium dioxide or zinc oxide in sunscreens also provide physical block against higher wavelengths of light.

*Hydroquinone.* The most frequently used topical skin-lightening agent is hydroquinone, a hydroxyphenol that inhibits the tyrosinase enzyme and impedes conversion of dopa to melanin. It is available in 2% over-the-counter formulations or higher concentrations by prescription in the United States. A double-blind, placebo-controlled study in Brazil of 48 patients treated with 4% hydroquinone twice daily versus placebo and utilizing only subjective outcome measures found hydroquinone to be effective in the treatment of melasma [26] (level of evidence II-iii). In 2006, the Food and Drug Administration (FDA) issued a proposed ruling to remove hydroquinone from over-the-counter products due to concern of ochronosis [27] and carcinogenesis from toxic metabolites [28]. The carcinogen benzene is metabolized into hydroquinone, and early studies in rodents suggested that hydroquinone had the potential to damage DNA. However, there are no reports of similar harmful findings in humans, and the data is insufficient to dismiss the use of hydroquinone from a safety standpoint [29]. At this time, the FDA ruling has not been upheld, and investigation is still under way. Meanwhile, hydroquinone continues to be the standard therapy for melasma throughout the world. Although hydroquinone has been banned as an over-the-counter or prescription product in many countries, dermatologists in those countries routinely compound formulations containing hydroquinone for melasma patients.

Hydroquinone is most effective in combination with other agents, as first reported by Kligman and Willis in 1975. The Kligman-Willis formula combines hydroquinone 5% with tretinoin 0.1% and dexamethasone 0.1% [30]. Steroids inhibit melanin synthesis, reduce pigmentation, and reduce irritation from tretinoin, while tretinoin decreases the atrophogenic effect of steroids and helps epidermal penetration of hydroquinone. A modern adaptation of the Kligman-Willis formula is a triple combination cream (Tri-Luma®, Galderma Laboratories) containing a class 6 steroid (fluocinolone acetonide 0.01%), hydroquinone 4%, and tretinoin 0.05%. This formula has been extensively studied in clinical trials. In two 8-week multicenter, randomized, investigator-blinded, controlled trials of 641 patients, Taylor et al. found 26.1% receiving triple combination cream versus 4.6% treated with any combination of two of the ingredients had complete clearing of melasma [31] (level of evidence I). A 12-month multicenter, open-label study of once-daily triple combination cream effectively showed minimal adverse effects, mostly application site reactions, and a positive safety profile [32] (level of evidence II-ii). An 8-week multicenter, open-label, community-based trial in 1,290 patients by Grimes et al. found a significant decrease in MASI score ($p < .0001$) and 75% of patients achieving a "clear" or "almost clear" rating with triple combination cream in patients with skin types I–VI [33] (level of evidence II-ii). Chan et al. studied the triple combination cream versus 4% hydroquinone in Asian patients with melasma and found superior efficacy and greater satisfaction with the triple combination cream, though it also had a greater incidence of mild adverse events [34] (level of evidence II-ii).

*Azelaic Acid.* Azelaic acid is a naturally occurring dicarboxylic acid that functions as a depigmenting agent through inhibition of tyrosinase activity [35]. A 6-month study of 155 patients of Indo-Malay-Hispanic ethnicity treated with either 20% azelaic acid or 2% hydroquinone demonstrated that azelaic acid produced "good to excellent" overall results in 73% of patients versus 19% with hydroquinone [36] (level of evidence I). A subsequent 24-week study of Argentinian women showed that 20% azelaic acid was as efficacious as 4% hydroquinone [37] (level of evidence I). Optimal efficacy may be achieved through a combination of 20% azelaic acid, 0.05% tretinoin, and 15–20% glycolic acid [38]. Undesired side effects with azelaic acid use included allergic sensitization, pruritus, erythema, and scaling.

*Kojic Acid.* Also functioning as a tyrosinase inhibitor to lighten skin, kojic acid, a fungal metabolic product, is a potent antioxidant available in preparations of 1–4%. A split-face study of 39 patients treated with 2% kojic acid gel and 2% hydroquinone gel twice daily for 3 months produced equivocal results: 51% had equal response, 28% experienced improvement with kojic acid, and 21% improved with hydroquinone [39] (level of evidence II-i). Of note, many patients found the kojic acid preparation irritating and reduced their frequency of application to every other day. A second split-face trial of 10% glycolic acid and 2% hydroquinone with and without kojic acid showed synergistic action and 60% improvement with the three agents versus 47.5% without kojic acid [40] (level of evidence II-i).

## Peeling Agents

Chemical peels, both alone and in conjunction with bleaching agents, are often used to treat melasma. Superficial peels function to remove stratum corneum and accelerate penetration of topical agents, while deep peels remove undesired melanin pigmentation. All peeling agents have the potential to cause postinflammatory hyperpigmentation, of particular concern in darker-skinned individuals. Other side effects from chemical peels include atrophy, telangiectasias, bacterial and viral infections, desquamation, milia, and erythema.

*Glycolic Acid Peels.* Glycolic acid (GA) is an alpha-hydroxy acid found naturally in sugarcane juice. An early study of glycolic acid peels for melasma demonstrated maximal benefit with 52.5% GA peels for 3 min [41] (level of evidence II-ii). Subsequent studies of glycolic acid peels were conducted with various topical regimens. The efficacy of glycolic acid peels with a modified Kligman's formula (2% hydroquinone, 0.05% tretinoin, and 1% hydrocortisone cream) was evaluated in 40 Indian women who were treated with the combination versus topical agent alone for 5 months [42]. The glycolic acid peel and modified Kligman's formula together produced greater improvement (79.9% vs. 63.1%) by MASI scoring (level of evidence I). Another prospective trial studied patients with epidermal melasma who were treated with 20% azelaic acid and 0.1% adapalene with or without additional glycolic acid peels for 20 weeks [43]. The group treated with glycolic acid peels and topical agents demonstrated an 83% decrease in MASI score versus 69% with topical treatment alone (level of evidence I). In a similar study of glycolic acid peels plus hydroquinone in Hispanic women with epidermal melasma, no benefit was noted using objective and subjective assessment methods [44] (level of evidence I). However, a recent study by Garg et al. determined that pretreatment with 2% hydroquinone versus 0.025% tretinoin prior to glycolic acid peels enhanced results and reduced the likelihood of postinflammatory hyperpigmentation [45] (level of evidence I). From the available data, it appears that intense therapy with multiple sequential peels and progressively higher concentrations may have some benefit in patients with melasma.

*Salicylic Acid Peels.* In addition to its role for postinflammatory hyperpigmentation, salicylic acid peels have been found to have mixed results in the treatment of melasma. A small study of 25 patients, six with melasma, who underwent 20–30% salicylic acid peels every 2 weeks for 5 sessions and pretreatment with 4% hydroquinone showed moderate to significant improvement in 66% of participants [46] (level of evidence IV). An equal number of patients reported mild side effects, including crusting and dryness.

*Other Peels and Dermabrasion.* A trial of Jessner's solution (salicylic acid, lactic acid, resorcinol, and ethanol) versus glycolic acid peels showed equal efficacy using both agents [47]. A nonrandomized, split-face trial of Jessner's solution against lactic acid found no significant benefit by MASI score between the two treatments and recurrence of disease upon discontinuation [48] (level of evidence II-i). The use of dermabrasion has been limited to recalcitrant melasma due to the potential for adverse effects, such as keloids and postinflammatory hyperpigmentation, especially in darker skin types. A study by Kunachak et al. found 97% clearance of melasma in patients with skin types III–V who underwent mechanical dermabrasion [49] (level of evidence II-iii). However, unfavorable side effects associated with the procedure included hyperpigmentation, erythema, pruritus, milia formation, and hypertrophic scarring. While dermabrasion is not a first-line therapy for melasma, many dermatologists do perform microdermabrasion for this condition. A prospective, open, randomized trial of 12 patients with melasma found 5–15% improvement in pigmentation with weekly microdermabrasion (30–40% with the addition of a topical retinoid) [50]. The technique is relatively safe, with reports of minor erythema and pain [51].

## Laser and Light Therapy

Recent advances in laser and light therapies are promising for the treatment of melasma. However, data is limited for these fairly new modalities, and their use should be reserved for recalcitrant melasma after other treatments have been ineffective. Low doses and test spots should be utilized in order to prevent side effects in patients with darker skin.

*Q-switched Ruby or Nd:YAG Laser.* The Q-switched ruby and Nd:YAG (neodymium:yttrium-aluminum-garnet) lasers utilize a red light at 532 nm that penetrates to 2–3-mm skin depth and damages melanosomes. These lasers have been used with success for hyperpigmentation, such as lentigines. In melasma, however, they were found to induce unacceptable postinflammatory hyperpigmentation and worsen existing melasma in one small study [52]. Two recent case reports of refractory dermal melasma treated with the MedLite C6 Q-switched Nd:YAG laser demonstrated 80% reduction with 10 weekly laser treatments, along with sunscreen and 7% alpha-arbutin [53] (level of evidence IV). This study demonstrates the potential for treating recalcitrant melasma with a combination of laser and topical therapy.

*Er:YAG Resurfacing Laser.* The erbium:yttrium-aluminum-garnet laser, which emits at 2,940 nm and targets water molecules, has shown immediate postprocedure improvement of refractory melasma in a study of 10 female patients [54]. However, all participants developed postinflammatory hyperpigmentation 3–6 weeks after laser therapy and required further treatment with glycolic acid peels and azelaic acid for months (level of evidence II-iii). A retrospective analysis of 218 Asian patients who underwent er:YAG laser treatment found that erythema persisted for several months as well as postinflammatory hyperpigmentation in 38.1% after the procedure [55] (level of evidence II-iii).

*Fractional Photothermolysis.* A recent addition to the world of laser therapy for melasma involves fractional laser resurfacing of the epidermis and dermis. Fractional photothermolysis employs thermal radiation to cause damage to microscopic zones of lesional skin while maintaining viability of surrounding healthy skin. These lasers are FDA-cleared for the treatment of melasma and other skin conditions, including acne and surgical scars, pigmented lesions, and periorbital rhytides. A pilot study of 10 females with recalcitrant melasma and skin types III–V who underwent 4–6 treatments of fractional photothermolysis using initially the 1,535-nm and later the 1,550-nm erbium:glass Fraxel laser showed 75–100% clearing in 6 patients [56] (level of evidence IV). Postprocedure erythema was noted in several patients, and one developed postinflammatory hyperpigmentation. However, adverse effects of nonablative fractional photothermolysis have been minimal, as determined by a recent retrospective evaluation of 961 patients who have undergone this procedure for various indications. Only 7.6% developed complications, which included postinflammatory hyperpigmentation, acneiform eruptions in 1.87%, and herpes simplex outbreaks in 1.77% [57] (level of evidence II-iii). Ultrastructural analysis of 10 patients with epidermal melasma (skin types III–IV) who received 4 treatments with the commercially available 1,550-nm erbium:glass Fraxel laser and pre- and postprocedure biopsies revealed fewer melanocytes and less epidermal melanin in lesional skin [58] (level of evidence II-iii). There was no correlation, however, between these histologic changes and investigator-rated improvement.

*Intense Pulsed Light.* IPL therapy was first used for vascular anomalies by utilizing high-intensity visible light (range 515–1,200 nm dependent on skin type and desired depth) for photothermolysis of target lesions [20]. Treatment of melasma with intense pulsed light has demonstrated efficacy in several studies in Asia. Wang et al.

compared treatment with topical hydroquinone plus sunscreen alone against topical therapy with 4 IPL sessions and found a reduction in Mexameter readings of 11.6% versus 39.8% [59] (level of evidence I). A trial of 89 Chinese females with refractory mixed melasma demonstrated improvement by MASI score and Mexameter after 4 treatments with IPL over 12 weeks [60] (level of evidence II-iii). Patients did not receive pretreatment with depigmenting agents. Disadvantages of intense pulsed light therapy include transient erythema and edema, postinflammatory hyperpigmentation, postprocedure skin sloughing, and the need for multiple treatment sessions. The expertise required for accurate and successful administration of IPL as well as the large handpiece required for this form of light causes difficulty in achieving precise pulsing of affected areas.

## *Recommendations for Skin of Color*

Melasma remains a challenge to treat, as clinical trials are limited by subjective methods of evaluation and variability in controls and patient population. Based on the trials noted above, the following are recommendations for the management of melasma in skin of color (Table 8.1). Table 8.2 provides the guidelines for grading strength of recommendations and quality of evidence.

1. Sun protection with an oil-free, noncomedogenic, broad-spectrum, UVA- and UVB-blocking sunscreen with minimum SPF 15 and sun avoidance are keys to preventing further lesions. A physical block may be added in order to reduce exposure to visible light (grade A recommendation).
2. Triple combination cream (fluocinolone acetonide 0.01%, hydroquinone 4%, and tretinoin 0.05%) has been clinically proven to be a safe and effective topical agent for long-term treatment of melasma (grade A recommendation). Extemporaneously compounded combination creams can also be used. Patients who are unable to tolerate combination creams may be treated with hydroquinone alone. Azelaic acid may be used in cases of hydroquinone intolerance (grade B recommendation).
3. Although the evidence is mixed, glycolic acid peels (initially 30%, with increasing concentration as tolerated) and pretreatment with 2% hydroquinone may be useful if given multiple times every 4–6 weeks for the treatment of recalcitrant melasma (grade B recommendation). Salicylic acid peels have not yet been shown to be effective in the treatment of melasma in controlled studies but have demonstrated efficacy in a small, open-label study (grade D recommendation).
4. Q-switched ruby, Nd:YAG, and Er:YAG resurfacing lasers have shown negative effects, particularly postinflammatory hyperpigmentation, in melasma therapy (grade E recommendation). Nonablative fractional photothermolysis is a promising treatment but remains a third-line approach in refractory patients (grade C recommendation).
5. Intense pulsed light therapy demonstrates modest efficacy in patients with mixed melasma and should only be used as adjunctive therapy (grade B recommendation).

**Table 8.1** Recommendations for melasma in skin of color

| Clinical recommendation | Evidence rating | References | Comments |
|---|---|---|---|
| Sun protection with oil-free, broad-spectrum, UVA-/UVB-blocking, minimum SPF 15 sunscreen and sun avoidance are key | A | [21–23] | A physical block may be added to reduce exposure to visible light |
| Triple combination cream (fluocinolone acetonide 0.01%, hydroquinone 4%, and tretinoin 0.05%) is beneficial for long-term treatment | A | [31–34] | Combination cream can be used once daily |
| Treatment outcomes should be assessed with both objective and subjective measures, including MASI score, colorimetry, and MELASQOL | A | [17–19] | The psychological impact of melasma can be greater than the physical findings. There is a validated MELASQOL available in Spanish and Portuguese |
| Use azelaic acid in cases of hydroquinone intolerance | B | [36, 37] | |
| Glycolic acid peels with 2% hydroquinone pretreatment may be used in recalcitrant melasma | B | [42, 43, 45] | Begin with 30% GA and increase concentration as tolerated. Treatment may be repeated Q 4–6 weeks |
| Intense pulsed light demonstrates modest efficacy in patients with mixed melasma and should only be used as adjunctive therapy | B | [59, 60] | |
| Fractional photothermolysis should be a third-line approach in refractory patients | C | [56, 57] | |
| Salicylic acid peels are not effective | D | [46] | |
| Q-switched ruby, Nd:YAG, and Er:YAG lasers have shown negative effects, such as PIH, in melasma therapy | E | [50, 54, 55] | |

Strength of recommendations (US Preventive Services Task Force evidence rating system)
A There is good evidence to support the use of the procedure
B There is fair evidence to support the use of the procedure
C There is poor evidence to support the use of the procedure
D There is fair evidence to support the rejection of the use of the procedure
E There is good evidence to support the rejection of the use of the procedure

6. Investigational studies on treatment modalities for melasma should be assessed with both objective and subjective measures, such as MASI scoring and colorimetry. Quality-of-life scores, such as the MELASQOL, should be considered as well since the psychological impact of melasma can be greater than physical findings (grade A recommendation). The availability of a validated MELASQOL in Spanish and Portuguese helps facilitate the study of melasma in various populations.

**Table 8.2** US preventive services task force grade definitions after May 2007

| | |
|---|---|
| *Strength of recommendations* | |
| A | There is good evidence to support the use of the procedure |
| B | There is fair evidence to support the use of the procedure |
| C | There is poor evidence to support the use of the procedure |
| D | There is fair evidence to support the rejection of the use of the procedure |
| E | There is good evidence to support the rejection of the use of the procedure |
| *Quality of evidence* | |
| I | Evidence obtained from at least one properly designed randomized controlled trial |
| II-i | Evidence obtained from well-designed controlled trials without randomization |
| II-ii | Evidence obtained from well-designed cohort or case-control analytical studies, preferably from more than one center or research group |
| II-iii | Evidence obtained from multiple time series with or without the intervention. Dramatic results in uncontrolled experiments could also be regarded as this type of evidence |
| III | Opinions of respected authorities based on clinical experience, descriptive studies, or reports of expert committees |
| IV | Evidence inadequate owing to problems of methodology (e.g., sample size, or length of comprehensiveness of follow-up or conflicts in evidence) |

Source: http://www.ahrq.gov/clinic/uspstf/gradespost.htm

## Postinflammatory Hyperpigmentation

Postinflammatory hyperpigmentation (PIH) is an acquired, transient excess of skin pigment that occurs following inflammation or injury. It is seen with many disorders, including contact dermatitis, acne vulgaris, lichen planus, papulosquamous disorders, vesiculobullous diseases, and drug reactions. The hyperpigmentation predominantly affects skin types IV–VI and is often frustrating, taking months to years to resolve.

### *Etiology*

Postinflammatory hyperpigmentation is thought to be due to the stimulation of melanocytes by inflammatory mediators, such as IL-1$\alpha$, endothelin-1, and reactive oxygen species, which increase the synthesis of melanin [61, 62]. The melanin pigment remains in the cytoplasm of keratinocytes until the cells are sloughed off [63], so deeper involvement takes longer to resolve. Thus, hyperpigmentation is difficult to treat with follicular, basal layer, or basement membrane involvement.

### *Clinical Diagnosis and Histopathology*

Diagnosis of postinflammatory hyperpigmentation is easily made in an individual with a preceding history of inflammatory dermatosis in the same distribution.

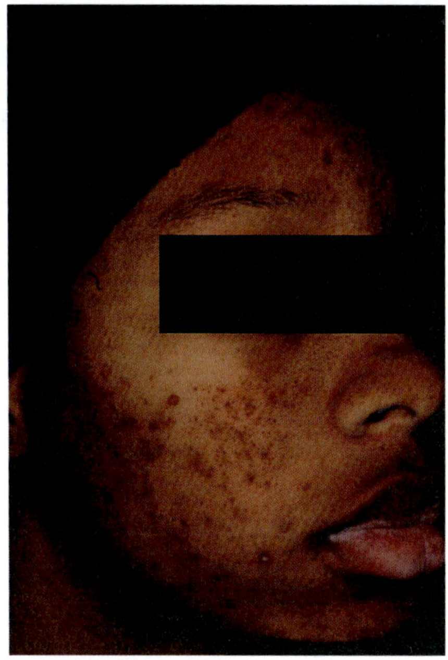

**Fig. 8.2** Postinflammatory hyperpigmentation associated with acne vulgaris

Lesions are light brown to black, may be diffuse or localized, and follow the distribution of underlying inflammation (Fig. 8.2). Epidermal lesions are brown, well circumscribed, with borders enhanced by Wood's lamp exam, while dermal lesions are dark gray to blue and do not accentuate [64].

## *Treatment*

The treatment of PIH is similar to that of melasma presented above. Mainstays of treatment include topical and peeling agents.

### Topical Agents

The earliest recognition of tretinoin for treatment of hyperpigmentation in skin of color was a study by Bulengo-Ransby et al. in 1993, in which 54 African American patients were treated with 0.1% tretinoin cream versus vehicle for 40 weeks and assessed by colorimetry and biopsy [65] (level of evidence I). Statistically significant results (40% vs. 18%) indicated that tretinoin was effective for PIH in dark-skinned patients. However, 50% of the tretinoin-treated patients developed retinoid dermatitis. Recent studies have investigated the use of combination agents with retinol to improve efficacy and minimize adverse effects. An open-label study of 28 patients, 12 with PIH, treated twice daily for 12 weeks with a microsponge formulation of 4% hydroquinone and 0.15% retinol (Epiquin Micro®) showed improvement over baseline [66] (level of evidence IV). The microentrapped 4% hydroquinone formulation was also well tolerated. A large, multicenter, randomized, investigator-blinded trial of a triple combination cream (fluocinolone acetonide 0.01%, hydroquinone 4%, and tretinoin 0.05%) versus a combination of two of the individual components found that 45% of patients were clear or almost clear in 8 weeks versus 35% with two components [67] (level of evidence II-ii). The triple combination cream has been efficacious in the treatment of melasma and shows promise for PIH.

The potential use of tazarotene, a retinoid derivative, was studied in a randomized, double-blind, controlled trial of 74 patients with postinflammatory hyperpigmentation and acne who were treated with daily 0.1% tazarotene versus vehicle for 18 weeks [68] (level of evidence I). Tazarotene had the additional benefit of treating the acne. Patients who received tazarotene demonstrated significant reductions of PIH with only mild side effects, such as dryness, erythema, or burning.

### Peeling Agents

A study of glycolic acid peels, combined with 0.05% tretinoin and 2% hydroquinone, produced clinical improvement of PIH with few side effects in darker-skinned patients but without statistically significant improvement [69] (level of evidence II-i). Similarly, in a split-face study of 10 patients with skin types IV–VI treated with salicylic acid peels, Joshi et al. found no statistically significant difference using visual analog scales between those treated with salicylic acid peels versus no treatment [70] (level of evidence I). However, a study of 24 Korean patients with PIH from acne treated with 30% salicylic acid peels biweekly for 3 months noted improvement using colorimetry to measure pigmentation [71] (level of evidence II-iii). A recent study by Garg et al. comparing 35% glycolic acid peels to 20% salicylic acid-10% mandelic acid peels (SMPs) in Indian patients with PIH found both agents to be safe and effective, with SMPs preferred by patients [72] (level of evidence II-iii).

## *Recommendations for Skin of Color*

The following are recommendations for the management of postinflammatory hyperpigmentation in skin of color (Table 8.3):

1. First and foremost, treat the underlying inflammatory disorder (grade A recommendation).
2. Sun protection with broad-spectrum, minimum SPF 15 sunscreen and sun avoidance can prevent exacerbation of pigmented lesions (grade A recommendation).

**Table 8.3** Recommendations for postinflammatory hyperpigmentation in skin of color

| Clinical recommendation | Evidence rating | References | Comments |
|---|---|---|---|
| Treat the underlying inflammatory disorder | A | | |
| Sun protection with oil-free, broad-spectrum, minimum SPF 15 sunscreen and sun avoidance are critical | A | | |
| Retinoids and hydroquinone are effective bleaching agents and are the first-line treatment for PIH | A | [65–67] | Resolution may take months to years. Combination creams have shown additional benefit over monotherapy |
| Use glycolic acid and salicylic acid peels with caution, as results are equivocal on these treatment approaches | C | [69–71] | May be used in refractory cases of PIH |

Strength of recommendations (US Preventive Services Task Force evidence rating system)
A There is good evidence to support the use of the procedure
B There is fair evidence to support the use of the procedure
C There is poor evidence to support the use of the procedure
D There is fair evidence to support the rejection of the use of the procedure
E There is good evidence to support the rejection of the use of the procedure

3. Both retinoids and hydroquinone are efficacious depigmenting agents and the first-line of treatment for PIH but may take months for complete resolution. Combination creams have shown additional benefit over monotherapy (grade A recommendation).
4. Although glycolic acid and salicylic acid peels may be beneficial, they should be used with caution, as PIH may result from the peel and results are equivocal with these treatment approaches (grade C recommendation).

## Nevus of Ota/Ito

Nevus of Ota, also called oculodermal melanocytosis and nevus fuscoceruleus ophthalmomaxillaris, refers to a unilateral dermal nevus with blue-black pigmentation in the distribution of the first and second branches of the trigeminal nerve of the face. It is bilateral in up to 10% of patients and often involves ocular and mucosal membranes [73]. Though Asian females are predominantly affected, with an incidence of up to 0.4% in Japan, it has also been reported in those of African, Indian, and European descent [74]. Nevus of Ito (nevus fuscoceruleus acromiodeltoides) was first reported in 1954 and is histologically identical to nevus of Ota. However, its distribution includes the shoulder, lateral neck, and scapular areas [75].

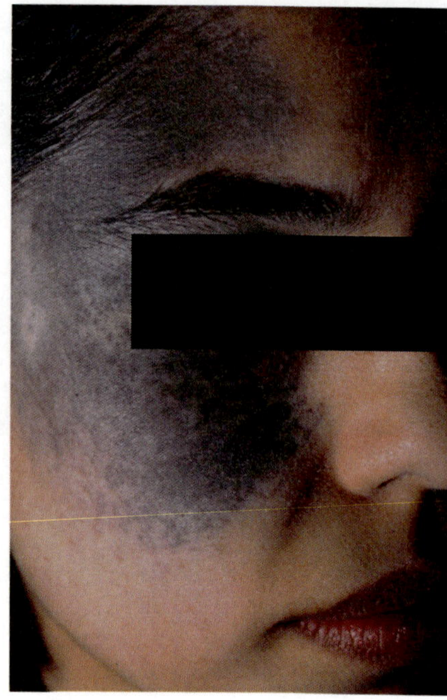

**Fig. 8.3** Nevus of Ota

## *Etiology*

Nevus of Ota is present at birth (60% of cases) or appears shortly thereafter in infancy [76]. It is not thought to be hereditary, and only six cases of familial nevus of Ota have been reported worldwide to date [77]. The precise mechanism for its development is unknown, but the most widely accepted theory involves defective migration from the neural crest of melanoblasts in the skin [78].

## *Clinical Diagnosis and Histopathology*

Nevus of Ota is determined by the presence of macules ranging from blue and gray to brown along the facial innervations of the ophthalmic and maxillary branches of cranial nerve V (eyelids, eyebrow, temple, forehead, and nose) (Fig. 8.3). The differential diagnosis includes Hori's nevus (acquired bilateral nevus of Ota-like macules – ABNOM), a bilateral dermal facial melanocytosis that primarily affects middle-aged Japanese women but does not extend to mucosal or ocular surfaces (Fig. 8.4). Nevus of Ito appears in the lateral brachial nerve and supraclavicular distribution (shoulder, neck, arm, scapular regions). The two conditions may, in rare cases, be found together in the same patient. Unlike other disorders of hyperpigmentation which frequently

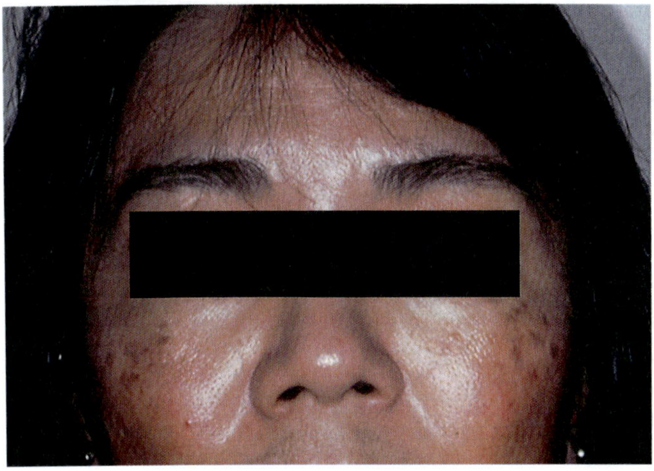

**Fig. 8.4** Hori's nevus (acquired bilateral nevus of Ota-like macules, or ABNOM)

**Table 8.4** Classification of nevus of Ota

| Class | Tanino | Hirayama et al. |
|---|---|---|
| I | A: upper/lower eyelid; periorbital and temporal | Superficial |
| | B: infrapalpebral fold, nasolabial fold, and zygomatic region | |
| | C: forehead | |
| | D: nasal | |
| II | Over upper and lower lids, periocular, zygomatic, cheek, and temple | Superficial dominant |
| III | Scalp, forehead, eyebrow, and nose | Diffuse |
| IV | Bilateral | Deep dominant |
| V | – | Deep |

Adapted from [79], with permission. This material is reproduced with permission of John Wiley & Sons, Inc

improve with time, nevus of Ota/Ito does not fade with age, and the intensity can vary with menstrual or environmental changes. Clinical diagnosis can be organized according to Tanino's system, which classifies the patient into type I through IV depending on area of involvement (Table 8.4) [79]. If diagnosis is uncertain, proper identification may be made by biopsy.

Histopathologically, nevus of Ota can be classified according to Hirayama et al. (Table 8.4) [80]. The lesion is categorized as superficial, superficial dominant, diffuse, deep dominant, or deep. Biopsies demonstrate an abundance of bipolar dendritic melanocytes with melanin scattered throughout the dermis. The melanocytes are surrounded by an extracellular sheath [81]. Due to the possible development of malignant melanoma or uveal melanoma with underlying nevus of Ota, the clinician should maintain a low threshold for obtaining a biopsy.

## Treatment

Laser therapy is the mainstay of treatment for nevus of Ota/Ito. Watanabe et al. successfully treated 114 Japanese patients with pulsed Q-switched ruby laser therapy and produced depigmentation without damage to surrounding healthy skin [82] (level of evidence II-iii). In a retrospective study, Kagami et al. found good to excellent results following Q-switched alexandrite laser treatment of patients with nevus of Ota and Ito [83] (level of evidence III). Wang et al. also retrospectively evaluated the outcomes of 602 Chinese patients who received Q-switched alexandrite treatment and found that it was an effective and safe therapy with results correlating with Tanino's classification and number of treatments received [84] (level of evidence II-ii). A trial of 55 Korean patients treated with Q-switched alexandrite laser for three sessions every three months produced 80% with excellent or good clearing [85] (level of evidence II-iii). Prognosis was dependent on depth of the lesion, with depth less than 1 mm producing the best results.

More than half (55%) of patients in this study developed postinflammatory hyperpigmentation, but this resolved within four months. Another disadvantage of laser therapy is the recurrence of pigmentation within a few years after alexandrite or Nd:YAG treatment [86]. A case report by Trindade et al. explored the surgical management of a patient with nevus of Ota [87]. The patient received reconstructive surgery and was successfully cured of her lesions with the use of skin grafts (level of evidence IV). This may be a potential therapeutic modality for patients with recurrent nevus of Ota or lesions with strong malignant potential but is not recommended due to prohibitive costs, scarring, and procedural risks.

## Recommendations for Skin of Color

The following are recommendations for the management of nevus of Ota/Ito in skin of color:

1. Classify the lesion according to Tanino's system (Table 8.4). If the diagnosis is uncertain, maintain a low threshold for biopsy (grade A recommendation).
2. If ocular involvement is noted, refer to ophthalmology for melanoma and glaucoma screening (grade A recommendation).
3. Check for underlying neurocutaneous conditions, especially in children (grade A recommendation).
4. Schedule regular follow-ups with the patient to check for malignant transformation (grade A recommendation).
5. Studies have demonstrated the efficacy and safety of Q-switched ruby, Nd:YAG, and alexandrite lasers as treatments of choice, with particular recent emphasis on alexandrite laser therapy (grade A recommendation).
6. Consider surgical options if malignant potential is high or if lesion is refractory to laser therapy (grade C recommendation).

## Periorbital Hypermelanosis

Periorbital melanosis, infraorbital darkening, and dark circles under the eyes are all phrases used to refer to bilaterally symmetric hyperpigmented patches encircling the eyes [88]. This condition is of great cosmetic concern, especially in those with skin of color.

### *Etiology*

Theories of melanocytosis include deposition of dermal melanin, infraorbital edema, and postinflammatory hyperpigmentation from contact dermatitis. Identifiable triggers, such as pregnancy and viral illness, have been associated with the condition. A recent investigation of 100 Indian patients with periorbital melanosis concluded that the hyperpigmentation was an extension of pigmentary demarcation line-F (PDL-F) in 92% of the patients [89]. Also known as Futcher's or Voigt's lines, pigmentary demarcation lines separate physiologic areas of pigment transition. Types A–E have been well described in the literature, including in darker-skinned individuals of African and Japanese descent [90]. PDL types F–H were identified in Indian patients. PDL-F presents as bilateral, symmetric hyperpigmented patches in a triangular shape on the lateral face from the temple to malar prominence [91].

### *Clinical Diagnosis and Histopathology*

The uniform, gray-brown patches of periorbital melanosis extend from the eyebrows to the upper cheeks. The hyperpigmentation does not enhance by Wood's lamp examination. Biopsy of the lesion demonstrates melanophages in the upper dermis with dermal and epidermal melanin.

### *Treatment*

Current treatment modalities focus on laser therapy to remove pigmentation. Pulsed carbon dioxide laser resurfacing has shown subjective reduction of under-eye hyperpigmentation, but reflectance spectrophotometer readings did not support these changes [92] (level of evidence IV). A study of 18 Asian patients who received combination therapy with Q-switched ruby laser and tretinoin plus hydroquinone was unconvincing in its proof of efficacy [93] (level of evidence IV). Improvement was noted only after 6–7 weeks of pretreatment with the topical depigmenting agents, and patients suffered a long posttreatment recovery phase (5–7 days) with extended duration of treatment. However, the combination treatment reduced the number of adverse effects, with postinflammatory hyperpigmentation reported in only 11.1% of patients. A previous study of Q-switched ruby laser therapy in Caucasians with infraorbital pigmentation reported 29.4% of patients with PIH after treatment [94].

### *Recommendations for Skin of Color*

Combination therapy of Q-switched ruby laser with tretinoin and hydroquinone pretreatment may provide reduction of pigmentation with minimal postinflammatory hyperpigmentation but requires a long treatment period (grade B recommendation).

## References

1. Halder RM. Ethnic skin disorders overview. J Am Acad Dermatol. 2003;48 suppl 6:143–8.
2. Alexis AF, Sergay AB, Taylor SC. Common dermatologic disorders in skin of color: a comparative practice survey. Cutis. 2007;80:387–94.
3. Sivayathorn A. Melasma in orientals. Clin Drug Invest. 1995;10 suppl 2:34–40.
4. Hann SK, Im S, Chung WS, et al. Pigmentary disorders in the South East. Dermatol Clin. 2007;25:431–8.
5. Moin A, et al. Prevalence and awareness of melasma during pregnancy. Int J Dermatol. 2006;45:285.
6. Werlinger KD, Jabery Z, Fallah N. Prevalence of self-diagnosed melasma among premenopausal Latino women in Dallas and Fort Worth, Tex. Arch Dermatol. 2007;143:424–5.
7. Goh CL, Dlova CN. A retrospective study on the clinical presentation and treatment outcome of melasma in a tertiary dermatological referral centre in Singapore. Singap Med J. 1999;40: 455–8.
8. Vasquez M, Maldonado H, Benmaman C, et al. Melasma in men: a clinical and histologic study. Int J Dermatol. 1988;27:25.
9. Resnik S. Melasma induced by oral contraceptive drugs. JAMA. 1967;199:95.
10. Lieberman R, Moy L. Estrogen receptor expression in melasma: results from facial skin of affected patients. J Drugs Dermatol. 2008;7(5):463–5.
11. Jee SH, Lee SY, Chiu HC, et al. Effects of estrogen and estrogen receptor in normal human melanocytes. Biochem Biophys Res Commun. 1994;199:1407–12.
12. Im S, Kim J, On WY, et al. Increased expression of α-melanocyte-stimulating hormone in the lesional skin of melasma. Br J Dermatol. 2007;146:165–7.
13. Pandya AG, Guevara IL. Disorders of hyperpigmentation. Dermatol Clin. 2000;18:91–7.
14. Rigopoulos D, Gregoriou S, Katsambas A. Hyperpigmentation and melasma. J Cosmet Dermatol. 2007;6:195–202.
15. Sanchez NP, Pathak MA, Sato S, et al. Melasma: a clinical, light microscopic, ultrastructural and immunofluorescence study. J Am Acad Dermatol. 1981;4(6):698–709.
16. Grimes PE, Yamada N, Bhawan J. Light microscopic, immunohistochemical, and ultrastructural alterations in patients with melasma. Am J Dermatopathol. 2005;27:96–101.
17. Balkrishnan R, McMichael AJ, Camacho FT, et al. Development and validation of a health-related quality of life instrument for women with melasma. Br J Dermatol. 2003;149:572.

18. Dominguez AR, Balkrishnan R, Ellzey AR, et al. Melasma in Latina patients: cross-cultural adaptation and validation of a quality-of-life questionnaire in Spanish language. J Am Acad Dermatol. 2006;55:59–66.
19. Cestari TF, Hexsel D, Viegas ML, et al. Validation of a melasma quality of life questionnaire for Brazilian Portuguese language: the MelasQoL-BP study and improvement of QoL of melasma patients after triple combination therapy. Br J Dermatol. 2007;156:13–20.
20. Pathak MA, Riley FC, Fitzpatrick TB, et al. Melanogenesis in human skin following exposure to long-wave ultraviolet and visible light. J Invest Dermatol. 1962;39:435.
21. Mahmoud BH, Hexsel CL, Hamzavi IH, et al. Effects of visible light on the skin. Photochem Photobiol. 2008;84:450–62.
22. Mahmoud BH, et al. Photobiologic effects of long wavelength UVA and visible light on melanocompetent skin. J Invest Dermatol. 2009;129 suppl 1:125.
23. Lakhdar H, Zouhair K, Khadir K, et al. Evaluation of the effectiveness of a broad-spectrum sunscreen in the prevention of chloasma in pregnant women. J Eur Acad Dermatol Venereol. 2007;21:738–42.
24. Benchikhi H, Razoki H, Lakhdar H. Sunscreens: use in pregnant women at Casablanca. Ann Dermatol Venereol. 2002;129:387–90.
25. Vazquez M, Sanchez JL. The efficacy of a broad-spectrum sunscreen in the treatment of melasma. Cutis. 1983;32:92.
26. Ennes SBP, et al. A double-blind, comparative, placebo-controlled study of the efficacy and tolerability of hydroquinone as a depigmenting agent in melasma. J Dermatol Treat. 2000;11:173–9.
27. Charlin R, Barcaui CB, Kac BK, et al. Hydroquinone-induced exogenous ochronosis: a report of four cases and usefulness of dermoscopy. Int J Dermatol. 2008;47:19–23.
28. Nordlund JJ, Grimes P, Ortonne JP, et al. The safety of hydroquinone. J Eur Acad Dermatol Venereol. 2006;20:781–7.
29. Draelos ZD. Skin lightening preparations and the hydroquinone controversy. Dermatol Ther. 2007;20:308–13.
30. Kligman AM, Willis I. A new formula for depigmenting human skin. Arch Dermatol. 1975;111:40–8.
31. Taylor S, Torok H, Jones T, et al. Efficacy and safety of a new triple combination agent for the treatment of facial melasma. Cutis. 2003;72:67–72.
32. Torok H, Jones T, Rich P, et al. Hydroquinone 4%, tretinoin 0.05%, fluocinolone acetonide 0.01%: a safe and efficacious 12-month treatment for melasma. Cutis. 2005;75:57–62.
33. Grimes P, Kelly AP, Torok H, et al. Community-based trial of a triple-combination agent for the treatment of facial melasma. Cutis. 2006;77:177–84.
34. Chan R, Park KC, Lee MH, et al. A randomized controlled trial of the efficacy and safety of a fixed triple combination (fluocinolone acetonide 0.01%, hydroquinone 4%, tretinoin 0.05%) compared with hydroquinone 4% cream in Asian patients with moderate to severe melasma. Br J Dermatol. 2008;159:697–703.
35. Del Rosso JQ. The use of topical azelaic acid for common skin disorders other than inflammatory rosacea. Cutis. 2006;77((2 suppl)):22–4.
36. Verallo-Rowell VM, Verallo V, Graupe K, et al. Double-blind comparison of azelaic acid and hydroquinone in the treatment of melasma. Acta Derm Venereol (Stockh). 1989;143((suppl)):58–61.
37. Balina LM, Graupe K, et al. The treatment of melasma: 20% azelaic acid versus 4% hydroquinone cream. Int J Dermatol. 1991;30:893.
38. Graupe K, Verallo-Rowell VM, Verallo V, et al. Combined use of 20% azelaic acid cream and 0.05% tretinoin in topical treatment of melasma. J Dermatol Treat. 1996;7:235–7.
39. Garcia A, Fulton JE. The combination of glycolic acid and hydroquinone or kojic acid for the treatment of melasma and related conditions. Dermatol Surg. 1996;22:443.
40. Lim JT. Treatment of melasma using kojic acid in a gel containing hydroquinone and glycolic acid. Dermatol Surg. 1999;25:282–4.

41. Gupta RR, Mahajan BB, Garg G, et al. Chemical peeling – evaluation of glycolic acid in varying concentrations and time intervals. Cosmetol. 2001;67:28–9.
42. Sarkar R, Kaur C, Ghalla M, et al. The combination of glycolic acid peels with a topical regimen in the treatment of melasma in dark-skinned patients: a comparative study. Dermatol Surg. 2002;28:828–32.
43. Erbil H, Sezer E, Tastan B, et al. Efficacy and safety of serial glycolic acid peels and a topical regimen in the treatment of recalcitrant melasma. J Dermatol. 2007;34:25–30.
44. Hurley ME, Guevara IL, Gonzales RM, et al. Efficacy of glycolic acid peels in the treatment of melasma. Arch Dermatol. 2002;138:1578.
45. Garg VK, Sarkar R, Agarwal R, et al. Comparative evaluation of beneficiary effects of priming agents (2% hydroquinone and 0.025% retinoic acid) in the treatment of melasma with glycolic acid peels. Dermatol Surg. 2008;34:1032–9.
46. Grimes P. The safety and efficacy of salicylic acid chemical peels in darker racial-ethnic groups. Dermatol Surg. 1999;25:18.
47. Lawrence N, Cox SE, Brody HJ. Treatment of melasma with Jessner's solution versus glycolic acid: a comparison of clinical efficacy and evaluation of the predictive ability of Wood's light examination. J Am Acad Dermatol. 1997;36:589–93.
48. Sharquie KE, Al-Tikreety MM, Al-Mashhadani SA. Lactic acid chemical peels as a new therapeutic modality in melasma in comparison to Jessner's solution chemical peels. Dermatol Surg. 2006;32:1429–36.
49. Kunachak S, Leelaudomlipi P, Wongwaisayawan S. Dermabrasion: a curative treatment for melasma. Aesthetic Plast Surg. 2001;25:114–7.
50. Bhalla M, Thami G. Microdermabrasion: reappraisal and brief review of literature. Dermatol Surg. 2006;32:809–14.
51. Karimipour DJ, Karimipour G, Orringer JS. Microdermabrasion: an evidence-based review. Plast Reconstr Surg. 2010;125:372.
52. Tse Y, Levine VJ, McClain SA, et al. The removal of cutaneous pigmented lesions with the Q-switched ruby laser and the Q-switched neodymium:yttrium-aluminum-garnet laser: a comparative study. J Dermatol Surg Oncol. 1994;20:795.
53. Polnikorn N. Treatment of refractory dermal melasma with the MedLite C6 Q-switched Nd:YAG laser: two case reports. J Cosmet Laser Ther. 2008;10:167–73.
54. Manaloto RMP, Alster T. Erbium:YAG laser resurfacing for refractory melasma. Dermatol Surg. 1999;25:121.
55. Ko NY, Ahn HH, Kim SN, et al. Analysis of erythema after Er:YAG laser skin resurfacing. Dermatol Surg. 2007;33:1322–7.
56. Rokhsar CK, Fitzpatrick RE. The treatment of melasma with fractional photothermolysis: a pilot study. Dermatol Surg. 2005;31:1645–50.
57. Graber EM, Tanzi EL, Alster TS. Side effects and complications of fractional laser photothermolysis: experience with 961 treatments. Dermatol Surg. 2008;34:301–5.
58. Goldberg DJ, Berlin AL, Phelps R. Histologic and ultrastructural analysis of melasma after fractional resurfacing. Lasers Surg Med. 2008;40:134–8.
59. Wang CC, Hui CY, Sue YM, et al. Intense pulsed light for the treatment of refractory melasma in Asian patients. Dermatol Surg. 2004;30:1196–200.
60. Li YH, Chen JZ, Wei HC, et al. Efficacy and safety of intense pulsed light in treatment of melasma in Chinese patients. Dermatol Surg. 2008;34:693–701.
61. Sriwiriyanont P, Ohuchi A, Hachiya A, et al. Interaction between stem cell factor and endothelin-1: effects on melanogenesis in human skin xenografts. Lab Invest. 2006;86:1115–25.
62. Ruiz-Maldonado R, Orozco-Covarrubias ML. Postinflammatory hypopigmentation and hyperpigmentation. Semin Cutan Med Surg. 1997;16:36–43.
63. Nordlund JJ. Postinflammatory hyperpigmentation. Dermatol Clin. 1988;6:185.
64. Kim NY, Pandya AG. Pigmentary diseases. Office Dermatol. 1998;82:1185–207.
65. Bulengo-Ransby S, Griffiths CD, Kimbrough-Green CK, et al. Topical tretinoin (retinoic acid) therapy for hyperpigmented lesions caused by inflammation of the skin in black patients. N Engl J Med. 1993;328:1438–43.

66. Grimes P. A microsponge formulation of hydroquinone 4% and retinol 0.15% in the treatment of melasma and postinflammatory hyperpigmentation. Cutis. 2004;74:362–8.
67. Baumann L, Grimes P, Pandya AG, Rendon M, Taylor S. Poster #1887, World congress of dermatology. Buenos Aires; 30 Sept–5 Oct 2007.
68. Grimes P, Callender V. Tazarotene cream for postinflammatory hyperpigmentation and acne vulgaris in darker skin: a double-blind, randomized, vehicle-controlled study. Cutis. 2006;77:45–50.
69. Burns RL, Prevost-Blank PL, Lawry MA, et al. Glycolic acid peels for postinflammatory hyperpigmentation in black patients. Dermatol Surg. 1997;23:171–5.
70. Joshi SS, Boone SL, Alam M, et al. Effectiveness, safety, and effect on quality of life of topical salicylic acid peels for treatment of postinflammatory hyperpigmentation in dark skin. Dermatol Surg. 2009;35:638–44.
71. Ahn HH, Kim IH. Whitening effect of salicylic acid peels in Asian patients. Dermatol Surg. 2006;32:372–5.
72. Garg VK, Sinha S, Sarkar R. Glycolic acid peels versus salicylic-mandelic acid peels in active acne vulgaris and post-acne scarring and hyperpigmentation: a comparative study. Dermatol Surg. 2009;35:59–65.
73. Qian Y, Zakov ZN, Schoenfield L, et al. Iris melanoma arising in iris nevus in oculo (dermal) melanocytosis. Surv Ophthalmol. 2008;53:411–5.
74. Sekar S, Kuruvila M, Pai HS. Nevus of Ota: a series of 15 cases. Indian J Dermatol Venereol Leprol. 2008;74:125–7.
75. Torres JE, Sanchez JL. Melasma and other disorders of hyperpigmentation. In: Arndt KA, LeBoit PE, Robinson JK, Wintroub BU, editors. Cutaneous medicine and surgery, vol. 2. Philadelphia: W.B. Saunders; 1996. p. 1239–40.
76. Hidano A, Kajima H, Ikeda S, et al. Natural history of nevus of Ota. Arch Dermatol. 1967;95:187–95.
77. Agero AL, Lahmar JJ, Holzborn RM, et al. Naevus of Ota presenting in two generations: a mother and daughter. J Eur Acad Dermatol Venereol. 2009;23:102–4.
78. Sinha S, Cohen PJ, Schwartz RA. Nevus of ota in children. Cutis. 2008;82:25–9.
79. Chan HH, Lam LK, Wong DS, et al. Nevus of ota: a new classification based on the response to laser treatment. Lasers Surg Med. 2001;28:267–72.
80. Hirayama T, Suzuki T. A new classification of Ota's nevus based on histopathological features. Dermatologica. 1991;183:169–72.
81. Mosher DB, Fitzpatrick TB, Ortonne J-P, Hori Y. Hypomelanoses and hypermelanoses. In: Freedberg IM, Eisen AZ, Wolff K, Austen KF, Goldsmith LA, Katz SI, Fitzpatrick TB, editors. Fitzpatrick's dermatology in general medicine. 5th ed. New York: McGraw-Hill; 1999. p. 1004.
82. Watanabe S. Basics of laser application to dermatology. Arch Dermatol Res. 2008;300 suppl 1:S21–30.
83. Kagami S, Asahina A, Watanabe R, et al. Treatment of 153 Japanese patients with Q-switched alexandrite laser. Lasers Med Sci. 2007;22:159–63.
84. Wang HW, Liu UH, Zhang GK, et al. Analysis of 602 Chinese cases of nevus of Ota and the treatment results treated by Q-switched alexandrite laser. Dermatol Surg. 2007;33:455–60.
85. Kang W, Lee E, Choi GS. Treatment of Ota's nevus by Q-switched alexandrite laser: therapeutic outcome in relation to clinical and histopathological findings. Eur J Dermatol. 1999;9:639–43.
86. Chan HH, Leung RS, Ying SY, et al. Recurrence of nevus of Ota after successful treatment with Q-switched lasers. Arch Dermatol. 2000;136:1175–6.
87. Trindade F, Cabecadas J, Rosa J. Surgical management of the eyelid and bulbar conjunctiva in a patient with nevus of Ota. J Eur Acad Dermatol Venereol. 2008;22:618–20.
88. Goodman RM, Belcher RW. Periorbital hyperpigmentation. Arch Dermatol. 1969;100:169–74.
89. Malakar S, Lahiri K, Banerjee U, et al. Periorbital melanosis is an extension of pigmentary demarcation line-F on face. Indian J Dermatol Venereol Leprol. 2007;73:323–5.

90. Selmanowitz VJ, Krivo JM. Pigmentary demarcation lines: comparison of Negroes with Japanese. Br J Dermatol. 1975;93:371–7.
91. Somani VK, Razvi F, Sita VN. Pigmentary demarcation lines over the face. Indian J Dermatol Venereol Leprol. 2005;70:336–41.
92. West TB, Alster TS. Improvement of infraorbital hyperpigmentation following carbon dioxide laser resurfacing. Dermatol Surg. 1998;24:615–6.
93. Momosawa A, Kurita M, Miyamoto S, et al. Combined therapy using Q-switched ruby laser and bleaching treatment with tretinoin and hydroquinone for periorbital skin hyperpigmentation in Asians. Plast Reconstr Surg. 2008;121:282–8.
94. Lowe NJ, Wieder JM, Shorr N, et al. Infraorbital pigmented skin: preliminary observations of laser therapy. Dermatol Surg. 1995;21:767.

# Chapter 9
# Disorders of Hypopigmentation and Depigmentation

**Ife J. Rodney and Rebat M. Halder**

Disorders of hypopigmentation and depigmentation are of great concern to patients of skin of color because of the marked contrast between the affected skin and normal skin. These disorders can be psychologically devastating in this patient group. There are a number of disorders of hypopigmentation and depigmentation that are clinically relevant. Those that will be discussed in this chapter are idiopathic guttate hypomelanosis, pityriasis alba, progressive macular hypomelanosis, postinflammatory hypopigmentation, oculocutaneous albinism 2B, piebaldism and vitiligo.

## Idiopathic Guttate Hypomelanosis

Idiopathic guttate hypomelanosis presents as multiple, discrete, circumscribed, porcelain white macules on the extensor arms and legs. No consistently effective treatment is yet available. Idiopathic guttate hypomelanosis (IGH) is a very common, acquired leukoderma that occurs in all races and skin types, but is very apparent in persons of color [1]. The number of lesions increases with age and may be seen in up to 80% of patients over the age of 70 years [2]. An apparent female predominance is possibly the result of heightened cosmetic concern.

I.J. Rodney, M.D. (✉)
Department of Dermatology and Pathology, Howard University College of Medicine, 2041 Georgia Avenue, NW, Washington, DC 20060, USA
e-mail: ife.rodney@howard.edu

R.M. Halder, M.D.
Department of Dermatology, Howard University College of Medicine, 2041 Georgia Avenue, NW, Washington, DC 20060, USA
e-mail: rhalder@howard.edu

A.F. Alexis and V.H. Barbosa (eds.), *Skin of Color: A Practical Guide to Dermatologic Diagnosis and Treatment*, DOI 10.1007/978-0-387-84929-4_9,

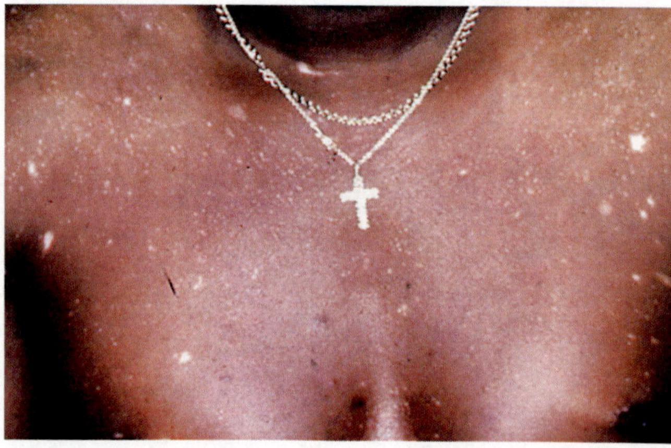

**Fig. 9.1** Idiopathic guttate hypomelanosis

IGH is characterized by multiple, discrete, circumscribed, asymptomatic porcelain white macules [3], usually on the extensor surfaces of the arms and legs. The surface is smooth, not scaly or atrophic. IGH occasionally affects the trunk and rarely the face. Lesions are usually 0.5–6 mm in diameter, but may be up to 2.5 cm (Fig. 9.1). Once formed, they do not enlarge or coalesce [4]; spontaneous repigmentation has not been observed. Vellus hairs within the lesions are usually not depigmented [5].

Histologically, there is flattening of the dermal–epidermal junction, with a marked reduction of melanin granules in the basal and suprabasal layers. The melanin granules that are present are irregularly distributed [3]. There is also a significant reduction in the number of DOPA-positive melanocytes [6].

The differential diagnosis includes other causes of guttate leukoderma of the extremities, such as chemical hypomelanosis, pityriasis lichenoides chronica, and disseminated hypopigmented keratoses that follow PUVA therapy.

The exact pathogenesis of IGH is unclear, but genetic factors, trauma, and autoimmunity have been suggested as causative factors. Also, because lesions mostly develop on sun-exposed parts of the extremities, ultraviolet light is thought to play a role. Kaya et al. describe a case of a patient with mycosis fungoides in whom widespread IGH occurred during narrowband ultraviolet B (NBUVB) therapy [7].

Patients with pigmented skins may request treatment for IGH because of the psychological effects of the disease. However, patients should be reassured that the lesions usually remain small in size and do not coalesce. As sunlight is possibly a precipitating factor, sunbathing is discouraged, and sunscreens and physical barriers should be used. No consistently effective treatment is yet available, but options include cryotherapy, intralesional corticosteroids, topical and oral PUVA, skin grafts, and localized superficial dermabrasion [8–10].

Cryotherapy is the most frequently used procedure for IGH. It is thought that destruction of the epidermal melanin units in IGH lesions by cryotherapy may allow keratinocytes and melanocytes of the surrounding normally pigmented skin to migrate into the affected skin, thus causing repigmentation [10]. As melanocytes are sensitive to freezing by liquid nitrogen, the risk of leukoderma, as well as postinflammatory hyperpigmentation, should be discussed with the patient. However, 3–5 second cryotherapy with liquid nitrogen has been shown to be effective in IGH [11]. Histologic examination of the repigmenting lesions demonstrated the reappearance of DOPA-positive melanocytes. The number of DOPA-positive melanocytes was significantly greater in the repigmented areas than in untreated lesions but less than in normal skin [9].

The method of localized superficial dermabrasion for IGH is also effective, fast, and inexpensive. It does not require anesthesia, and patients return immediately to their regular activities. The objective is to put pressure on the dermabrader so that it reaches the papillary dermis, without causing bleeding. It is then recommended that the skin be exposed to sunlight after the procedure. This stimulates migration of melanocytes from the follicular epithelium to the healing skin, favoring regimentation [10].

Falabella et al. [2] described the treatment of IGH with skin grafts and intralesional triamcinolone with limited success. The follow-up evaluations did not extend beyond 6 months. Also, in some cases, when normally pigmented skin was grafted onto the IGH lesions, the grafts then became depigmented.

## Pityriasis Alba

Pityriasis alba presents as ill-defined, hypopigmented, round patches on the face, neck, and trunk. It occurs most commonly in children of African, Hispanic, or Asian origin. It usually resolves spontaneously at puberty. Management includes limiting sun exposure and hot baths, liberal use of emollients, topical corticosteroids, phototherapy, topical calcineurin inhibitors, and topical tar.

Pityriasis alba, first described by Fox [12] in 1923, is a common eczematous disorder that presents as ill-defined, hypopigmented, slightly scaly, round to oval patches usually on the face, neck, and trunk [13]. It is a disease of childhood and adolescence that occurs in all races, but is most common in black children and children of Hispanic or Asian origin [14]. Both genders are equally affected. It is more noticeable in darkly pigmented individuals and becomes more apparent during the summer months.

The relationship between pityriasis alba and atopic dermatitis was first suggested by Watkins in 1961 [15]. It is now regarded as a minor feature of atopic dermatitis. In the general population, the prevalence is estimated at 1%, but in atopic individuals, it is 32% [16].

The pathogenesis of pityriasis alba is unclear, but several mechanisms have been proposed. It may be best characterized as an eczematous dermatitis related to atopy [17, 18], which results in hypomelanosis after the inflammation has subsided. This hypomelanosis may be related to impaired pigment transfer from melanocytes to keratinocytes. Also, light and electron microscopy demonstrate reduced numbers of melanocytes and a decrease in the size and number of melanosomes within both melanocytes and keratinocytes [19].

Xerosis, which may result from frequent bathing and hot baths, is often associated with both pityriasis alba and atopic dermatitis [20]. This is explained by the reduced water-holding capacity of the stratum corneum in pityriasis alba, compared to healthy skin [21].

Other proposed mechanisms include nutritional and vitamin deficiencies [16, 22, 23]. In particular, patients with pityriasis alba have been shown to have low serum levels of copper [24], which is a cofactor for the enzyme tyrosinase, needed for melanin synthesis. Thus, a copper deficiency may play a role.

Initially, lesions consist of erythematous macules or patches, which then fade over a few weeks, and result in ill-defined hypopigmented patches with a whitish, dry, scaly surface. The border of these lesions may be slightly raised and erythematous. However, most patients present after the erythema has already faded and all that remains is hypopigmentation with scaling. Although generally asymptomatic, some patients complain of pruritis or burning. Lesions are frequently symmetrically distributed on the malar region of the face and vary in size from 5 to 30 mm. Less often, they may be found on the upper extremities and shoulders. Although most patients have only 2 or 3 lesions, some patients may have as many as 20 lesions.

There are several variations of pityriasis alba. Extensive pityriasis alba consists of widespread and symmetric involvement of the skin of the trunk by numerous, round, nonscaly hypopigmented patches [20, 25]. It is an asymptomatic dermatosis that is usually seen in adults. Because there is no preceding erythema and patients give no history of atopy, some authors consider this to be a distinct entity.

Pigmenting pityriasis alba may present as bluish hyperpigmentation surrounded by scaly hypopigmentation. The bluish pigment is due to melanin deposition in the dermis. These lesions appear on the face and may be associated with a superficial dermatophyte infection, in up to 65% of affected patients [26].

Pityriasis alba can imitate an array of other inflammatory skin conditions that are associated with postinflammatory hypopigmentation. However, these can usually be easily distinguished based on clinical presentation, histologic examination, or simple procedures like potassium hydroxide preparation or examination under a Wood's lamp.

The differential diagnosis includes tinea versicolor, tinea faciei, vitiligo, nevus depigmentosus, nevus anemicus, hypopigmented mycosis fungoides, and hypopigmentation secondary to leprosy, nummular eczema, psoriasis, or use of a topical steroid. When lesions are extrafacial, pityriasis lichenoides chronica should be considered.

Pityriasis alba is a self-limiting disease [27] that usually remains stable for months or years, but then resolves spontaneously at puberty. However, treatment should be attempted, particularly in dark-skinned races as the hypopigmentation may be striking. Patients should be advised to limit sun exposure and avoid hot baths. Use of emollients should be encouraged, as they lessen dryness and irritation of the skin. Topical corticosteroids, with low potency for the face and medium potency for the body, have been used with limited improvement. As pityriasis alba is considered a mild eczematous dermatitis, it is logical that topical corticosteroids may relieve the pruritus and inflammation associated with the disorder. Topical and oral PUVA are treatment alternatives. Topical PUVA [28] is performed once weekly.

Thirty minutes after application of 0.1% Oxsoralen cream, the patient is exposed to UVA light at a starting dose of 0.5 J and increased by 0.3 J on a weekly basis until repigmentation occurs, but without resulting erythema or burning of the lesions. Oral PUVA is used for more widespread lesions.

311 nm NB-UVB phototherapy may also be used with starting doses varying from 75 to 200 mJ/cm$^2$, depending on skin phototype. This is subsequently increased by 20% at each treatment. Treatments are given two to three times per week. Also, topical calcineurin inhibitors such as pimecrolimus and tacrolimus are used off label for treatment [29].

Tar emulsions, applied twice daily, may be very beneficial. Tar is itself melanogenic, without having to use ultraviolet light [27]. It is available commercially as a 6% cream and may also be compounded as 5% liquor carbonis detergens (LCD) in any variety of vehicles such as acid mantle cream, aquaphor, or with a low-potency topical steroid. Patients, particularly children, should be cautious of sun exposure with the use of tar. Controlled trials have yet to prove the effectiveness of these agents.

## Progressive Macular Hypomelanosis

Progressive macular hypomelanosis (PMH) is a common skin disorder, observed most frequently in young women with darkly pigmented skin who originate from tropical climates. While it can be seen in all ethnicities, PMH may be more noticeable in darker skin.

PMH presents with symetrically distributed hypopigmented macules on the trunk. Treatment of choice is once daily 5% benzoyl peroxide gel and once-daily 1% clindamycin, combined with UVA light therapy. Other proposed treatments include topical and systemic antifungals, topical corticosteroids, and PUVA treatment.

Patients present with ill-defined hypopigmented macules that are symmetrically located on the trunk and rarely extend to the extremities and head/neck region (Fig. 9.2). Characteristically, there is no preceding pruritus, pain, or inflammation. In many patients, there may be confluence of lesions centrally [30], resulting in large hypopigmented patches (5–20 cm), with round solitary macules on the lateral trunk.

Under Wood's lamp, there is accentuation of the hypopigmented macules, and red follicular fluorescence is also visible within hypopigmented skin. This is absent in adjacent normal skin and is a key diagnostic sign of PMH [30]. It is thought that Propionibacterium acnes within the hair follicles may produce a porphyrin that causes this red follicular fluorescence [31]. Although P. acnes also causes acne vulgaris, preliminary analysis has shown that different subtypes of the species are related to the two diseases [30].

The differential diagnosis consists of other disorders with acquired hypopigmentation, particularly on the trunk. This includes pityriasis versicolor, seborrheic dermatitis, hypopigmented mycosis fungoides, tuberculoid or borderline tuberculoid leprosy, and postinflammatory hypopigmentation. Historically, extensive pityriasis

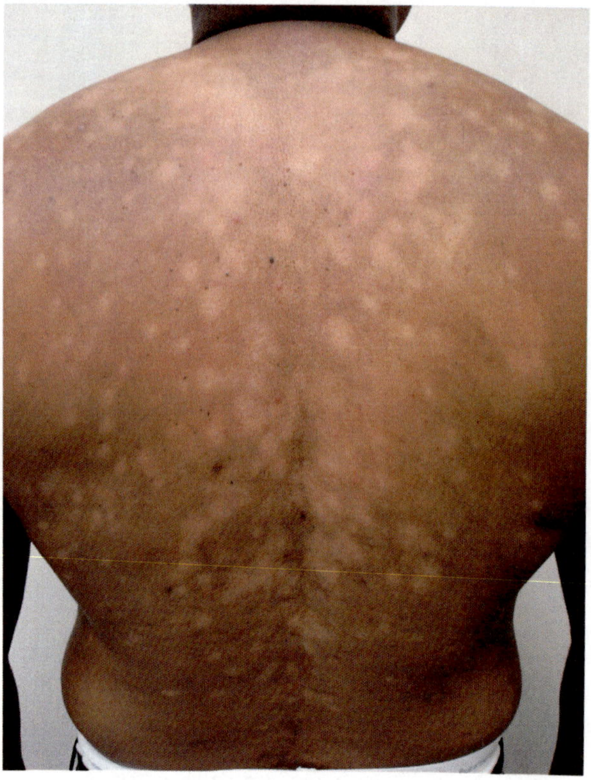

**Fig. 9.2** Progressive macular hypomelanosis, generalized lesions

alba was considered in the differential for PMH, but more recently, some authors have proposed that they are, indeed, the same disease [32]. However, there are some electron microscopic differences between EPA and PMH [33].

On hematoxylin–eosin stain, there is decreased melanin content in the epidermis of hypopigmented skin compared to the adjacent normal skin. The number of melanocytes is unchanged and the dermis is normal. No spongiosis, inflammation, spores, or hyphae are seen [31]. Electron microscopy (of patients with Fitzpatrick skin types V and VI) shows a shift from large stage IV single melanosomes in keratinocytes of normal skin to small, stage I–III aggregated, membrane-bound melanosomes in hypopigmented skin [30, 34, 35].

The natural history of PMH, although not known with certainty, appears to be stable disease, sometimes with very slow progression over decades and spontaneous disappearance after midlife [30]. This is supported by the observation that PMH has never been reported in the elderly.

Several treatment modalities have been attempted for PMH. These include topical and systemic antifungals and topical corticosteroids, all yielding poor results [36]. Resolution of the hypopigmentation was noted with psoralen plus UVA treatment (PUVA). Unfortunately, after the PUVA was discontinued, the hypopigmentation returned in the exact same distribution [36].

The hypothesis that P. acnes is the pathogenic factor in PMH was supported by a study conducted by Relyveld et al. [37]. This showed that when both antibacterial and anti-inflammatory treatments were combined with UVA irradiation, the antibacterial treatment was significantly superior. Therefore, the treatment of choice is once-daily 5% benzoyl peroxide hydrogel and once-daily 1% clindamycin, in combination with broadband UVA irradiation (230 J/m$^2$) without the use of psoralens, three times a week (for 12 weeks). However, this high UVA dose is not our recommendation. We recommend starting at 20 J/m$^2$. UVB irradiation, both broadband and narrowband UVB, may also be used. However, the response rates of these treatments are variable. Maintenance treatments are recommended for patients with multiple recurrences over 1 year, or within 3 months of cessation of therapy [37].

## Postinflammatory Hypopigmentation

Postinflammatory hypopigmentation is a common end result of inflammatory cutaneous disorders due to a decrease in melanin production, resulting in hypopigmented lesions. Management includes treatment of the underlying disease, topical or oral PUVA therapy, narrowband UVB phototherapy, topical corticosteroids, and skin grafts.

Postinflammatory hypopigmentation (PIH) is a very common end result of inflammatory cutaneous disorders, such as psoriasis, seborrheic dermatitis, atopic dermatitis, lichen planus, pityriasis lichenoides chronica, vesiculobullous diseases, and acne vulgaris. It may also be due to irritation from therapeutic interventions such as topical retinoids or benzoyl peroxide. This normal biological response in human skin is more noticeable and distressing in darker-skinned individuals and accounts for a significant number of visits to dermatologists.

In postinflammatory hypopigmentation, there is a decrease in melanin production, resulting in clinically apparent light areas [38] (Fig. 9.3). PIH can be distinguished from melanocytopenic conditions, such as vitiligo and piebaldism, with use of a Wood's lamp. In these melanocytopenic diseases, the hypopigmentation is accentuated with the Wood's lamp. However, this technique is sometimes not helpful in persons of color because of optical factors [39].

Although the exact pathogenesis of postinflammatory hypopigmentation is unknown, it is thought that inflammation leads to the release of cytokines and inflammatory mediators such as interferon-gamma, tumor necrosis factor (TNF)-alpha, TNF-beta, interleukin (IL)-6, and IL-7 from keratinocytes and melanocytes [40]. Also, there may be melanocyte cell-surface expression of intercellular adhesion molecule (ICAM)-1 induced by these mediators. The theory is that this may lead to leukocyte–melanocyte attachments, with the final result being innocent bystander destruction of melanocytes.

Treatment modalities for postinflammatory hypopigmentation include phototherapy with topical or oral PUVA or narrowband UVB light. For topical PUVA, 8-methoxypsoralen is applied to the hypopigmented skin at concentrations of 0.1% or lower. Thirty minutes after application, the patient is exposed to the UVA light at a starting dose of 0.5 J/cm$^2$ and increased by 0.5 J/cm$^2$ on each treatment.

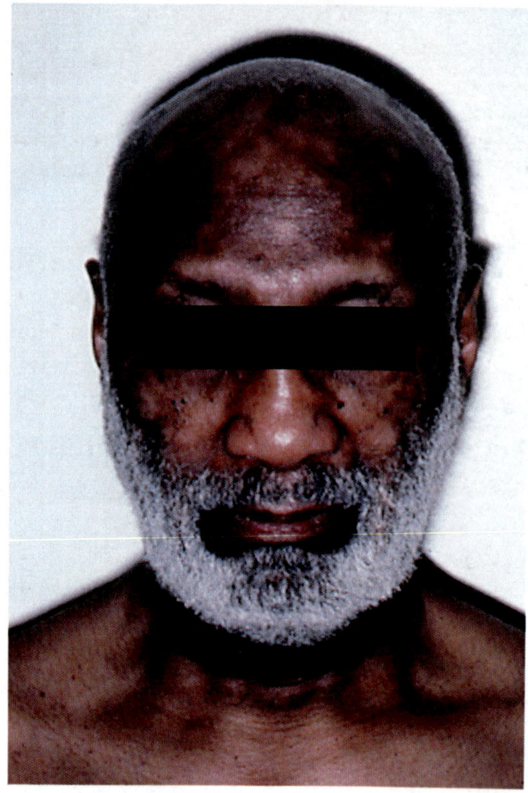

**Fig. 9.3** Postinflammatory hypopigmentation from seborrheic dermatitis

Oral PUVA is used when lesions are more generalized. Oral 8-MOP is given at a dose of 0.3 mg/kg, and treatments are administered twice weekly. The initial dose of UVA is usually 0.5–1.0 J/cm$^2$. NB-UVB phototherapy is administered twice weekly, with starting doses varying from 75 to 200 mJ/cm$^2$. The dose is then increased by 10–20% on each treatment. For all of the previously described treatments, the dose of phototherapy is gradually increased until minimal asymptomatic erythema occurs.

Other treatment options consist of cosmetic cover-ups, topical corticosteroids, and skin grafts [41]. However, treating the underlying cause of the hypopigmentation is imperative in preventing further dyschromia. The efficacies of the previously mentioned treatment modalities are variable.

## Oculocutaneous Albinism 2B

Oculocutaneous albinism 2B is an autosomal recessive genetic disorder that presents as diffuse pigmentary dilution due to decreased or absent melanin within melanocytes. Individuals are at increased risk of non-melanoma skin cancers, particularly squamous cell carcinoma. No specific treatment is available. Photoprotection is mandatory and includes sun avoidance, protective clothing, and broad-spectrum sunscreens.

Oculocutaneous albinism (OCA) consists of a group of autosomal recessive genetic disorders characterized by diffuse pigmentary dilution due to a partial or total absence of melanin pigment within melanocytes of the skin, hair follicles, and eyes [42]. It is the most commonly inherited disorder that leads to diffuse hypomelanosis. There may also be nystagmus and reduced visual acuity [43].

Four different types of OCA have been defined. OCA type 1 results from reduced or absent tyrosinase activity, due to mutations in the tyrosinase gene [44]. OCA type 2 is due to mutations in the P gene [45] on chromosome segment 15q11–q13 [46, 47]. The function of the P protein is still debated, but several mechanisms have been proposed. For example, a membrane transporter of a substrate [48], a sorter of tyrosinase to the melanosome [49], a stabilizer of a melanosomal protein complex [50], a regulator of melanosomal pH [45], and a controller of the processing of tyrosinase, arsenic sensitivity, and, most recently, cellular glutathione metabolism [51–53].

About 1% of patients with Prader–Willi syndrome (PWS) and Angelman syndrome (AS) also have OCA2. This is because the 15q chromosomal deletion seen in PWS and AS includes the P gene. Therefore, OCA2 occurs when a deletion of one copy of the P gene is accompanied by a mutation in the second copy [54].

OCA type 3 results from mutations in the tyrosinase-related protein 1 [55]. A fourth type of OCA, OCA4, was identified more recently [56]. The gene involved is MATP (membrane-associated transporter protein). In Africans and African–Americans, OCA2 is the most common type of OCA. In the Ibo people of Nigeria, the frequency is 1 in 1,100 [57], while it is 1 in10,000 among African-Americans, compared to 1 in 36,000 among Caucasians [58].

In OCA2, eumelanin is almost completely absent. However, there is cutaneous and ocular pigmentation, due to pheomelanin, that often increases with time. Also, darkly pigmented nevi may develop in sun-exposed areas. These occur at rates similar to that of unaffected white subjects [59]. The clinical phenotype of OCA2 is broad, ranging from minimal to moderate pigmentary dilution of the hair, skin, and iris, with minimal ability to tan. Affected individuals are at increased susceptibility to non-melanoma skin cancers, with squamous cell carcinoma being the most common in this population [60, 61]. This is a significant cause of morbidity and mortality in tropical regions.

Another phenotypic subtype more commonly seen in patients of African descent is called "brown OCA." Like classic OCA2, it is due to mutations in the P gene. At birth, these patients have light brown skin and hair, and gray to tan irides. They do not usually develop sunburns.

The ocular manifestations of OCA reflect a reduction in melanin in the iris, retina, and fovea that are associated with photophobia and reduced visual acuity. There is also misrouting of optic nerve fibers during development resulting in the characteristic strabismus, nystagmus, and lack of binocular vision.

On histopathology, the number of epidermal and follicular melanocytes is normal, but there is a reduction in melanin content.

The differential diagnoses of OCA2 consist of diseases with diffuse pigmentary dilution with onset at birth or during infancy. These include the other types of oculocutaneous albinism (OCA 1, 3, 4), Hermansky–Pudlak syndrome, Chédiak–Higashi syndrome, Cross syndrome, Tietz syndrome, Menkes syndrome, Griscelli syndrome, phenylketonuria, histidinemia, and homocystinuria.

There is no specific treatment available for oculocutaneous albinism. However, as these patients are at increased risk for photocarcinogenesis, specifically squamous cell carcinoma, photoprotection is mandatory. This includes sun avoidance and the use of hats and protective clothing. Broad-spectrum sunscreens should be used daily and should be reapplied at least every 2 h if the patient is outdoors.

## Piebaldism

Piebaldism is a rare, autosomal dominant disorder resulting from mutations in the c-kit proto-oncogene that presents with white forelock on the anterior midline scalp and stable leukoderma on the central forehead, central anterior trunk, and anterior mid-extremities. Treatments include liberal sunscreen and protective clothing, split thickness skin grafts, and melanocyte transplantation. Piebaldism is a rare autosomal dominant disorder, characterized by congenital poliosis and stable leukoderma. Although the exact prevalence is unknown, all races and genders are affected.

The most characteristic manifestation of piebaldism is the white forelock, which is present at birth and may be the only sign in most patients [62]. About 80–90% of affected individuals have this manifestation. All of the hairs in the forelock, along with the underlying skin, are depigmented. It is located on the anterior midline scalp, is symmetrical, and may have a triangular or diamond shape. In severe cases of piebaldism, the medial third of the eyebrows and eyelashes may also be depigmented [63].

The leukoderma of piebaldism is characteristically nonprogressive and distributed on the central forehead, the central anterior trunk, and anterior mid-extremities. It presents as irregularly shaped, well-circumscribed, milk white patches, with hyperpigmented macules and patches within the depigmented skin and also on adjacent normal skin (Fig. 9.4).

Most patients are otherwise healthy and have no systemic symptoms, but piebaldism may rarely be associated with other disorders such as Hirschsprung's disease, neurofibromatosis type 1, Grover's disease, and deafness [64–67]. Also, because the depigmentation of piebaldism is striking in dark-skinned races, there is significant emotional burden.

Piebaldism results from mutations in the c-kit proto-oncogene [54], which encodes the tyrosine kinase transmembrane receptors that are found on the surface of melanocytes. It is critical for melanoblast migration from the neural crest and also proliferation and differentiation. These c-kit mutations are found in 75% of patients with piebaldism [68]. Patients without the c-kit mutation have been reported to have a mutation in the slug gene, which is a zinc-finger neural crest transcription factor [69].

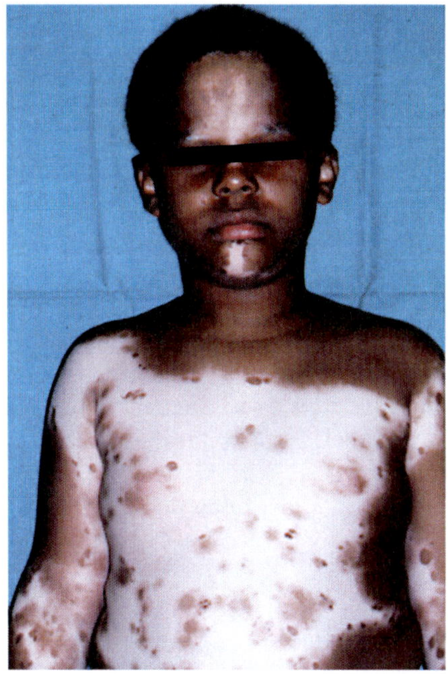

**Fig. 9.4** Piebaldism. Note midline depigmentation with islands of pigmentation

There are numerous different mutation sites in c-kit that result in piebaldism of varying severity. Interestingly, a Val620Ala mutation results in progression of the depigmented patches [70], unlike classic piebaldism.

Histopathologic examination reveals an absence of melanocytes in the amelanotic skin [71]. The hyperpigmented macules are characterized by an abundance of melanosomes in the melanocytes and keratinocytes [63].

The differential diagnosis of piebaldism consists of any condition that presents with a depigmented lesion or white forelock. This includes vitiligo, Vogt–Koyanagi–Harada syndrome, postinflammatory hypopigmentation, Alezzandrini syndrome, alopecia areata, tuberous sclerosis, and, very importantly, Waardenburg syndrome. This differential diagnosis should be further explored via ocular and auditory examinations. Less common syndromes that should be considered are Ziprkowski–Margolis syndrome and Woolf syndrome.

Piebaldism is unresponsive to agents typically used for vitiligo, such as topical corticosteroids and phototherapy (PUVA or narrowband UVB). Surgical techniques attempted include autografts of normal skin into amelanotic areas, split thickness grafts, and transplantation of autologous cultured melanocytes. These may require multiple procedures, with variable success [72, 73]. More recently, Guerra et al. [74] reported permanent repigmentation of piebaldism via destruction of amelanotic epidermis with the erbium:YAG laser, followed by transplantation of autologous cultured epidermal grafts. The mean percentage repigmentation was 95.45% [72–74]. In all patients, liberal sunscreen use and protection against sunburn is necessary. Also, cosmetic cover-up may be used as a means of camouflage.

## Vitiligo

Vitiligo is a result of autoimmune destruction of melanocytes and presents as well demarcated, depigmented macules and patches. Treatments include topical corticosteroids, topical immunomodulators, UVB, narrowband UVB, PUVA/PUVASOL, excimer laser, skin grafts, melanocyte transplantation, cosmetics, and depigmentation with 20% monobenzylether of hydroquinone.

Vitiligo is an acquired, idiopathic disorder that causes destruction of melanocytes not only in the skin but also in mucous membranes, eyes, hair bulbs, and in the ears [75]. It presents as well demarcated, depigmented macules and patches with variable progression. This can be more psychologically devastating in people of color due to marked contrast between normal and affected skin [76]. Vitiligo can occur at any age, but it usually occurs before 20 years in nearly 50% of patients and affects nearly 1–2% of the world population [77, 78]. The distribution is equal regardless of race, ethnicity, or gender [79, 80].

The exact etiology is not clearly understood. However, an autoimmune pathogenesis is preferred [76]. This is supported by the association of vitiligo with autoimmune endocrinopathies such as hypo- and hyperthyroidism and, less often, pernicious anemia and Addison's disease. Other proposed mechanisms include an intrinsic defect in the structure and function of melanocytes, dysregulation in melanocyte apoptosis, defective free radical defenses, viral infection, or a combination of these. There is also a genetic component to vitiligo that is characterized by genetic heterogeneity, incomplete penetrance, and multiple susceptibility loci.

Diagnosis of vitiligo is based almost exclusively on the clinical examination. Lesions may be found anywhere on the body. However, initial lesions are most frequently found on the hands, forearms, feet, face, and lips [81].

There are four main types of vitiligo: generalized, acrofacial, segmental, and universal. Generalized is the most common type. Patients present with bilateral symmetric lesions involving the periorofacial areas, neck, torso, bony prominences of hands, wrists, and legs, extensor surfaces, orifices, axillae, and mucosal areas [75] (Fig. 9.5). Acrofacial vitiligo presents with lesions on distal fingers and on the facial orifices. Segmental vitiligo presents in an asymmetric dermatomal distribution. It has an earlier age of onset and is not associated with autoimmune diseases. Universal vitiligo, which has been associated with multiple endocrinopathies, presents with depigmented macules and patches involving almost the entire body [75].

Clinical variants of vitiligo include vitiligo ponctué and trichrome vitiligo. Vitiligo ponctué is characterized by small, discrete, confetti-like amelanotic macules. Trichrome vitiligo is a term used to describe lesions that show a tan intermediate zone between normal and totally depigmented skin. In this zone, melanocytes are reduced in number but not completely absent [82]. In quadrichrome vitiligo, there is perifollicular hyperpigmentation at sites of repigmentation. Other uncommon variants include vitiligo with raised inflammatory borders and blue vitiligo macules, which occur when vitiligo develops in skin already affected by postinflammatory hyperpigmentation. Depending on the distribution and percentage of body surface

**Fig. 9.5** Generalized vitiligo

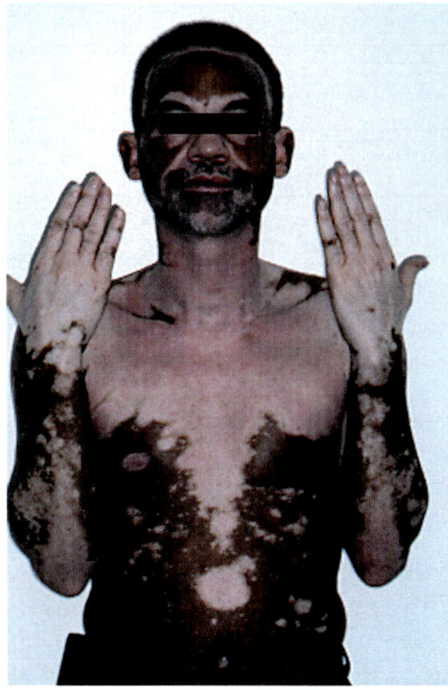

area involved, the differential diagnosis may include nevus depigmentosus, nevus anemicus, piebaldism, chemical leukoderma, the leukodermas associated with melanoma or scleroderma, or postinflammatory depigmentation.

There are various modalities for treating vitiligo [77, 78]. They include, but are not limited to, topical corticosteroids, UVB, narrowband UVB, PUVA, PUVASOL, excimer laser, topical immunomodulators, skin grafts, melanocyte transplantation, and cosmetics [83–89]. However, color matching with cosmetics may not be ideal for darker-skinned individuals. Topical corticosteroids are a first-line therapy for small localized lesions. Class III steroids are the most effective while minimizing potential side effects. This therapy should be discontinued after 2 months if no improvement is seen. Tacrolimus ointment 0.1% is a topical immunomodulator that may function as a steroid-sparing agent. It may be used in conjunction with topical steroids and other therapies such as excimer laser [90, 91].

NB-UVB, at a wavelength of 311 nm, has become the treatment of choice for adults and children (over 6 years of age) with generalized vitiligo. It is very effective as monotherapy [89, 92], with starting doses varying from 75 to 200 mJ/cm$^2$. If the patient tolerates treatment, with no burning or peeling of skin, the dose is increased by 10–20% at each treatment until asymptomatic erythema is achieved. Treatments are given two to three times per week [89]. NB-UVB may be considered superior to PUVA therapy because of the shorter treatment times, no additional cost of oral medication, or the limitations for patients with hepatic or renal disease associated with the 8-MOP.

Psoralen photochemotherapy involves the use of psoralens combined with UVA light (PUVA). PUVA acts to repigment via stimulation of melanocytes in the outer root sheath of the hair follicle through the action of immune cytokines and inflammatory mediators released by keratinocytes [93–95]. The areas that respond most favorably to PUVA are the face and trunk [96].

The psoralen most commonly used in the United States is 8-methoxypsoralen (8-MOP). Psoralens can be applied either topically or orally, followed by exposure to either artificial UV light or natural sunlight (PUVASOL). For oral PUVA, 8-MOP is given at a dose of 0.3 mg/kg. Treatments are usually administered two times per week. For vitiligo patients, the initial dose of UVA is usually 0.5–1.0 J/cm$^2$. This is gradually increased until minimal asymptomatic erythema occurs.

Topical PUVA is more difficult to administer because of the high risk of phototoxicity from topical psoralen. Therefore, concentrations of 0.1% or lower of 8-MOP should be used. Thirty minutes after the topical psoralen is applied to the depigmented lesions, the patient is exposed to the UVA light. This should be started at 0.3 J/cm$^2$ and increased by 0.3 J/cm$^2$ on each treatment until mild erythema is observed.

Excimer laser therapy also known as targeted phototherapy, a new promising treatment, delivers high doses of light to depigmented lesions. The wavelength of this laser, 308 nm, is close to that of NB-UVB. Localized lesions are treated twice weekly for 24–48 sessions [97].

There are surgical treatments for vitiligo. However, they should only be used on patients in whom vitiligo has been stable for approximately 4–6 months [85]. Autologous minigrafts involve harvesting 1.2–2.0-mm punch grafts from a donor site on the lower back below the waistline and placing them 3–4 mm apart on the recipient site, which has been prepared with a similar-sized punch. Another technique termed autologous thin Thiersch grafting allows grafting of large areas in a relatively short time, prepared by a process similar to dermabrasion, with minimal scarring in treated areas [98]. However, the disadvantage of this technique is that it requires general anesthesia. Suction blister grafting is another technique used to cover depigmented areas, prepared by denuding them with liquid nitrogen blisters or dermabrasion [83]. Suction blister grafts are obtained using negative pressure at 200 mmHg for nearly 4 h. The tops of the donor blisters are harvested and applied directly to the depigmented areas in a mosaic pattern, taking approximately 3–6 months for regimentation [83].

Lastly, autologous, noncultured, melanocyte–keratinocyte cell transplantation is effective in the repigmentation of recalcitrant leukodermic lesions in patients with stable, segmental, or focal vitiligo. This technique involves injecting an epidermal suspension of melanocytes and keratinocytes from normally pigmented donor skin onto dermabraded, depigmented skin and covered with a collagen dressing.

Depigmentation is sometimes considered when patients have widespread recalcitrant disease. Patients must understand that their appearance will be altered significantly and that strict lifelong photoprotection is necessary. Depigmentation is commonly accomplished with the use of 20% monobenzylether of hydroquinone (MBEH) [77, 78]. This is applied to the affected areas, twice daily, for 6–12 months [99].

**Table 9.1** Response rates for individual therapies

| Therapy | Duration | Response rate (%) |
|---|---|---|
| Topical corticosteroids | 4–6 months | 45 |
| Topical immunomodulators | 4–6 months | 45 |
| Topical PUVA | 4–6 months | 45 |
| Oral PUVA | 12–18 months | 50–60 |
| Narrow band UVB | 12–18 months | 60–65 |
| Excimer laser | 8–10 weeks | 70 |
| Surgical grafting procedures | 1 week | 90 |
| Melanocyte transplantation | 1 week | 95 |

A response may be seen in up to 3 months. Depigmentation may also be achieved with the Q-switched ruby laser therapy. This may give faster results than the topical bleaching agents [100]. There is great variability in response rates from patient to patient with the aforementioned therapies. In general, response rates for therapies are listed in Table 9.1.

## References


1. Falabella R. Idiopathic guttate hypomelanosis. Dermatologic Clin. 1988;6(2):241–7.
2. Falabella R, Escobar C, Giraldo N, Rovetto P, Gil J, Barona MI, Acosta F, Alzate A. On the pathogenesis of idiopathic guttate hypomelanosis. J Am Acad Dermatol. 1987;16(pt 1): 35–44.
3. Ortonne JP, Perrot H. Idiopathic guttate hypomelanosis. Arch Dermatol. 1980;116:664–8.
4. Cummings KI, Cottel WI. Idiopathic guttate hypomelanosis. Arch Dermatol. 1966;93:184.
5. Bolognia J, Pawelek J. Biology of hypopigmentation. J Am Acad Dermatol. 1988;19:217–55.
6. Wallace ML, Grichnik JM, Prieto VG, et al. Numbers and differentiation status of melanocytes in idiopathic guttate hypomelanosis. J Cutan Pathol. 1998;25:375–9.
7. Kaya TI, Yazici AC, Tursen U, Ikizoglu G. Idiopatihic guttate hypomelanosis: idiopathic or ultraviolet induced? Photodermatol Photoimmunol Photomed. 2005;21:270–1.
8. Golhar A, Pillar T, Eidelman S, Etzioni A. Vitiligo and idiopathic guttate hypomelanosis. Repigmentation of skin following engraftment onto nude mice. Arch Dermatol. 1989;125(10): 1363–6.
9. Ploysangam T, Dee-Ananlap S, Suvanprakorn P. Treatment of idiopathic guttate hypomelanosis with liquid nitrogen: light and electron microscopic studies. J Am Acad Dermatol. 1990;23(4 Pt 1):681–4.
10. Hexsel DM. Treatment of idiopathic guttate hypomelanosis by localized superficial dermabrasion. Dermatol Surg. 1999;25(11):917–8.
11. Kumarasinghe SP. 3-5 second cryotherapy is effective in idiopathic guttate hypomelanosis. J Dermatol. 2004;31(5):437–9.
12. Fox H. Partial depigmentation: chiefly on the face in Negro children. Arch Dermatol Syphilol. 1923;7:268–9.
13. O'Farrell MM. Pityriasis alba. Arch Dermatol. 1956;73:376–8.
14. Halder RM. Pigmentary disorders in pigmented skins. In: Halder RM, editor. Dermatology and dermatological therapy of pigmented skins. Boca Raton: Taylor and Francis; 2006.

15. Watkins DB. Pityriasis alba: a form of atopic dermatitis. A preliminary report. Arch Dermatol. 1961;83:915–9.
16. Diepgen TL, Fartasch M, Hornstein OP. Evaluation and relevance of atopic basic and minor features in patients with atopic dermatitis and in the general population. Acta Derm Venereol Suppl (Stockh). 1989;144:50–4.
17. Bassaly M, Miale Jr A, Prasad AS. Studies on pityriasis alba: a common facial skin lesion in Egyptian children. Arch Dermatol. 1963;88:272–5.
18. Martin RF, Lugo-Somolinos A, Sanchez JL. Clinicopathologic study on pityriasis alba. Bol Asoc Med PR. 1990;82:463–5.
19. Zaynoun ST, Aftimos BG, Tenekjian KK, et al. Extensive pityriasis alba: a histological, histochemical and ultrastructural study. Br J Dermatol. 1983;108:83–90.
20. Blessmann Weber M, Sponchiado deAvila LG, Albaneze R, et al. Pityriasis alba: a study of pathogenic factors. J Eur Acad Dermatol Venereol. 2002;16:463–8.
21. Urano-Suehisa S, Tagami H. Functional and morphological analysis of the horny layer of pityriasis alba. Acta Derm Venereol. 1985;65:164–7.
22. Wells BT, Whyte HJ, Kierland RR. Pityriasis alba: a ten year survey and review of the literature. Arch Dermatol. 1960;82:183–9.
23. Galan EB, Janniger CK. Pityriasis alba. Cutis. 1998;61:11–3.
24. Galadari E, Helmy M, Ahmed M. Trace elements in serum of pityriasis alba patients. Int J Dermatol. 1992;31:525–6.
25. Zaynoun S, Jaber LA, Kurban AK. Oral methoxsalen photochemotherapy of extensive pityriasis alba. Preliminary report. J Am Acad Dermatol. 1986;15:61–5.
26. Dhar S, Kanwar AJ, Dawn G. Pigmenting pityriasis alba. Pediatr Dermatol. 1995;12:197–8.
27. Shah AS, Supapannachart N, Nordlund JJ. Acquired hypomelanotic disorders. In: Levine N, editor. Pigmentation and pigmentary disorders. Boca Raton: CRC Press; 1993. p. 352–3.
28. Zaynoun ST, Aftimos BG, Tenekjian KK, Bahuth N, Kurban AK. Extensive pityriasis alba: a histological, histochemical and ultrastructural study. Br J Dermatol. 1983;108:83–6.
29. Lin A. Topical immunotherapy. In: Wolverton SE, editor. Comprehensive dermatological therapy. Philadelphia: Saunders; 2001. p. 617–9.
30. Relyveld GN, Menke HE, Westerhof W. Progressive macular hypomelanosis: an overview. Am J Clin Dermatol. 2007;8(1):13–9.
31. Westerhof W, Relyveld GN, Kingswijk M, et al. Propionibacterium acnes and the pathogenesis of progressive macular hypomelanosis. Arch Dermatol. 2004;140:210–4.
32. Di Lernia V, Ricci C. Progressive and extensive hypomelanosis and extensive pityriasis alba: same disease, different names? J Eur Acad Dermatol Venereol. 2005;19:370–2.
33. Relyveld G, Menke H, Westerhof W. Letter to the editor: progressive and extensive hypomelanosis and extensive pityriasis alba: same disease, different names? J Eur Acad Dermatol Venereol. 2006;20(10):1363–4.
34. Guillet G, Helenon R, Gauthier Y, et al. Progressive macular hypomelanosis of the trunk: primary acquired hypopigmentation. J Cutan Pathol. 1988;15:286–9.
35. Guillet G, Helenon R, Guillet MH, et al. Hypomelanose maculeuse confluente et progressive du metis melanoderme. Ann Dermatol Venereol. 1992;119(1):19–24.
36. Menke HE, Ossekoppele R, Dekker SK, et al. Nummulaire en confluerende hypomelanosis van de romp. Ned Tijdsch Dermatol Venereol. 1997;7:117–22.
37. Relyveld GN, Kingswijk M, Reitsma JB, et al. Benzoyl peroxide/clindamycin/ultraviolet A is more effective than fluticasone/ultraviolet A in progressive macular hypomelanosis: a randomized study. J Am Acad Dermatol. 2006;55(5):836–43.
38. Morelli JG, Norris DA. Influence of inflammatory mediators and cytokines on human melanocyte function. J Invest Dermatol. 1993;100(2):191S–5. Review. PubMed PMID: 8381839.
39. Grover R, Morgan BD. Management of hypopigmentation following burn injury. Burns. 1996;22(8):627–30. Review. PubMed PMID: 8982542.
40. Ellis DA, Tan AK. How we do it: management of facial hyperpigmentation. J Otolaryngol. 1997;26(4):286–9.

41. Johnston GA, Sviland L, McLelland J. Melasma of the arms associated with hormone replacement therapy. Br J Dermatol. 1998;139(5):932.
42. Passeron T, Mantoux F, Ortonne JP. Genetic disorders of pigmentation. Clin Dermatol. 2005;23:56–67.
43. Witkop Jr CJ, Hill CW, Desnick S, Theis JK, Thorn HL, Jenkins M. Ophthalmologic, biochemical, platelet and ultrastructural defects in the various types of oculocutaneous albinism. J Invest Dermatol. 1973;60:443–56.
44. Toyofuku K, Wada I, Spritz RA, Hearing VJ. The molecular basis of oculocutaneous albinism type 1 (OCA1): sorting failure and degradation of mutant tyrosinases results in a lack of pigmentation. Biochem J. 2001;355:259–69.
45. Brilliant MH. The mouse p (pink-eyed dilution) and human P genes, oculocutaneous albinism type 2 (OCA2), and melanosomal pH. Pigment Cell Res. 2001;14:86–93.
46. Rinchik EM, Bultman SJ, Horsthemke B, Lee ST, Strunk KM, Spritz RA, Avidano KM, Jong MTC, Nicholls RD. A gene for the mouse pink-eyed dilution locus and for human type II oculocutaneous albinism. Nature. 1993;361:72–6.
47. Lee ST, Nicholls RD, Bundey S, Laxova R, Musarella M, Spritz RA. Mutations of the P gene in oculocutaneous albinism, ocular albinism, and Prader-Willi syndrome plus albinism. N Engl J Med. 1994;330:529–34.
48. Rosemblat S, Sviderskaya EV, Easty DJ, Wilson A, Kwon BS, Bennett DC, Orlow SJ. Melanosomal defects in melanocytes from mice lacking expression of the pink-eyed dilution gene: correction by culture in the presence of excess tyrosine. Exp Cell Res. 1998;239:344–52.
49. Puri N, Gardner JM, Brilliant MH. Aberrant pH of melanosomes in pink-eyed dilution (p) mutant melanocytes. J Invest Dermatol. 2000;115:607–13.
50. Manga P, Orlow SJ. Inverse correlation between pink-eyed dilution protein expression and induction of melanogenesis by bafilomycin A1. Pigment Cell Res. 2001;14:362–7.
51. Chen K, Manga P, Orlow SJ. Pink-eyed dilution protein controls the processing of tyrosinase. Mol Biol Cell. 2002;13:1953–64.
52. Staleva L, Manga P, Orlow SJ. The pink-eyed dilution gene product controls arsenic sensitivity and cellular glutathione metabolism. Mol Biol Cell. 2002;13:4206–20.
53. Toyofuku K, Valencia JC, Kushimoto T, et al. The etiology of oculocutaneous albinism (OCA) type II: the pink protein modulates the processing and transport of tyrosinase. Pigment Cell Res. 2002;15:217–24.
54. Spritz RA. The molecular basis of human piebaldism. Pigment Cell Res. 1992;5:340–3.
55. Sarangarajan R, Boissy RE. Tyrp1 and oculocutaneous albinism type 3. Pigment Cell Res. 2001;14:437–44.
56. Newton JM, Cohen-Barak O, Hagiwara N, et al. Mutations in the human orthologue of the mouse underwhite gene (uw) underlie a new form of oculocutaneous albinism, OCA4. Am J Hum Genet. 2001;69:981–8.
57. Okoro AN. Albinism in Nigeria. Br J Dermatol. 1975;92:485–92.
58. Witkop CJ, Jr, Quevedo WC, Jr, Fitzpatrick TB, King RA. Albinism. In: Scriver CR, Beaudet AL, Sly WS, Valle D, editors. The metabolic basis of inherited disease. 6th ed. Vol. 2. New York: McGraw-Hill; 1989. pp. 2905–2947.
59. Bothwell JE. Pigmented skin lesions in tyrosinase-positive oculocutaneous albinos: a study in black South Africans. Int J Dermatol. 1997;36(11):831–6.
60. Kromberg JGR, Castle D, Zwane EM, Jenkins T. Albinism and skin cancer in Southern Africa. Clin Genet. 1989;36:43–52.
61. Perry PK, Silverberg NB. Cutaneous malignancy in albinism. Cutis. 2001;67(5):427–30.
62. Ward KA, Moss C, Sanders DS. Human piebaldism: relationship between phenotype and site of kit gene mutation. Br J Dermatol. 1995;132:929–35.
63. Thomas I, Kihiczac GG, Fox MD, et al. Piebaldism: an update. Int J Dermatol. 2004;43: 716–9.
64. Mahakrishnan A, Srinivasan MS. Piebaldism with Hirschprung's disease. Arch Dermatol. 1980;116:1102.

65. Angelo C, Cianchini G, Grosso MG, et al. Association of piebaldism and neurofibromatosis type 1 in a girl. Pediatr Dermatol. 2001;18:490–3.
66. Kiwan RA, Mutasim DF. Grover disease (transient acantholytic dermatosis) and piebaldism. Cutis. 2002;69:451–3.
67. Spritz RA, Beighton P. Piebaldism with deafness: molecular evidence for an expanded syndrome. Am J Med Genet. 1998;75:101–3.
68. Ezoe K, Holmes SA, Ho L, et al. Novel mutations and deletions of the KIT (steel factor receptor) gene in human piebaldism. Am J Hum Genet. 1995;56:58–66.
69. Sanchez-Martin M, Perez-Losada J, Rodriguez-Garcia A, et al. Deletion of the SLUG(SNAI2) gene results in human piebaldism. Am J Med Genet A. 2003;122:125–32.
70. Richards KA, Fukai K, Oiso N, et al. A novel KIT mutation results in piebaldism with progressive depigmentation. J Am Acad Dermatol. 2001;44:288–92.
71. Jimbow K, Fitzpatrick TB, Szabo G, et al. Congenital circumscribed hypomelanosis: a characterization based on electron microscopy study of tuberous sclerosis, nevus depigmentosus and piebaldism. J Invest Dermatol. 1975;64:50–62.
72. Falabella R, Barona M, Escobar C, et al. Surgical combination therapy for vitiligo and piebaldism. Dermatol Surg. 1995;21:852–7.
73. Njoo MD, Nieuweboer-Krobotova L, Westerhof W. Repigmentation of leucodermic defects in piebaldism by dermabrasion and thin split-thickness skin grafting in combination with minigrafting. Br J Dermatol. 1998;139:829–33.
74. Guerra L, Primavera G, Raskovic D, et al. Permanent repigmentation of piebaldism by erbium: YAG laser and autologous cultured epidermis. Br J Dermatol. 2004;150:715–21.
75. Kovac S. Vitiligo. J Am Acad Dermatol. 1998;38:647–66.
76. Kent G, Al'Abadie M. Psychologic effects of vitiligo: a critical incident analysis. J Am Acad Dermatol. 1996;35(6):895–8.
77. Halder RM, Chappell JL. Vitiligo update. Semin Cutan Med Surg. 2009;28(2):86–92.
78. Halder RM, Brooks HL. Medical therapies for vitiligo. Dermatol Ther. 2001;14:1–6.
79. Boisseau-Garsaud AM, Garsaud P, Calès-Quist D, Hélénon R, Quénéhervé C, Claire RC. Epidemiology of vitiligo in the French West Indies (Isle of Martinique). Int J Dermatol. 2000;39(1):18–20.
80. Falabella R, Barona M, Escobar C, Borrero I, Arrunategui A. Surgical combination therapy for vitiligo and piebaldism. Dermatol Surg. 1995;21(10):852–7.
81. Nordlund JJ, Ortonne J. The normal color of human skin. In: Nordlund JJ, Boissy RE, Hearing VJ, King RA, Ortonne J, editors. The pigmentary system. Physiology and pathophysiology. New York: Oxford University Press; 1988. p. 475–84.
82. Hann SK, Kim Y-S, Yoo JH, Chun YS. Clinical and histopathologic characteristics of trichrome vitiligo. J Am Acad Dermatol. 2000;42:589–96.
83. Falabella R. Surgical therapies for vitiligo. Clin Dermatol. 1997;15(6):927–39. Review.
84. Grimes PE. Melasma. Etiologic and therapeutic considerations. Arch Dermatol. 1995;131(12):1453–7. Review.
85. Halder RM, Young CM. New and emerging therapies for vitiligo. Dermatol Clin. 2000;18(1): 79–89.
86. Vitiligo JK. Therapeutic advances. Dermatol Clin. 1998;16(2):399–407.
87. Scherschun L, Kim JJ, Lim HW. Narrow-band ultraviolet B is a useful and well-tolerated treatment for vitiligo. J Am Acad Dermatol. 2001;44(6):999–1003.
88. Spencer JM, Nossa R, Ajmeri J. Treatment of vitiligo with the 30-nm excimer laser: a pilot study. J Am Acad Dermatol. 2002;46(5):727–31.
89. Westerhof W, Nieuweboer-Krobotova L. Treatment of vitiligo with UVB radiation vs topical psoralen plus UVA. Arch Dermatol. 1997;133(12):1525–8.
90. Passeron T, Ortonne JP. Use of the 308-nm excimer laser for psoriasis and vitiligo. Clin Dermatol. 2006;24:33–42.
91. Ortonne JP, Passeron T. Melanin pigmentary disorders: treatment update. Dermatol Clin. 2005;23:209–26.

92. Scherschun L, Kim JJ, Lim HW. Narrow-band ultraviolet B is a useful and well-tolerated treatment for vitiligo. J Am Acad Dermatol. 2001;44:999–1003.
93. Scherschun L, Kim JJ, Lim H. Narrow-band UVB is a useful and well-tolerated treatment for vitiligo. J Am Acad Dermatol. 2001;44:999–1003.
94. Arrunátegui A, Arroyo C, Garcia L, Covelli C, Escobar C, Carrascal E, Falabella R. Melanocyte reservoir in vitiligo. Int J Dermatol. 1994;33(7):484–7.
95. Halder RM, Grimes PE, McLaurin CI, Kress MA, Kenney Jr JA. Incidence of common dermatoses in a predominantly black dermatologic practice. Cutis. 1983;32(4):388–90.
96. Halder RM. Topical PUVA therapy for vitiligo. Dermatol Nurs. 1991;3(3):178–80, 98.
97. Halder RM, Taliaferro SJ. Vitiligo. In: Wolff K, Goldsmith LA, Katz SI, Gilchrest B, Paller A, Lefell D, editors. Fitzpatrick's dermatology in general medicine. 7th ed. New York: McGraw-Hill; 2008.
98. Bose SK. Modified Thiersch grafting in stable vitiligo. J Dermatol. 1996;23(5):362–4.
99. Mosher DB, Parrish JA, Fitzpatrick TB. Monobenzylether of hydroquinone. A retrospective study of treatment of 18 vitiligo patients and a review of the literature. Br J Dermatol. 1977;77(97):669–79.
100. Thissen M, Westerhof W. Laser treatment for further depigmentation in vitiligo. Int J Dermatol. 1997;36:386–8.

# Chapter 10
# Keloids

**Hilary Baldwin**

Keloidal scarring has been described by many cultures dating back as far as the Smith Papyrus in 3000 BC [1]. The Yoruba tribe of Western Africa gives us perhaps the most complete record of ancient knowledge with their painting and sculpture of keloids circa 1600 AD [2]. Despite this long history of knowledge and the explosion of medical care in other arenas, we have made minimal progress since the Yorubas toward understanding keloid prevention and eradication. No small measure of our current lack of consistently reliable, safe treatment measures is grounded in our ignorance of keloid pathogenesis. Prevention, too, is hampered by aspects of keloid occurrence that are out of our control. One can avoid trauma resulting from voluntary and elective procedures to adorn, augment, or improve. Aggressive prevention of keloids after accidental trauma and necessary surgery is also potentially within our abilities. However, most aspects of keloid formation are out of our control: ethnicity, skin pigmentation, age, gender, and genetic makeup. This chapter briefly reviews what is known about keloid epidemiology and pathogenesis in an effort to gain insight into the development of a rational treatment and prevention plan for these unsightly lesions.

## Epidemiology

The reported incidence of keloid formation is dependent on the population studied. It has been reported to range from a low of 0.09% in England to a high of 16% in Zaire [3]. Such variation is explained by numerous variables including race and

H. Baldwin, M.D. (✉)
State University of New York, 450 Clarkson Avenue, Box 46, Brooklyn, NY 11203, USA
e-mail: hbaldwin@downstate.edu

A.F. Alexis and V.H. Barbosa (eds.), *Skin of Color: A Practical Guide to Dermatologic Diagnosis and Treatment*, DOI 10.1007/978-0-387-84929-4_10,

**Table 10.1** Potential etiology factors for keloid formation

| |
|---|
| Trauma |
| Increased skin tension |
| Infectious skin diseases |
| Wound infections |
| Endocrine factors |
| Genetic predisposition |

degree of skin pigmentation. In predominately black and Hispanic populations, incidences between 4.5% and 16% have been reported [4]. Darkly pigmented individuals form keloids 2 to 19 times more frequently than Caucasians [5, 6]. But ethnicity, regardless of pigment intensity, is also a factor. In Aruba, more children of the lighter-skinned Polynesian population form keloids than those of African descent [7]. In Malaysia, those of Chinese descent are more prone to keloid formation than are the darker-skinned Indians and Malays [8]. Although Caucasians form keloids less frequently, those who do so can be very lightly complected; these patients are often among the most difficult to treat.

Older textbooks claim that keloids are rare in the young. However, keloids are reported at any age. In young children, the low incidence may be explainable by the rarity of significant skin trauma. Cosman et al. reported a median age of onset of 22.3 years and 22.6 years in women and men, respectively [9]. Keloid regression has been reported in postmenopausal women [9]. New keloid formation is relatively less common in the elderly. Aging fibroblasts may be less capable of collagen overproduction [10, 11]. In an unpublished study of 212 Caribbean-American and African-American keloid formers at Kings County Hospital, we found that age as an isolated factor did not correlate with keloid frequency. Rather, the timing of the pierce relative to puberty was predictive of keloid incidence.

Reporting bias and cultural practices are perhaps responsible for gender differences that have been reported in the literature. Multiple ear piercings are far more common in women than men as are the resulting keloids. Additionally, women may more readily seek medical attention for cosmetic improvement.

## Etiology

Theories regarding keloid etiology abound, and this is a reflection of our lack of understanding of the condition. The concept that is most enduring is that keloids occur following some form of skin trauma occurring in an individual with a genetic predisposition. Increased wound tension at the time of closure and trauma resulting from wound infection may also play a role (Table 10.1).

## *Trauma*

Although the concept of *spontaneous* keloiding has found its way into textbooks, trauma is probably a requisite for keloid formation. It may be that the severity of the trauma is sometimes so insignificant as to go unnoticed by the patient. Minor abrasions and burns, insect bites, varicella and zoster, vaccinations, and tattoos can result in significant keloiding. Acne lesions of the jaw, anterior chest, and deltoid areas often morph imperceptibly into keloids. Isotretinoin treatment in these patients can prevent additional keloids from forming even when the acne lesions are not readily identifiable.

However, trauma only serves as a potential *precipitating* etiologic factor. Deep and significant surgical wounds are often less likely to keloid than are the minor insults described above. We see drain site keloids next to the larger surgical wound that failed to keloid. Areas prone to trauma such as the hands and feet rarely keloid; this may be explained by evidence of a phenotypic difference between fibroblasts taken from earlobe keloids and palmar skin [12]. Interpatient variation is marked; patients experiencing the same trauma keloid differently. Less easy to explain is individual patient variability. It is a common observation that acne lesions immediately adjacent to each other heal differently and bilateral pierces or adjacent pierces often have different scar outcomes.

## *Skin Tension*

Keloids appear most commonly on the lateral jaw, anterior chest, upper back, and deltoid areas where skin tension is the highest. As they progress, they tend to stretch along skin tension lines, forming linear or bow tie-shaped lesions.

Closing a wound against the relaxed skin tension lines results in a wound with twice the tension of one closed along Langer's lines [13]. Postsurgical wound tension has been implicated as a contributing factor in keloid formation [14, 15]. Clearly, the loss of tissue that results from surgical excisions increases wound tension. Skin grafts may be preferable to primary closure of a tight wound; however, donor site keloids may occur. The use of tissue expanders to stretch the skin preoperatively offers an alternative that both reduces wound closure tension and applies pressure preoperatively that one could posit might help reduce postoperative fibroblast function.

Wound tension as a primary etiologic factor in keloid formation loses credibility when one considers the high incidence of earlobe keloids following piercing. The only tension in this loose, fleshy area is that created by the minor edema resulting from the trauma of the pierce. Chronic edema has been reported to increase glycosaminoglycans (GAGs) in the dermis [16]. It is unknown if the chronic edema caused by the pierce (and subsequent reaction to the presence of a metal foreign body) could result in increased incidence of keloid formation.

## Infection

There is no evidence to support the supposition that infectious agents themselves cause keloids. Previous case reports of keloids following infections with varicella, smallpox, syphilis, and tuberculosis were probably related to the trauma, edema, and increased skin tension that occurred as a result of wound infection [16, 17]. These reports still highlight the importance of assiduous avoidance and aggressive treatment of infectious diseases of the skin and wound infections, especially in the keloid-prone individual.

## Endocrine Factors

Multiple and diverse endocrine factors have been associated with keloid incidence, although causality is unproven. Keloids have been reported to grow more readily or to appear de novo during pregnancy [11, 14]. Keloids have been shown to be more common after puberty than before. This was well known by the Yorubas in the 1600s who knew how to pierce ears early in life to prevent keloiding. This has been demonstrated twice in more recent times. In a study at Kings County Hospital, ear pierces that resulted in keloids occurred at a median age of 6.4 years postmenarche, whereas those that did not keloid were pierced at a median age of 4.25 years premenarche [18]. Lane et al. found that earlobe keloids were far more likely to form in patients who were pierced after the age of 11 (80%) than before (23.5%) [19].

Melanocyte-stimulating hormone (MSH) has been postulated to play a role in keloid formation. This hypothesis is based on the observation that keloids are more common in patients with hyperpigmentation associated with pregnancy, puberty, and hyperthyroidism. Melanocytes in patients with skin of color may be more reactive to MSH than Caucasians, explaining the higher incidence of keloids in darker-skinned patients. Additionally, keloids are rare on the melanocyte-poor regions of the palms and soles. However, following the same logic, it is hard to explain why the highly pigmented skin of the genitalia so infrequently keloid. A final observation that defies explanation is that there has never been a reported case of keloid development in an albino patient, even one of African descent.

## Genetic Predisposition

There is no clear pattern of inheritance, but keloids are widely believed to have a familial predisposition [3, 20]. In our study at Kings County Hospital, we found a familial history in 32% of keloid formers [18]. It remains to be seen if the familial tendency to keloid is genetically inherited or if it is merely related to the similarity of skin coloration between family members.

## Pathogenesis

Our understanding of keloid pathogenesis is composed of numerous isolated facts that as yet fail to form a cohesive picture. The simple answer to the pathogenesis puzzle is that keloid formation is caused by an increase in anabolic activity; why this happens is not known.

After wounding takes place, various signals are sent to the neighboring fibroblasts, triggering an increase in collagen and glycosaminoglycan (GAG) production. Upon completion of the rebuilding task, the fibroblasts are signaled to return to prewound status. Abnormalities in these signals, particularly those that indicate reduction in collagen production, are believed to be responsible for keloid growth. Interferons may be one of those "stop" signals. In normal wounds, there is regression of connective tissue elements after the third week. In keloid tissue, however, fibroblasts proliferate around the plentiful new and dilated capillaries. Collagen synthesis and GAG synthesis are markedly increased; collagen synthesis is 20 times greater in keloids than in normal skin [21, 22]. The absolute number of fibroblasts within the entire keloid is not increased, and they appear histologically normal, but the activity of proline hydroxylase is markedly elevated, suggesting that the rate of collagen biosynthesis is increased in a normally sized fibroblast population [21, 23].

Although collagenase is also increased, collagen degradation is not, possibly due to an increased deposition of alpha globulins within the keloid [24, 25]. Serum alpha globulins are known inhibitors of collagenase [24]. Estrogens increase the level of serum alpha globulins which may help to explain the increased incidence of keloids in pregnant women [24]. Corticosteroids, in contrast, have been shown to reduce the alpha globulin deposits within keloids [24]. They too may act by increasing activation of collagenase with subsequent breakdown and resorption of the excessive collagen and subsequent clinical flattening [25].

Keloid fibroblasts also appear to resist programmed cell death [26, 27]. Defective apoptosis within keloids may be due to a dysfunctional p53 gene. Injectable interferon may be effective in treating keloids by its enhancement of native p53.

## Clinical Manifestations

Keloids rarely represent a clinical diagnostic dilemma except for the occasional challenge posed by the differential diagnosis between a hypertrophic scar and a newly forming keloid (Table 10.2). This is not simply an academic debate; the two lesions respond quite differently to therapy. A mature, aged keloid presents little clinical confusion. It is the early, pruritic, relatively flat, red keloid that can be a difficult diagnosis. Hypertrophic scars generally develop rapidly after surgery, whereas keloids may occur months after the inciting trauma. Hypertrophic scars tend to subside with time, while keloids generally progress, most eventually reaching a size or time when they cease growing and become stable. Keloids rarely, if

**Table 10.2** Clinical differences between keloids and hypertrophic scars

| Hypertrophic scars | Keloids |
|---|---|
| Develop rapidly after trauma | May develop years after inciting trauma |
| Often spontaneously subside with time | Rarely regress but eventually stabilize |
| Shape commensurate with trauma | Exceeds footprint of original trauma |
| Common in mobile skin/across joints | Common in areas with limited mobility |
| Respond more readily to therapy | Often recur/may worsen after surgery |

ever, regress. Hypertrophic scars achieve a shape that is commensurate with the size and shape of the preceding trauma, whereas keloids exceed – sometimes greatly – the extent of the initial trauma. Hypertrophic scars are more likely to occur in areas prone to excessive motion such as those across joints. Keloids are most often found in areas in which there is limited motion such as the chest and back. Careful and thoughtful surgical and therapeutic planning often results in resolution of the hypertrophic scar. Keloids (except perhaps on the earlobe) nearly always recur following excisional surgery unless adjunctive therapy is implemented. The postoperative keloid recurrence is frequently worse than the initial lesion.

During their active growth phase, keloids are generally symptomatic. Patients complain of itching, burning, pain, and pulling. The sensation of pain can be the result of a lesion that is, in itself, tender or because of rubbing of the keloid against other body parts or external objects. Most patients seek care for keloids for cosmetic improvement. However, some are concerned primarily or solely with relief of itch and pain. Older, mature, and stable keloids are less symptomatic except when rubbed or manipulated. Pain can be used to determine lesion activity as increased symptomatology is often a clinical sign of lesion progression. Resolution of symptoms during treatment is often rapid and can be used as a guide to treatment success. Once the symptoms are alleviated, the patient may choose to discontinue therapy.

Keloids of the jaw, neck, and anterior chest can also cause dysfunction. Patients with large lesions of the jaw and neck may be unable to fully turn the head from side to side or to extend or flex the neck (Fig. 10.1). Keloids of the midchest often pull breast or adipose tissue toward the center of the chest, creating the sensation of tightness and/or the appearance of cleavage (Fig. 10.2). The latter is particularly troublesome to male patients. Complete lesion eradication is often not necessary to alleviate the dysfunction. Portions of the lesions tethering the skin can be excised to improve mobility, or high-dose corticosteroid injections can be used to intentionally cause atrophy with resultant skin relaxation.

Large keloids of hair-bearing areas often trap terminal hairs beneath them. Periodically, the patient will present with sudden swelling and pain. The keloid will be fluctuant or ballottable with evident drainage. Over time, a sinus tract may develop, often with numerous orifices. Excision of, at minimum, the immediate surrounding tissue is usually necessary, but these patients may respond temporarily to a short course of oral antibiotics.

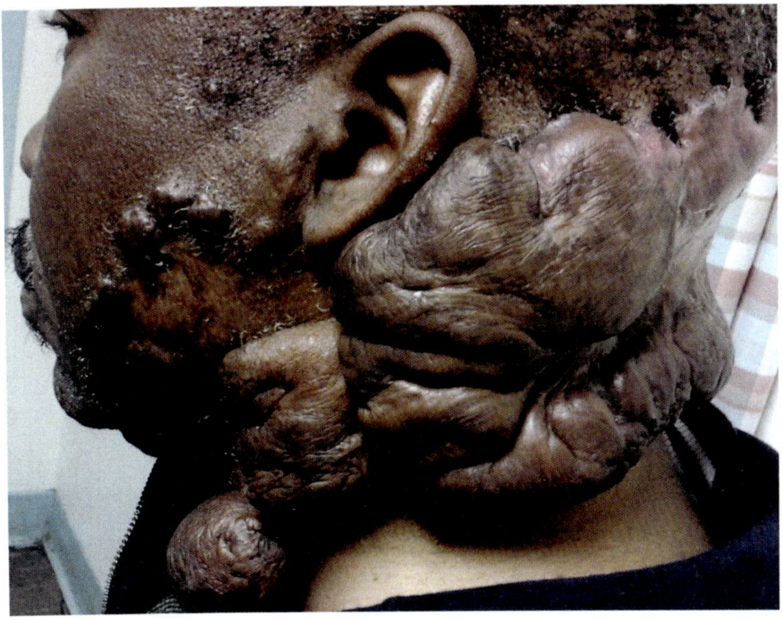

**Fig. 10.1** Mobility reduction resulting from keloids

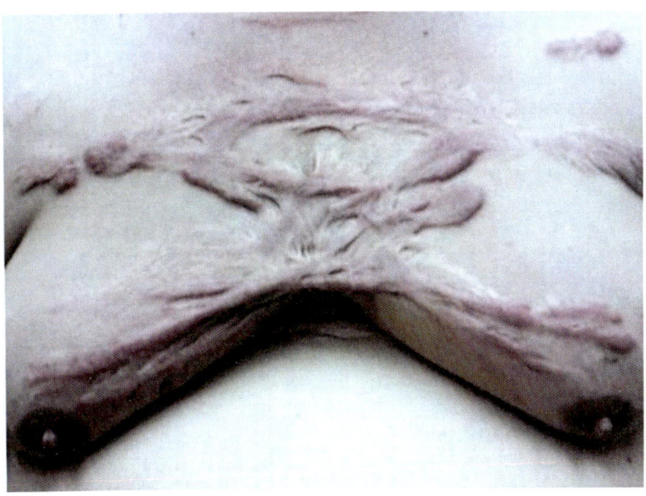

**Fig. 10.2** Tightening and pulling resulting from midchest keloid

Lastly, the morphology and location of the lesion will often dictate the therapeutic plan. Pedunculated lesions, particularly when they occur on soft, mobile skin such as the axilla or earlobe, are amenable to simple excisional surgery. Tight, flat, sessile keloids such as those on the anterior chest, upper back, and deltoid areas are

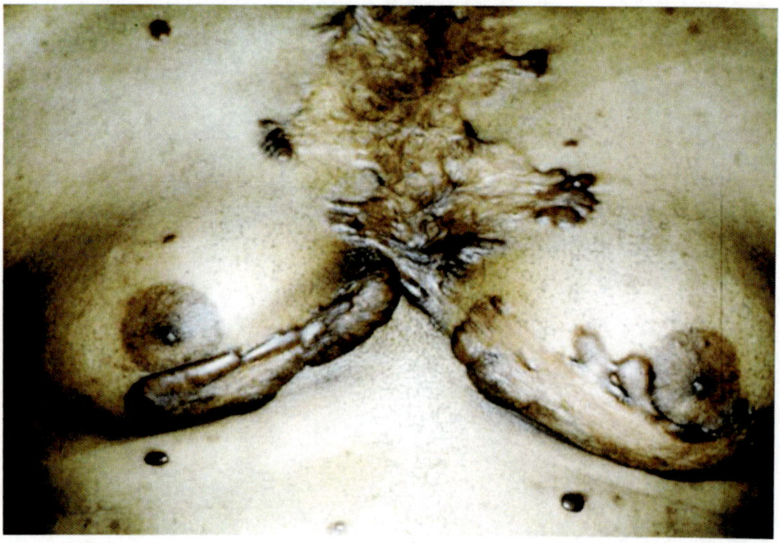

**Fig. 10.3** Flat, tight, sessile keloids

poor surgical candidates with high recurrence risk; these lesions will respond best to pharmacologic therapy (Fig. 10.3). Earlobe keloids come in five clinical varieties: anterior button, posterior button, dumbbell, wraparound, and lobular. Button keloids have small-diameter stalks and can be shaved off in their entirety. Dumbbell keloids have two buttons and a core component within the lobe. Wraparound keloids form a cuff around the lobe from one side to the other. Lobular keloids entirely replace the fatty lobe and frequently represent postoperative recurrences. Wraparound and lobular keloids often require wedge excisions for complete removal (see treatment techniques: surgery).

## Treatment Techniques

In any medical inquiry, a scholarly literature review of available therapeutic options demands attention to study design and validity of conclusions. This is nowhere more evident than in the field of keloidal scarring in which one must sift through large numbers of anecdotal reports and pure conjecture. The problem begins with the absence of the delineation of hypertrophic scars from keloids (Table 10.2). Many studies include both entities in the inclusion criteria yet fail to reveal which lesions ultimately responded to therapy. Other patient and lesion characteristics routinely omitted from these studies include such important factors as patient race and age, lesion age and symptomatology, lesion size and location, prior operative history, and lesion morphology (sessile vs. pedunculated or dome-shaped). Most reports also

**Table 10.3** Therapeutic options for keloids

| |
|---|
| **Treatment of existing keloids** |
| *Monotherapy* |
| Corticosteroid injections |
| 5-FU injections |
| *Polytherapy* |
| Surgical or laser removal followed by prevention techniques |
| **Prevention of occurrence/recurrence** |
| *Pharmacologic modalities* |
| Corticosteroid injections |
| Interferon injections |
| Imiquimod application |
| 5-Fluorouracil injections |
| Verapamil injections |
| Bleomycin injections |
| *Physical modalities* |
| Radiation therapy |
| Vascular lasers |
| Silicone products |
| Topical scar preparations |
| Cryotherapy |
| Compression techniques |

suffer from inadequate follow-up time of less than 6 months. It is an undisputable truth that keloid removal is easy; the art is found in preventing recurrence.

In a recent review article, Shaffer et al. concluded that despite a plethora of papers on the topic of keloids, "...there are no definitive treatment protocols" [28]. This is a result of studies that are uncontrolled and/or poorly designed in which the endpoint of therapy (cosmesis, function, or symptom reduction) is rarely identified. The only modality to meet their standards for evidence-based therapy was postsurgical radiation therapy. Mustoe et al. also lamented the absence of well-controlled studies and concluded that corticosteroid injection and silicone gel sheeting (SGS) are the "...only treatments for which sufficient evidence exists to make evidence-based recommendations" [29]. Durani and Bayat found SGS and laser therapy to have the highest level of support, albeit subpar [30]. Leventhal et al. noted that "most treatments for keloidal and hypertrophic scarring offer minimal likelihood of improvement" [31]. Other treatments at this time are still lacking the proof of efficacy that arises only from a well-designed, randomized, placebo-controlled trial with adequate patient numbers. The nature of keloid therapy is such that a comparison of various techniques is often not amenable to double-blinding. We therefore look forward to more studies in which single techniques are compared to controls, vehicles, or dummy therapy.

Regardless of the fact that most keloid treatment and prevention techniques are not evidence-based, we utilize what we have to treat the patients in our care. Presented below are the techniques that have become the standard of care in the field despite the lack of conclusive data (Table 10.3).

## *Corticosteroids*

Because of their ease of administration, low cost, and low side effect potential, intralesional corticosteroids alone and in combination are the workhorses of keloid therapy. Corticosteroids are one of the only agents that can be used to treat existing keloids as solo therapy without prior surgical removal. One of the most successful uses of corticosteroids, however, lies in its use postoperatively to prevent keloid occurrence or recurrence. Although no solid evidence-based literature supports its use in these roles, it has justifiably become the first-line approach of most physicians dealing with this condition worldwide.

The effect of corticosteroids on collagen synthesis and degradation is not completely understood. In young keloids, they have been shown to increase the production of collagenase and reduce the collagenase-inhibiting alpha globulins [24]. TNF-β may also play a role [32]. Corticosteroid injections postoperatively have been shown to downregulate the type I collagen gene expression [33].

### Solo Therapy for Existing Keloids

When used as solo therapy, corticosteroids are most useful in sessile, flat, and broad keloids. These lesions will flatten and soften, become less erythematous; symptoms will improve or resolve. However, the lesion will not be fully eradicated. It is important that the patient be cognizant of this as well as the fact that the appearance of the skin will never normalize. The overall lateral dimensions or "footprint" of the keloid will not improve; in fact, footprints often enlarge with therapy. When explaining realities of treatment to the patient, it is often helpful to use the modeling clay analogy: as a dome-shaped keloid is flattened, it will become wider. Although this does not always happen, it is a prudent concept to bring into the informed consent process.

Corticosteroids are less helpful as solo therapy in pedunculated or particularly thick lesions. Although they may be useful for palliation of symptoms, repeated injections into a pedunculated or high, dome-shaped keloid will soften and shrink the keloidal tissue, rendering it a saggy pouch that will eventually need to be excised. An argument can be made, however, that the saggy pouch is more amenable to surgical excision with relaxed closure than was the parent lesion.

Corticosteroids generally have an impressive *initial* effect on existing keloids; durability of response is not always a guarantee. Patients often report improvement in symptomatology within a week. Softening occurs more slowly, appearing after the second or third injection. This seemingly minor clinical improvement represents a therapeutic milestone and is almost never noted by the patient. It is worthwhile to bring to the patient's attention as it heralds a more rapid phase of clinical improvement; softer keloids allow more thorough infiltration of the steroid. Ultimately, after many injections, the lesion will appear flatter and/or smaller. Unfortunately, this response may prove to be temporary. Some patients may need to return after several months for repeat treatments. Completely flattened, soft, and non-erythematous lesions are less likely to recur than are partially treated keloids. Kiil [34] and Griffith [35] reported recurrences of 50% at 5 years and 11.2% at 4 years, respectively.

Depending on keloid size, shape, age, and location, various dilutions of triamcinolone acetonide (TAC) can be used. The most common cause of corticosteroid failure is insufficient concentration. A keloid occurring in thin skin is still a keloid and should be treated as such; the injection (at least in theory) is into the body of the keloid, not the skin upon which it arose. Concentrations less than 10 mg/cc are rarely effective in a mature keloid; most will require 40 mg/cc. This means that the total area treated in one session may be limited by total safe dose constraints. It is important not to spread the injections too thin but rather to deliver adequate amounts of corticosteroid to a smaller area, perhaps smaller than the full lesion. Exactly what constitutes a safe dose is unclear. The standard of care has always been to inject no more than 40 mg per monthly session. The source of this "rule" is not identifiable but is clearly based on the desire not to suppress the hypothalamic-pituitary axis. However, 40 mg of triamcinolone per month is the dosage equivalent of approximately 50 mg of prednisone per month. A higher dose delivered monthly would still be within most physicians' comfort zone, particularly in a heavier individual. This concept must be kept in mind when planning the surgical excision of an existing keloid. It is imprudent to remove more keloid volume than can be subsequently injected for recurrence prevention; partial, staged excisions may therefore be preferable.

When the keloid is particularly large, or when a patient presents with numerous lesions, choices must be made. Diluting the steroid to "get it all" is destined to failure. Spreading the injections too thin is similarly ineffective. Better to query the patient as to which lesion or which area of a large keloid is most symptomatic or bothersome. Utilize the entire allotment in the area chosen and save other areas for another day. With subsequent treatments, the strength of the steroid can be reduced in order to fine-tune the ultimate outcome. The remainder can be utilized in the next area of patient preference.

Injections can be repeated every 2–4 weeks, depending on the strength/total dose of steroid used and the size of the keloid. Although additional areas may be injected on the following weeks, it is best not to inject the same area with high concentrations at less than 2-week intervals. The depot effect of the steroids is such that repeat injections done too close together can result in too much thinning too fast, leaving an atrophic area. Hypopigmentation is also more likely in this setting.

Occasionally, mature keloids are so firm that injection is impossible. In this case, the deposition of steroid into the needle tract may be the only option. In order to be effective, multiple parallel tracts must be made with a large-bore (23 G or larger) needle. Luer-lock syringes are essential to avoid disconnect and backsplashes. Because of the high pressure within the firm keloid, the steroids will start to leak out the moment the needle is removed. This can be avoided by applying a small drop of cyanoacrylate glue to the hole *prior to injection* followed by rapid application of precut plastic tape immediately upon withdrawal of the needle.

Patients with very firm keloids generally require some form of anesthesia in order to make the requisite number of tracts. For pain control, topical eutectic mixtures of local anesthetics are unhelpful. The pain the patient experiences with these injections is not that of the needle passing through the epidermis; the pain is deeper and appears to be related to the displacement of the fibrotic tissue by the force of the liquid. Often a ripping sound is audible. This pain is beyond the scope of the topical anesthetics, even after hours of occlusion. However, they can be used to numb the skin *surrounding* the keloid in preparation for a lidocaine ring block. Mixing lidocaine with corticosteroid makes little difference as the pain of the injection is over before the lidocaine takes effect. Lidocaine will, however, help those uncommon patients who complain of persistent postinjection pain.

### Corticosteroids as Solo Therapy for Keloid Prevention

Corticosteroids are an integral part of keloid prevention – both for de novo occurrence in a new surgical wound in a known keloid former and for recurrence following keloid excision. This author follows the following injection schedule:

- On the day of surgery and then at 2, 4, and 6 weeks, the wound base and margins are injected with TAC 40 mg/cc regardless of the appearance of the wound.
- At 2 months and every month thereafter, injections are given as clinically necessary. At that point, dosage of the corticosteroids given at each session is determined clinically by the site, size, degree of firmness, and symptoms the patient is experiencing.
- Preventative therapy is best carried out for one full year; early discontinuation is associated with a higher incidence of unnecessary recurrences.

### Corticosteroids as Part of Polytherapy for Keloid Prevention

Corticosteroids can be combined with any other treatment modality to improve outcome. Following surgical excision, many authors have shown a reduction in recurrence rates with the addition of postoperative corticosteroids [36, 37]. Combinations with cryotherapy and silicone gel sheets have been shown to be superior to either modality alone [38]. Corticosteroids plus alpha interferon have been shown to be more effective than corticosteroids alone [39, 40]. Combinations with lasers and alpha interferon also have shown promise [41].

### Corticosteroid Side Effects

Common side effects of steroid injections include hypopigmentation and skin atrophy (Fig. 10.4). Although technically an adverse reaction, hypopigmentation is often a marker of clinical success, and skin atrophy is frequently a necessary consequence of adequate therapy. It is prudent to prepare patients for both sequelae. Hypopigmentation, when it occurs, can be pronounced and may last 6–12 months before resolving. In this authors' experience, patients are consistently less bothered by the dyspigmentation than the keloid that preceded it. The risk of both hypopigmentation and atrophy can

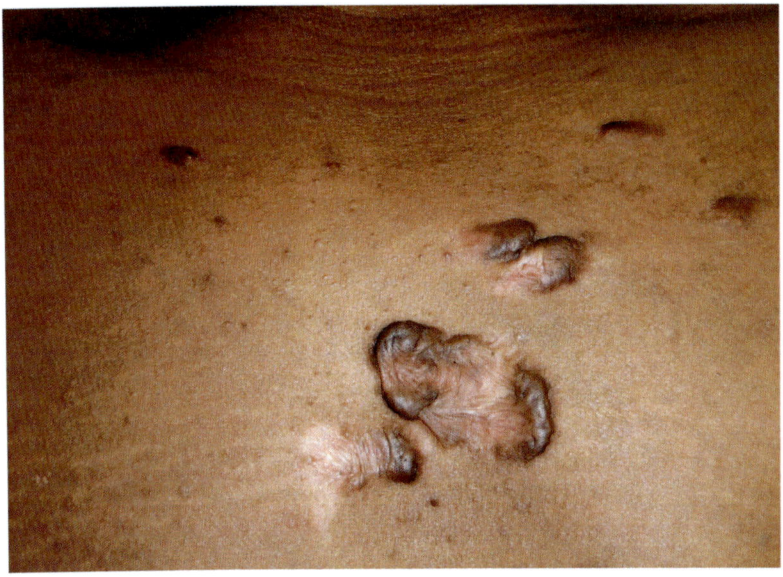

**Fig. 10.4** Corticosteroid side effect

be reduced by avoiding accidental injections into the surrounding normal tissue. This most often occurs when attempting to force steroids into a particularly firm keloid. A good rule of thumb is *either* to push harder *or* to redirect the needle but not both simultaneously. This helps to avoid the sudden dump of steroids into the softer subcutis or surrounding skin. Extensive misplacement of steroids can cause temporary linear hypopigmentation or atrophy extending out from the treatment site. After treatment, the atrophic footprint of the keloid may appear wrinkled or shiny, and telangiectasias are common. This appearance improves with time. Desiccation of prominent vessels is generally effective; alternatively, vascular lasers can be utilized to lessen the telangiectasias. Since pulsed dye lasers have been demonstrated to produce a small but perceptible improvement in relatively flat erythematous scars, they might have dual advantages in this regard (see laser therapy below).

## *Surgery*

Surgical removal of keloids is often necessary. Large, bulky keloids will respond poorly to solo treatment with corticosteroid injections. Surgical debridement also allows for the use of adjunctive techniques that are ineffective in preexisting keloids but useful postoperatively. Surgical techniques will vary according to the size, location, and shape of the keloid. Pedunculated keloids with narrow bases can be tangentially excised and closed primarily with little wound tension. Sessile keloids with broad bases are much more difficult to treat surgically. Wound closure will be a challenge, and healing by secondary intention may be preferable.

Surgical monotherapy results in a high incidence of recurrence, often 50–100% [37, 42]. The surgical removal of a keloid is easy; it is prevention of recurrence that is the art. Surgery must be combined with adjunctive techniques, often for prolonged periods of time. Several general rules of thumb are indicated:

- *Use the smallest incision possible*
  The smallest incision possible is made, minimizing trauma that might lead to the increased risk of recurrence and maximizing useful epidermis. This generally means extending the initial incision less than the entire length of the keloid. Dissect off any usable epidermis from the keloid for ease of closure.
- *Remove all keloidal tissue if possible*
  Unless it would result in gross deformity or loss of function, all of the keloidal material should be removed. Dogma has it that remaining keloid serves as a nidus for keloid reformation. Although data are scarce, this does appear to be a truism. Care should be taken to remove any trapped hairs. If left behind, they will in-grow, ultimately causing an inflammatory response that has no outlet. Patients will report repeated episodes of the sudden onset of tenderness and swelling followed by drainage.
- *Minimize wound tension*
  Closure should be done with the least amount of wound tension possible. In a large wound with significant tension, surgery followed by grafting alone may result in a superior nonrecurrence rate over primary closure [20]. However, donor site keloids are possible. Tissue expanders may be preferable in this situation.
- *Suture considerations*
  Whenever possible, nonreactive and monofilament suture should be used to reduce the incidence of wound infection, abscess formation, and inflammation along the suture line. It is said, but not supported by study, that buried sutures may serve as a nidus for keloid reformation. Underutilization of buried sutures, however, is likely to result in wound dehiscence; this seems to be especially true in keloid patients. In fact, superficial sutures often need to be left in longer than usual to prevent dehiscence. The injection of steroids postoperatively also increases the risk of dehiscence. If the resulting wound is fairly superficial or very broad and the patient is amenable, allowing the wound to heal by secondary intention often results in better cosmetic outcome and a lower incidence of recurrence. Some surgeons have recommended that if the lesion is too large to be closed primarily, a rim of keloid tissue should be left behind to act as a splint to prevent excessive central tensile contraction [43]. A full-thickness skin graft is placed on top.

## Earlobe Keloids

It behooves us to consider earlobe keloids as separate entities as they respond differently to intervention. Many authors have noted a lower rate of keloid recurrence in the earlobe [44–46]. Studies have shown a recurrence rate of only 41% after surgery alone [45]. Studies utilizing both surgery and corticosteroids have shown recurrence

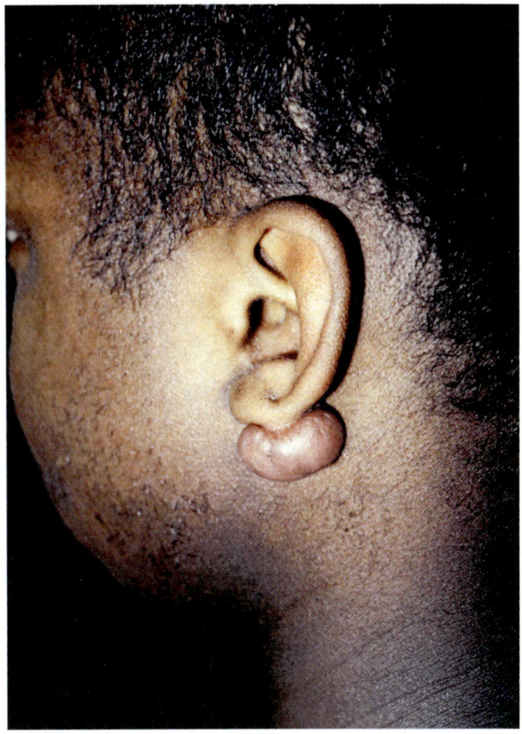

**Fig. 10.5** Button keloid

rates of 1–20% [47–49]. Surgery with adjunctive radiation therapy has resulted in recurrence rates of 0–8.6% [47, 50–52]. With careful, aggressive therapy and using multiple postoperative modalities, earlobe keloids rarely recur.

Better surgical results on earlobes probably result from several factors. First-time earlobe lesions tend to be very discrete and easily separated from the surrounding dermis and epidermis. Complete removal of all keloidal tissue is thus easily accomplished. Most earlobe keloids occur in women who are profoundly motivated to wear earrings again and are far more compliant than the average keloid patient. The fleshy tissue of the ear makes closure without tension easier to accomplish. Postoperative pressure, a highly effective but inconvenient adjunctive therapy elsewhere on the body, is easily applied with the use of pressure earrings. These earrings are not particularly cosmetically appealing, but the patients find them easy to wear and comfortable. They also make an ideal postoperative dressing, obviating the need for bulky, and often inadequate, pressure dressings.

As mentioned earlier, earlobe keloids come in five varieties, and the surgery for each is approached differently (Figs. 10.5, 10.6, and 10.7):

*Anterior and posterior buttons* – Posterior button keloids are by far the most common earlobe lesions that we see; both anterior and posterior buttons are the easiest to treat. Simple shave followed by secondary intention healing is often sufficient; however, the adjunctive use of postoperative corticosteroids is prudent.

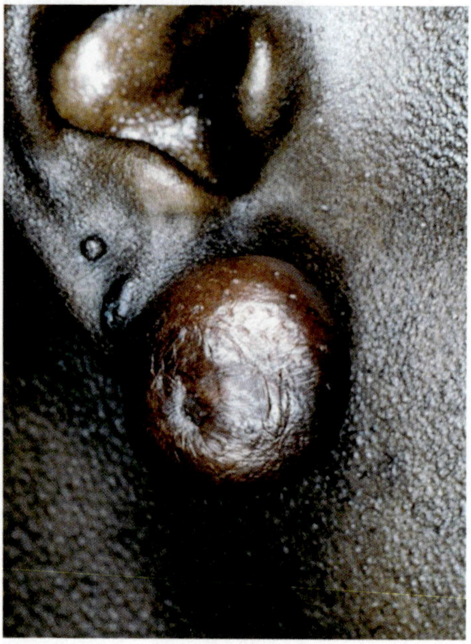

**Fig. 10.6** Anterior button keloid

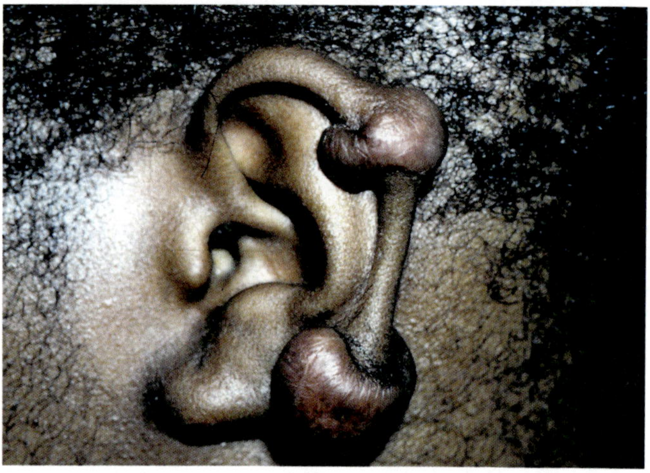

**Fig. 10.7** Wraparound keloid

*Dumbbell keloids* (anterior and posterior button keloids connected by a smaller intralobal core of keloid tissue) are more complicated to treat. In 1983, Salasche and Grabski reported a novel and elegant method for removing dumbbell keloids [53]. In this method, the anterior and posterior portions of the keloid were first dissected away from the earlobe. Then the core within the lobe was dissected from the normal lobular subcutis and the entire keloid removed en bloc through the posterior opening. An alternative and simpler method is to shave off the anterior and posterior buttons, allowing visualization and palpation of the firm tissue remaining within the adipose tissue of the earlobe. The diameter of the core is measured and punched out with a disposable punch at least 1 mm larger than the core itself. A useful trick is to close the defect horizontally on the anterior surface of the lobe and vertically on the posterior lobe to prevent a pointed lobe.

*Lobular and wraparound keloids* – Small lesions are best excised in a wedge with primary closure. Huge lobular keloids, wraparound, and multilobular recurrent keloids are the most difficult to manage. Removal of the entire keloid is preferable but may well leave no functioning lobe. A woman who chooses to adorn her earlobes will tell you that a perfectly keloid-free ear is not a successful outcome if earrings are not wearable. One option is to sculpt the lobe removing as much keloid as possible, leaving an earlobe-shaped keloid and relying on postoperative techniques to prevent recurrence. This is not a time for monotherapy or single adjunct therapy. Extensive postoperative treatment with radiation therapy *and* silicone gel *and* corticosteroid injections and interferon injection *and* pressure often prevents the regrowth of the keloid. Once the lobe-shaped keloid ages, it generally becomes stable and functional. Pressure earrings may be necessary for 6–18 months (or even permanently) after this technique, but the patients do not seem to mind as they have some adornment on a functioning lobe.

## Laser Surgery

After initial excitement over the demonstrated ability of the CO2 laser to decrease fibroblast activity in vitro, its use in keloid therapy was a disappointment [54, 55]. Used in the defocused mode, recurrence rate is extremely high [56]. In the focused mode, recurrence rate is similar to surgery alone (50–70%) [54, 57]. The Nd-YAG laser has been demonstrated to cause an in vitro selective bioinhibition of collagen production but recurrence rates of 53–100% in vivo [58]. The combination of UltraPulse CO2 laser and interferon injections was reported by Conejo-Mir [59]. Thirty lesions were treated with three million units thrice weekly for 9 weeks, resulting in 10/14 recurrences on the trunk and 0/16 recurrences on the ear at 3 years. This is similar to recurrence rates for conventional surgical removal.

The pulsed dye laser has been reported to improve HTS symptoms, decrease scar height, and improve skin texture. Alster and Williams showed a 57–83% improvement with the 585-nm flashlamp-pumped PDL in the prevention of keloids in sternotomy scars [60]. They noted the importance of starting therapy early for the best results. It has been proposed that the PDL decreases the microvasculature in early keloids and hypertrophic scars resulting in anoxia. Several combination studies have shown that PDL works better in combination with other modalities including corticosteroids, interferon, and carbon dioxide laser [61–64].

## *Radiation Therapy*

The mechanism of action of radiation therapy (RT) on keloidal tissue and prevention of keloids is unknown. Its preferential effectiveness in early keloids suggests that it may decrease fibroblast collagen synthesis [65]. Alternatively, it may act by decreasing vascular hyperplasia [66].

RT alone is ineffective in the eradication of existing keloids, although it may resolve the pruritus associated with the lesion [65, 67]. In a study of over 300 patients, RT alone at a total dose of 800–2,400 rads over 2–5 months was only effective in reducing keloids which were within 6 months of initiation [65–68]. Mature, thicker keloids require excision prior to radiation therapy [69, 70].

For prophylaxis in keloid-prone individuals, X-radiation, electron beam, and interstitial radiation have all been reported to be equally effective (recurrence rates near 20% – far superior to other modalities) [71–73]. Dosing schedule and fractionation vary greatly from one study to another, but outcomes are similar. A minimum of 1,000 rads or equivalent appears to be the common consensus for successful outcome, but the protocol seems to matter little [74]. Kal and Veen concluded that radiation therapy should be done within 2 days of surgical removal and that short treatment durations and "relatively high doses" are necessary [75]. In a study of earlobe keloids, surgery plus RT was compared to surgery plus corticosteroids [47]. Recurrence rates were 12.5% and of 33%, respectively. Recurrence rates of 4.7% with high-dose-rate brachytherapy [76], 21% with interstitial iridium-192 [77], and 16%, 19%, and 32% with electron beam [78–80] have been demonstrated. Recurrence rates have been shown to be higher in areas of high tension such as the chest, scapula, and suprapubic areas in three studies [79–81]. The short treatment plan required with RT may aid in patient compliance.

Despite its documented success in preventing keloid recurrence, RT is underutilized by many clinicians due to largely unfounded concerns regarding the long-term risks of malignancy of the skin or underlying structures. Numerous large studies report a carcinogenesis rate of 0% [74]. Literature review reveals only one reported case of squamous cell carcinoma arising in post-keloid radiation site, and the causality is unclear [82]. Botwood et al. attempted to put these concerns into perspective [74]. In more than 100 years in clinical use, there are only three case reports of internal malignancies occurring post-RT for a keloid. Breast cancer in a 57-year-old-woman occurring 29 years after RT to a chest keloid was reported in 1999 [74]. Breast cancer in a 36-year-old-woman 23 years after chest wall keloid radiation was reported in 1982 [83]. In both cases, confounding variables were also evident (7-year history of hormone replacement therapy and evidence of unusually high radiation doses, respectively). A single case report of thyroid cancer occurring in a 27-year-old-man 8 years after RT to a keloid of the chin has also been reported [84]. In this case, histopathology was consistent with a *medullary* carcinoma; radiation-induced carcinomas of the thyroid are primarily *papillary* carcinomas [85]. Based on dosimetry studies, RT in standard dosages to the ear with proper shielding would expose the ipsilateral thyroid lobe to only 2 rads [74].

The data therefore do not warrant a high level of concern with the use of RT. Common side effects to consider are skin atrophy, radiation dermatitis, abnormal skin pigmentation, and local alopecia. RT is not generally recommended in growing children. Alternatively, the metaphyses must be shielded to prevent retardation of bone growth which may occur at doses of 400 R and less [86].

## *Compression Therapy*

Compression therapy – applying pressure greater than that of capillary pressure (24 mmHg) – causes a reduction in soft tissue cellularity. Histopathology shows increased interstitial space and collagen bundles that are more widely dispersed [87]. It is theorized that pressure creates hypoxia resulting in fibroblast degeneration and subsequent collagen reduction.

Pressure alone is ineffective in the treatment of existing keloids. However, dressings which apply more than 24 mmHg, worn 24 h a day for 4–6 months, may be successful in reducing keloid recurrence rates postoperatively. Not all areas are amenable to pressure dressings, which in any event are uncomfortable, hot, and unsightly. As with all compression garments, they are difficult and time-consuming to don. Ears are the exception to this rule. Newer pressure earrings have large compression plates for improved comfort and are easily worn all day long. In order to accommodate the large surface area, the earrings are necessarily broad and bulky. Young patients are often dismayed by the cosmetic appearance of the "grandma earrings," and most males will not wear them at all in public. The earrings called "sleepers" are the same product without the adornments. They are intended to be more comfortable for nighttime use, but their smaller size makes them less conspicuous, and many patients prefer them for daytime use as well. Those intended for "heavy lobes" are always more appropriate postoperatively when the lobe is edematous from the procedure and the healing process. "Thin lobe" earrings may become necessary as the time goes on in order to provide continued consistent pressure.

The most complicated aspect of compression therapy is determining when it is safe to discontinue use. In this author's opinion, pressure can be stopped when overnight discontinuation fails to result in swelling of the affected area. This generally takes 4–6 months but may occur earlier. It is useful to remind the patient that this noninvasive technique is better used in overkill.

Kosaka and Kamiishi reported an interesting compression device for more difficult areas such as the trunk [87]. They created a vest into which was sewn the balloon and rubber tubing from a neonatal sphygmomanometer. The balloon was placed over the area to be compressed and inflated to the desired pressure. This was particularly good for the anterior chest as it fit well over the concave and uneven surfaces without the use of tape. There was minimal pain and overheating, and the balloon did not displace. Utilizing a spandex shirt allows for laundering and works equally well; the cost of the shirt, sphygmomanometer, and tailor fee is around $100.

## Silicone Products

Silicone gel sheeting (SGS) has been touted in many studies to be efficacious in preventing the development of hypertrophic scars and keloids [88–90]. These studies are marred by the absence of blinding and control, small patient numbers, retrospective design, inadequate follow-up time, and the inclusion of both keloids and hypertrophic scars within the same treatment group. Keeping these confounding factors in mind, these studies have shown that existing keloids may decrease in size by as much as 30% when the gels are applied 24 h a day consistently for 2 months [88]. SGS has been shown in small studies to reduce hypertrophic scar formation by as much as 70% when used consistently [90]. Consistency and duration are the key; they must be worn over a scar for 2–3 months, 12–24 h a day, to prevent scar development [91]. Sheets are available in varying thicknesses and consistency [92]. Although some are sticky, adhesive tape is necessary for consistent application and may be uncomfortable. A formulation of silicone gel that is self-drying has been reported [93]. It forms a flexible and transparent sheet after application, obviating the need for tape.

The mechanism of action of silicone gel sheeting is unknown, and many theories have been proposed. SGS is known to retard epidermal water loss. The drier agents have been shown to create static electricity which some believe to play a role in their effectiveness. In a controlled, prospective non-blinded study, SGS was compared to an occlusive dressing without silicone [94]. SGS was not found to be superior, leading the authors to conclude that it was wound hydration, not the presence of silicone that was responsible for the clinical effect. Occlusive dressings are markedly cheaper.

## Interferon

As discussed previously, fibroblast activity increases dramatically after wounding. Once the wound is adequately replenished, fibroblasts shut off their increased production of ground substance and collagen. Interferons are one of the signals that call for cessation of activity. Berman and Duncan reported that intralesional interferon alpha-2b treatment of a keloid resulted in a selective and persistent normalization of keloidal fibroblast collagen, GAG, and collagenase production in vitro and a rapid reduction in the area of the keloid [95]. Interferon has also been shown to upregulate native p53 that is dysfunctional in keloidal fibroblasts, promoting the natural cell death of overactive fibroblasts [96].

Both alpha and gamma interferons are available for use. Initial clinical trials with gamma interferon were disappointing, and it is no longer in use [97]. Granstein has reported that 18 of 19 keloid re-excisions were recurrence-free at 1 year following two postoperative injections of interferon alpha [98]. Berman reported response in 11/12 recurrent keloids of the head and neck after surgical excision and interferon alpha-2b [99]. Berman and Flores reported a recurrence rate of 51.5% following surgery alone, 58.4% after surgery and corticosteroids, and 18.7% when surgery was combined with both interferon and corticosteroid injections [39]. At Kings

County Hospital, we have found that interferon alpha injections can be used to decrease keloid recurrence after earlobe keloid excisions in which keloidal tissue was left behind.

We can predict from the in vitro findings highlighted above that interferon may work better in young, developing keloids and in keloid prevention than in mature, older keloids that are passed their active growth phase. Interferon injections are of limited or no use in existing mature and stable keloids.

The standard of care for this off-label indication is for injections of interferon alpha-2b to be done twice: on the day of surgery and then 1 week postoperatively. Injections of one million units/linear cm are performed directly into the wound base and walls. When allowing the wound to heal by secondary intention, injections can be given approximately every square centimeter. Side effects are reduced by limiting total dose to less than five million units per treatment.

Side effects of interferon alpha-2b include a flu-like syndrome which can be reduced or eliminated by the prophylactic use of acetaminophen: 1 g preoperatively, 3 h postoperatively, and every 4 h through the first 24 h. Timing of the procedure/injections late in the afternoon may allow mild febrile reactions to pass unnoticed during sleep. Patients should be told to plan to be free from work or caregiving obligations for 24 h. Occurrence of the flu-like reactions are unpredictable; precautions should be taken with the second round of injections even if the first round was uneventful.

## *Imiquimod Application*

Imiquimod 5% cream causes rapid and potent induction of interferon after topical application. Topical application of imiquimod to keloids has been shown to significantly alter the gene expression of markers of apoptosis [96]. As such, its use in keloid therapy was a logical continuance from injectable interferon. Berman and Kaufman reported its use postoperatively in an uncontrolled pilot study of 13 keloids removed from 12 patients [100]. Applications were done twice daily, beginning on the day of surgery and continuing for 8 weeks. At 24 weeks, none of 11 keloids (10 earlobe, 1 trunk) evaluated had recurred. The authors have subsequently reported one recurrence in the single truncal lesion.

Since then, several other small, uncontrolled trials have suggested that imiquimod is most effective on the earlobes. Stashower showed no recurrence at 12 months in four patients with eight earlobe keloids [101]. Martin-Garcia and Busquets reported a 25% recurrence rate in 8 earlobe keloids [102]. Chuangsuwanich and Gunjittisomram showed an overall 6-month recurrence rate of 28.6% in 35 patients [103]. Recurrences on the pinna were rare (2.9%) and those of the chest common (83.3%). Malhotra et al. showed an improvement after surgical excision of three presternal keloids in two patients over the 8-week treatment phase but 100% recurrence 4 weeks later [104]. In an ongoing study, we have found a modest reduction in keloid recurrence in non-earlobe keloids treated with imiquimod. In a placebo-controlled, double-blind unpublished study of 6 patients with 12 nonadjacent keloids, we found a 50%

reduction in keloid reformation. The recurrences in the imiquimod-treated areas occurred later and were more responsive to subsequent treatment than placebo-treated recurrences. More controlled studies need to be performed to assess the effectiveness of this treatment modality.

In all of the studies mentioned, there were few local and no systemic side effects noted, even when imiquimod was applied to open wounds healing by secondary intention. Application of imiquimod to open wounds was mostly well-tolerated with minimal stinging and burning.

Imiquimod application does not appear to result in an improvement in existing keloids or hypertrophic scars, even when applied under occlusion.

## *Cryotherapy*

Many publications applaud the use of cryotherapy alone and in combination with other products in the treatment of keloids and hypertrophic scars [105–107]. The proposed mechanism of action is cellular damage in combination with vascular damage that leads to anoxia and further cell death. Most authors propose 30-s freeze times repeated 2–3 times per cycle with a 60–75% "good results" outcome [105–107]. Younger lesions may respond better to treatment than more mature keloids [106].

Side effects of cryotherapy include pain and a prolonged healing phase of more than 1 month. Melanocytes are highly susceptible to cold damage, and the likelihood of hypopigmentation is pronounced. As a result, cryotherapy may be "…less applicable in dark-skinned patients" [106]. Unfortunately, this is the population most likely to present for therapy.

Several authors have reported unique cryosurgery techniques with good results in small case reports. Gupta and Kumar suggest inserting a lumbar puncture needle completely through the midsection of the keloid [107]. Liquid nitrogen is then passed through the needle utilizing an IV drip set for two freeze-thaw cycles of 20–30 s each. After 5–10 treatment sessions, 75% showed lesion flattening, although hypopigmentation was evident in all patients. Har-Shai et al. reported a 51.4% reduction in scar volume after only one session of cryotherapy utilizing a CryoProbe to completely freeze the keloid [108]. Other authors have suggested that the combination of cryotherapy and corticosteroids is superior to either modality alone [38, 109]. Pronounced, often permanent, hypopigmentation still remains a major issue in darker-skinned patients.

## *5-Fluorouracil (5-FU)*

Intralesional 5-FU has no evidence-based data to support its use but is the mainstay of therapy for one author who has extensive experience [110, 111]. Fitzpatrick reported on his use of 5-FU in more than 5,000 patients with hypertrophic scars and keloids [110]. Small amounts (0.05 ml of 50 mg/ml) were injected at 1-cm intervals along the scar. The total dose per session ranged from 2 mg to 50 mg and never exceeded 100 mg. Patients were treated once weekly on average but as high as thrice weekly in markedly indurated or symptomatic keloids. Fitzpatrick found that the younger, more symptomatic scars were the most amenable to the technique. Numerous additional small, uncontrolled studies have shown similar results: modest improvement and superiority in younger, smaller, virgin keloids. Side effects in all studies included ulceration, pain, and hyperpigmentation in virtually all patients [112–114].

Fitzpatrick further found that the addition of triamcinolone acetonide (TAC) (0.1 ml of TAC 10 mg/ml added to 0.9 ml of 5-FU mixture above) both improved efficacy and decreased the pain of injection [111]. Apikian also showed superior results when betamethasone was added [115].

As with the use of intralesional corticosteroids, the mechanism of action of 5-FU appears to be inhibition of fibroblast proliferation. Unlike corticosteroids, however, Fitzpatrick reports no side effect of telangiectasia formation. The further addition of pulsed dye laser therapy to TAC/5-FU injections was even more successful in Fitzpatrick's hands [62]. He hypothesizes that the pulsed dye laser causes selective damage to the microvasculature, resulting in a reduction of erythema and improved wound surface texture. Beranek and Masseyeff suggested that it is the prolonged angiogenesis that is the cause of hypertrophic scarring and that an interruption of this process results in lesion improvement [116].

## *Miscellaneous Therapies*

### Intralesional Verapamil

In vitro, verapamil increases procollagenase synthesis and drives fibroblasts toward extracellular matrix degradation [117]. Its low cost and good safety profile when used intralesionally lead to its use in keloid therapy. Two studies have shown it to be effective only in early HTS [117, 118]. It appears to be ineffective in sites other than earlobes.

### Mederma®

Mederma is a plant extract that has been shown to have a wide range of effects in biological systems. It has antioxidant and anti-inflammatory properties demonstrated in many in vitro studies [119]. However, there are no well-designed studies showing in vitro efficacy or clinical utility.

### Vitamin E

It is a popularly held belief by the lay public that the use of topical vitamin E on scars is highly effective. There is no evidence that vitamin E improves or prevents hypertrophic scars, although it may be a cause of local skin reactions. In one study, it was found to be ineffective in scar improvement and at the same time caused cutaneous adverse reactions in 33% of the patients [120].

### Bleomycin

Espana et al. describe the treatment of 13 patients with bleomycin [121]; 1.5 IU/ml was applied to the surface of the keloid that was then punctured repeatedly with a 25-gauge needle. A total of two to five treatments at 1–4-month interval resulted in complete flattening of three of seven keloids and a thinning of the rest. Side effects included pain necessitating lidocaine anesthesia and hyperpigmentation in all patients. There were two recurrences at 10 and 12 months.

### Combination Therapy

Most clinicians seem to rely on a single agent or modality for postoperative preventative therapy. This is an ill-advised oversight and a missed therapeutic opportunity. Prevention of keloid recurrence or occurrence can be greatly improved when all available modalities are utilized simultaneously. Interferon injections at day 1 and day 8 combined with radiation therapy can deliver two adjunctive therapies in the first 2 weeks post-op when patient compliance is at its peak. Pressure dressings if possible, imiquimod application, perhaps SGS, and continued corticosteroid injections as previously delineated can be used in conjunction to maximize outcome.

## Keloid Avoidance Behaviors

The first goal of preventative therapy is, of course, avoidance of unnecessary trauma. Cosmetic procedures should be discouraged in keloid-prone individuals. Ears from which keloids have been removed should not be re-pierced, a request that occurs with startling frequency. Alternatively, if re-piercing is planned against medical advice, it is perhaps prudent that it be performed by a professional rather than by a mall rent-a-piercer. A small amount of intralesional interferon into and around the re-pierce site is a recommendation grounded in personal experience with no supporting data.

Early and aggressive treatment of accidental wounds of nonelective surgeries is crucial in keloid-prone individuals. Necessary surgical procedures can generally be closed parallel to relaxed skin tension lines with minimal wound tension. Skin grafts, tissue expanders, and healing by secondary intention can also be considered to minimize wound tension. Wounds should be covered with silicone gel sheeting and/or pressure garments whenever possible. Postoperative radiation therapy is highly effective and should be considered and coordinated in advance with the

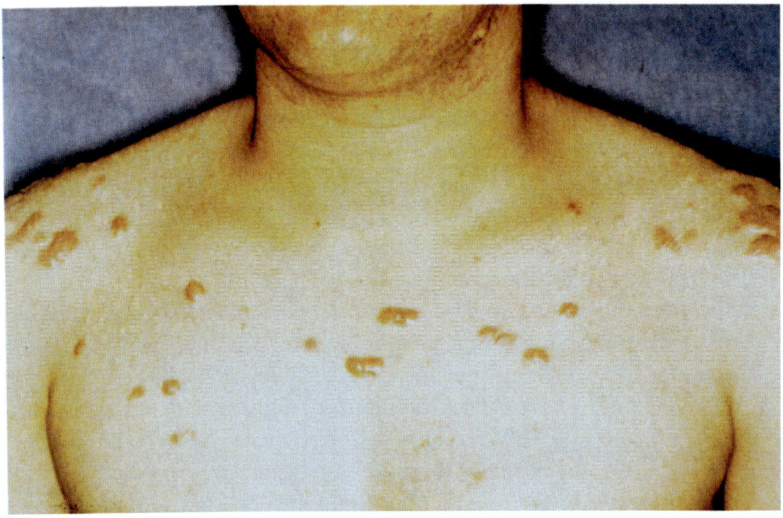

**Fig. 10.8** Acne morphing into keloids

general surgeon. Preventative intralesional corticosteroids should be injected at the time of the procedure or as soon as medically possible and regularly thereafter. Interferon injections postoperatively, although effective, are limited by the possibility of flu-like symptoms including pyrexia. Fevers within 24–48 h of surgery present diagnostic dilemmas that few surgeons are willing to risk. Although no data exists to confirm efficacy, injections done 3–4 days postoperatively and again 1 week later seem to work well. Interference with wound care and wound healing is often not appreciated by general surgeons. It is therefore prudent to elicit the help of the patient in discussing with the surgeon the importance of early intervention.

There are many patients in whom acne lesions morph imperceptibly into keloids, particularly on the chest, upper back, and deltoid areas. Indeed, the acne lesions themselves may be clinically unapparent, the presence of acne inferred by the distribution of the keloids. These patients must be carefully monitored and treated (Fig. 10.8). They should be educated to present at the first sign of an inflammatory lesion for intralesional corticosteroids. Multiple lesions are an indication for oral antibiotics or a course of isotretinoin. Similarly, in dark-skinned individuals with a family history of keloid formation, varicella, or zoster should be aggressively treated with antiviral agents.

## Summary

Keloids are challenging problems that have four distinct features: discomfort, bulk, discolor, and dysfunction. The relative importance of these features may differ from patient to patient or lesion to lesion. All of these issues need to be addressed with the patient prior to embarking on a treatment plan to assure that treatment is directed to the patient's optimal treatment goal, not the clinician's. Since therapy is generally slow, occasionally inadequate, and often fraught with complications, the patient must be fully prepared for what is inevitably a long treatment course. A variety of treatment modalities may be necessary, and patients find what is often a "trial and error" treatment plan to be off-putting. It is prudent to make no guarantees of treatment success since none is possible when dealing with keloids.

The future of keloid therapy rests with our better understanding of the pathogenesis of these fascinating lesions. Keloids can be envisioned as incomplete tumors, stuck in a proliferative phase and failing to proceed to a maturation phase. They share with malignancies several characteristics: poor regulation of growth, proliferation beyond the boundaries of the initial insult, and increased collagen synthesis. Yet literature searches fail to locate case reports of malignant degeneration of keloids. These factors predict that future advances in keloid therapy may lay in the direction of an immunologic approach rather than the slash and burn approach we currently pursue. Time will tell if interferons or other immune response modifiers will be the magic wand for which we and our patients are waiting.

## References


1. Breasted JH. The Edwin Smith surgical papyrus, vol I: hieroglyphic translation and commentary. Chicago: University of Chicago Press; 1930. p. 403–6.
2. Omo-Dare P. Yoruban contribution to literature on keloids. J Nat Med Assoc. 1973;65:367–406.
3. Bloom D. Heredity of keloids: review of the literature and report of a family with multiple keloids for five generations. N Y State J Med. 1956;56:511.
4. Abrahms B, Benedetto A, Humeniuk H. Exuberant keloidal formation. J AOAC Int. 1993;93:863–5.
5. Brenizer A. Keloid formation in the Negro. Ann Surg. 1915;61:87.
6. Fox H. Observations on skin diseases in the American Negro. J Cutan Dis. 1908;26:67.
7. Alhady SM, Sivanantharajah K. Keloids in various races; a review of 175 cases. Plast Reconstr Surg. 1969;44:564.
8. Arnold H, Graver F. Keloids: etiology and management. Arch Dermatol. 1959;80:772.
9. Kelly P. Keloids. Dermatol Clin. 1988;6:413–24.
10. Rockwell W, Cohen I, Erlich H. Keloids and hypertrophic scars. A comprehensive review. Plast Reconstr Surg. 1989;84:827–37.
11. Davies D. Scars, hypertrophic scars and keloids. Plast Reconstr Surg. 1985;290:1056–8.
12. Chipev C, Simman R, Hatch G, Katz A, Siegel D, Simon A. Myofibroblast phenotype and apoptosis in keloid and palmar fibroblasts in vitro. Cell Death Differ. 2000;7:166–7.
13. Flint M. The biological basis of Langer's lines. In: Longacre JJ, editor. The ultrastructure of collagen. Springfield: Charles C Thomas; 1976. p. 132–40.
14. Stucker F, Shaw G. An approach to management of keloids. Arch Otolaryngol Head Neck Surg. 1992;118:63–7.
15. Asboe-Hansen G. Hypertrophic scars and keloids; etiology, pathogenesis and dermatologic therapy. Dermatologia. 1960;120:178.
16. Kormoczy B. Enormous keloid(?) on a penis. Br J Plast Surg. 1978;31:268.
17. Garb J, Stone M. Keloids: review of the literature and a report of eighty cases. Am J Surg. 1942;58:315.

18. Baldwin H. Personal communication. 2000.
19. Lane J, Waller J, Davis L. Relationship between age of ear piercing and keloid formation. Pediatrics. 2005;115:1312–4.
20. Cosman B, Crikelair G, Ju M, Gaulin J, Lattes R. The surgical treatment of keloids. Plast Reconstr Surg. 1961;27:335–45.
21. Abergel R, Pizzurro D, Meeker C, et al. Biochemical composition of the connective tissue in keloids and analysis of collagen metabolism in keloid fibroblast cultures. J Invest Dermatol. 1985;84:384–90.
22. Cohen I, Keiser H, Sjoerdsma A. Collagen synthesis in human keloid patients. Plast Reconstr Surg. 1979;63:689.
23. Tan E, Rouda S, Greenbaum S, Moore J, Fox J, et al. Acidic and basic fibroblast growth factors down regulate collagen gene expression in keloid fibroblasts. Am J Pathol. 1993;142:463–70.
24. Diegelmann R, Bryant C, Cohen I. Tissue alpha globulins in keloid formation. Plast Reconstr Surg. 1977;59:481.
25. Bauer E, Eisen A, Jeffrey J. Regulation of vertebrate collagenase activity in vivo and in vitro. J Invest Dermatol. 1972;59:50–5.
26. Sayah DN, Soo C, Shaw WW, Watson J, Messadi D, et al. Downregulation of apoptosis-related genes in keloid tissues. J Surg Res. 1999;87:209–16.
27. AkasakaY FK, Ishikawa Y, Asuwa N, Inuzuka K, et al. Detection of apoptosis in keloids and a comparative study on apoptosis between keloids, hypertrophic scars, normal healed fibrotic scars, and dermatofibroma. Wound Repair Regen. 2001;9:501–6.
28. Shaffer J, Taylor S, Cook-Bolden F. Keloidal scars: a review with a critical look at therapeutic options. J Am Acad Dermatol. 2002;46:S63–97.
29. Mustoe T, Cooter R, Gold M, Hobbs F, Ramelet A, et al. International clinical recommendations on scar management. Plast Reconstr Surg. 2002;110:560–71.
30. Durani P, Bayat A. Levels of evidence for the treatment of keloid disease. J Plast Reconstr Aesthet Surg. 2008;61:4–17.
31. Lenventhal D, Furr M, Reiter D. Treatment of keloids and hypertrophic scars: a meta-analysis and review of the literature. Arch Facial Plast Surg. 2006;8:362–8.
32. Border W, Noble N. TGF-B. Sci Am Sci Med. 1995;2:68–77.
33. Kauh Y, Rouda S, Mondragon G, et al. Major suppression of pro-alpha 19(I) type I collagen gene expression in the dermis after keloid excision and immediate intrawound injection of triamcinolone acetonide. J Am Acad Dermatol. 1997;37:586–9.
34. Kiil J. Keloids treated with topical injections of triamcinolone acetonide (Kenalog): immediate and long term results. Scand J Plast Reconstr Surg. 1977;11:169–72.
35. Griffith B, Monroe C, McKinney P. A follow-up study on the treatment of keloids with triamcinolone acetonide. Plast Reconstr Surg. 1970;46:145–50.
36. Lahiri A, Tsiliboti D, Gaze N. Experience with difficult keloids. Br J Plast Surg. 2001;54:633–5.
37. Lawrence W. In search of the optimal treatment of keloids: report of a series and a review of the literature. Ann Plast Surg. 1991;27:164–78.
38. Yosipovitch G, Widijanti Sugene M, Goon A, Chan Y, Goh C. A Comparison of the combined effect of cryotherapy and corticosteroid injections versus corticosteroids and cryotherapy on keloids: a controlled study. J Dermatol Treat. 2001;12:87–90.
39. Berman B, Flores F. Recurrence rates of excised keloids treated with post operative triamcinolone injections of interferon alpha 2b. J Am Acad Dermatol. 1997;37:755–7.
40. Lee J, Kim S, Lee A. Effects of interferon-alpha2b on keloid treatment with triamcinolone acetonide intralesional injection. Int J Dermatol. 2008;47:183–6.
41. Akoz T, Gideroglu K, Akan M. Combination of different techniques for the treatment of earlobe keloids. Aesthetic Plast Surg. 2002;26:184–8.
42. Darzi M, Chowdi N, Kaul S, et al. Evaluation of various methods of treating keloids and hypertrophic scars: a 10 year follow-up study. Br J Plast Surg. 1992;45:374–9.
43. Cheng L. Keloid of the earlobe. Laryngoscope. 1974;82:673–81.

44. Ogawa R, Miyashita T, Hyakusoku H, Akaishi S, Kuribayashi S, et al. Postoperative radiation protocol for keloids and hypertrophic scars: statistical analysis of 370 sites followed for over 18 months. Ann Plast Surg. 2007;59:688–91.
45. Narkwong L, Thirakhupt P. Postoperative radiotherapy with high dose rate iridium 192 mould for prevention of earlobe keloids. J Med Assoc Thai. 2006;89:428–33.
46. Rauscher G, Kolmer W. Treatment of recurrent earlobe keloids. Cutis. 1996;38:67–8.
47. Sclafani A, Gordon L, Chadha M, Romo T. Prevention of earlobe keloid recurrence with postoperative corticosteroid injections versus radiation therapy. Dermatol Surg. 1996;22:569–74.
48. Shons A, Press B. The treatment of earlobe keloids by surgical excision and postoperative triamcinolone injection. Ann Plast Surg. 1983;10:480–2.
49. Rosen D, Patel M, Freeman K, Weiss P. A primary protocol for the management of ear keloids: results of excision combined with intraoperative and postoperative steroid injections. Plast Reconstr Surg. 2007;120:1395–400.
50. Akita S, Akino K, Yakabe A, Imaizumi T, Tanaka K, et al. Combined surgical excision and radiation therapy for keloid treatment. J Craniofac Surg. 2007;18:1164–9.
51. Ragoowansi R, Cornes P, Glees J, Powell B, Moss A. Earlobe keloids: treatment by a protocol of surgical excision and immediate postoperative adjuvant radiotherapy. Br J Plast Surg. 2001;54:504–8.
52. Chaudhry M, Akhtar S, Duvalsaint F, Garner L, Lucente F. Earlobe keloids, surgical excision followed by radiation therapy: a 10-year experience. Ear Nose Throat J. 1994;73:779–81.
53. Salasche S, Grabski W. Keloids of the earlobe: a surgical technique. J Dermatol Surg Oncol. 1983;9:552–6.
54. Kantor G, Wheeland R, Bailin P, Walker N, Ratz J. Treatment of earlobe keloids with carbon dioxide laser excision: a report of 16 cases. J Dermatol Surg Oncol. 1985;11:1063–7.
55. Driscoll B. Treating keloids with carbon dioxide lasers. Arch Otolaryngol Head Neck Surg. 2001;127:1145.
56. Alster T. Laser treatment of hypertrophic scars, keloids and striae. Dermatol Clin. 1997;15:419–29.
57. ApfelbergD MM, White D, Lash H. Failure of carbon dioxide laser excision of keloids. Lasers Surg Med. 1989;9:382–8.
58. Sherman R, Rosenfeld H. Experience with the NDYAG laser in the treatment of keloid scars. Ann Plast Surg. 1988;24:231–3.
59. Conejo-Mir JS. Carbon dioxide laser ablation in association with interferon alfa-2b injections reduces the recurrence of keloids. J Am Acad Dermatol. 1998;39:1039–40.
60. Alster T, Williams C. Treatment of keloid sternotomy scars with 585 nm flashlamp-pumped pulsed-dye laser. Lancet. 1995;345:118–200.
61. Connell P, Harland C. Treatment of keloid scars with pulsed dye laser and intralesional steroids. J Cutan Laser Ther. 2000;2:147–59.
62. Maniskiatti W, Fitzpatrick R. Treatment response of keloidal and hypertrophic, sternotomy scars: comparison among intralesional corticosteroid, 5-fluorouracil, and 585-nm flashlamp-pumped pulsed-dye laser treatments. Arch Dermatol. 2002;138:1149–55.
63. Asilian A, Darougheh A, Shariati F. New combination of triamcinolone, 5-fluorouracil, and pulsed-dye laser for treatment of keloid and hypertrophic scars. Dermatol Surg. 2006;32:907–15.
64. Alster T, Handrick C. Laser treatment of hypertrophic scars, keloids and striae. Semin Cutan Med Surg. 2000;19:287–92.
65. Order S, Donaldsen S. Radiation therapy for benign disease. Berlin: Springer; 1990. p. 147–53.
66. Borok T, Brav M, Sinclair I, Plafker J, LaBirth L. Role of ionizing irradiation for 393 keloids. Int J Radiat Oncol Biol Phys. 1988;15:865–70.
67. Brown J, Bromberg JH. Preliminary studies on the effect of time-dose patterns in the treatment of keloids. Radiology. 1963;80:298–302.
68. Edsmyr F, Larsoon L, Onyango J, Wanguru S, Wood M. Radiotherapy in the treatment of keloids in East Africa. East Afr Med J. 1973;50:457–61.

69. Garth J, Stone M. Keloids: review of literature and a report of 80 cases. Am J Surg. 1942;58:315–35.
70. Lo T, Seckel B, Salzman F, et al. Single-dose electron beam irradiation in treatment and prevention of keloids and hypertrophic scars. Radiother Oncol. 1990;19:267–72.
71. Ollstein R, Siegel H, Gillooley J, et al. Treatment of keloids by combined surgical excision and immediate post-operative X-ray therapy. Ann Plast Surg. 1981;7:281–5.
72. Khumpar D, Murray J, Anscher M. Keloids treated with excision followed by radiation therapy. J Am Acad Dermatol. 1994;31:225–31.
73. Darzi M, Chowdi N, Kaul S, Kahn M. Evaluation of various methods of treating keloids and hypertrophic scars: a 10-year experience. Int J Radiat Oncol Biol Phys. 1989;17:77–80.
74. Botwood N, Lewanski C, Lowdell C. The risks of treating keloids with radiotherapy. Br J Radiol. 1999;72:1222–4.
75. Kal H, Veen R. Biologically effective doses of postoperative radiotherapy in the prevention of keloids. Dose-effect relationship. Strahlenther Onkol. 2005;181:717–23.
76. Guix B, Henriquez I, Andres A, Finestres F, Tello J, et al. Treatment of keloids by high-dose-rate brachytherapy. Int J Radiat Oncol Biol Phys. 2001;50:167–72.
77. Escarmant P, Zimmerman S, Amar A, et al. The treatment of 783 keloid scars by iridium 192 interstitial radiation after surgical excision. Int J Radiat Oncol Biol Phys. 1993;26:245–51.
78. Maarouf M, Schleicher U, Schmachtenberg A, Ammon J. Radiotherapy in the management of keloids. Clinical experience with electron beam irradiation and comparison with X-ray therapy. Strahlenther Onkol. 2002;178:330–5.
79. Bischof M, Krempien R, Debus J, Treiber M. Postoperative electron beam radiotherapy for keloids: objective findings and patient satisfaction in self-assessment. Int J Dermatol. 2007;46:971–5.
80. Ogawa R, Mitsuhashi K, Hyakusoku H, Miyashita T. Postoperative electron-beam irradiation therapy for keloids and hypertrophic scars: retrospective study of 147 cases followed for more than 18 months. Plast Reconstr Surg. 2003;111:547–53.
81. Wagner W, Alfrink M, Micke O, Schafer U, Schuller P, et al. Results of prophylactic irradiation in patients with resected keloids: a retrospective analysis. Acta Oncol. 2000;39:217–20.
82. Mizuno H, Cagri Uysal A, Koike S, Hyakusoku H. Squamous cell carcinoma of the auricle arising from keloid after radium needle therapy. J Craniofac Surg. 2006;17:360–2.
83. Bilbey J, Muller N, Miller R, Nelemus B. Localised fibrous mesothelioma of pleura following external ionising radiation therapy. Chest. 1988;94:1291–2.
84. Hoffman S. Radiotherapy for keloids? Ann Plast Surg. 1982;9:265.
85. Sampson R, Kev C, Buschler C, Iijima S. Thyroid carcinoma and radiation. JAMA. 1969;209:65.
86. Doornbos J, Stoffel T, Hass A, Hussey D, Vigliotti A, et al. The role of kilovoltage irradiation in the treatment of keloids. Int J Radiat Oncol Biol Phys. 1990;18:833–8.
87. Kosaka M, Kamiishi H. New concept of balloon-compression wear for the treatment of keloids and hypertrophic scars. Plast Reconstr Surg. 2001;108:1454–5.
88. Gold M. A controlled clinical trial of topical silicone gel sheeting in the treatment of hypertrophic scars and keloids. J Am Acad Dermatol. 1994;30:506–7.
89. Fulton J. Silicone gel sheeting for the prevention and management of evolving hypertrophic and keloid scars. Dermatol Surg. 1995;21:947–51.
90. Ahn S, Monafo W, Mustoe T. Topical silicone gel: a new treatment for hypertrophic scars. Surgery. 1989;106:781–6.
91. Berman B, Perez O, Konda S, et al. A review of the biologic effects, clinical efficacy, and safety of silicone elastomer sheeting for hypertrophic and keloid scar treatment and management. Dermatol Surg. 2007;33:1291–302.
92. Mustoe T. Evolution of silicone therapy and mechanism of action in scar management. Aesthetic Plast Surg. 2008;32:82–92.
93. Signorini M, Clementoni M. Clinical evaluation of a new self-drying silicone gel in the treatment of scars: a preliminary report. Aesthetic Plast Surg. 2007;31(2):183–7.
94. Viana de Oliveira G, Nunes T, Magna L, Cintra M, Kitten G, et al. Silicone versus nonsilicone gel dressings: a controlled trial. Dermatol Surg. 2001;27:721–6.

95. Berman N, Duncan M. Short-term keloid treatment in vivo with human interferon alfa-2b results in a selective and persistent normalization of keloidal fibroblast collagen glycosaminoglycans and collagenase production in vitro. J Am Acad Dermatol. 1989;21:L694.
96. Jacob S, Berman B, Vincek V. Topical application of imiquimod 5% cream to keloids alters expression genes associated with apoptosis. Br J Dermatol. 2008;149:62–5.
97. Granstein R, Rook A, Flotte T, et al. Intralesional interferon gamma treatment for keloids and hypertrophic scars. Arch Otolaryngol Head Neck Surg. 1990;118:1159–62.
98. Granstein R. personal communication. New York Academy of Science; 1996.
99. Berman B, Bieley H. Adjunct therapies of surgical management of keloids. Dermatol Surg. 1996;22:126–30.
100. Berman B, Kaufman J. Pilot study of the effect of postoperative imiquimod 5 % cream recurrence rate of excised keloids. J Am Acad Dermatol. 2002;47:S209–11.
101. Stashower M. Successful treatment of earlobe keloids with imiquimod after tangential shave excision. Dermatol Surg. 2006;32:380–6.
102. Martin-Garcia R, Busquets A. Postsurgical use of imiquimod 5 % cream in the prevention of earlobe keloid recurrences: results of an open-label, pilot study. Dermatol Surg. 2005;31:1394–8.
103. Chuangsuwanich A, Gunjittisomram S. The efficacy of 5% imiquimod cream in the prevention of recurrence of excised keloids. J Med Assoc Thai. 2007;90:1363–7.
104. Malhotra A, Gupta S, Khaitan B, Sharma V. Imiquimod 5% cream for the prevention of recurrence after excision of presternal keloids. Dermatology. 2007;215:63–5.
105. Rusciani L, Rossi G, Bono R. Use of cryotherapy in the treatment of keloids. J Dermatol Surg Oncol. 1993;19:529–34.
106. Zouboulis C, Blume U, Buttner P, Orfanos C. Outcomes of cryosurgery in keloids and hypertrophic scars. Arch Dermatol. 1993;129:1146–51.
107. Gupta S, Kumar B. Intralesional cryosurgery using lumbar puncture and/or hypodermic needles for large, bulky, recalcitrant keloids. Int J Dermatol. 2001;40:349–53.
108. Har-Shai Y, Amar M, Sabo E. Intralesional cryotherapy for enhancing the involution of hypertrophic scars and keloids. Plast Reconstr Surg. 2003;111:1841–52.
109. Chowdri N, Masarat M, Mattoo A, Darzi M. Keloids and hypertrophic scars: results with intraoperative and serial postoperative corticosteroid injection therapy. Aust NZJ Surg. 1999;69:655–9.
110. Fitzpatrick R. Treatment of inflamed hypertrophic scars using intralesional 5-FU. Dermatol Surg. 1999;25:224–32.
111. Lebwohl M. From the literature. J Am Acad Dermatol. 1999;42:677.
112. Gupta S, Kalra A. Efficacy and safety of intralesional 5-FU in the treatment of keloids. Dermatology. 2002;204:130.
113. Kontochristopoulos K, et al. Intralesional 5-FU in the treatment of keloids: an open clinical and histopathologic study. J Am Acad Dermatol. 2005;52:474–9.
114. Nanda R. Intralesional 5-FU as a treatment modality of keloids. Dermatol Surg. 2004;30:54–6.
115. Apikian M, Goodman G. Intralesional 5-FU in the treatment of keloid scars. Australas J Dermatol. 2004;45:140–3.
116. Beranek J, Masseyeff R. Hyperplastic capillaries and their possible involvement in the pathogenesis of fibrosis. Histopathology. 1992;10:543–51.
117. Lawrence W. Treatment of earlobe keloids with surgery plus adjuvant intralesional verapamil and pressure earrings. Ann Plast Surg. 1996;37:167–9.
118. Lee R, Dwong J, Jellema A. The response of burn scars to intralesional verapamil: report of five cases. Arch Surg. 1994;129:107–11.
119. Phan T, See P, Tran E, Nguyen T, Chan S, et al. Suppression of insulin-like growth factor signaling pathway and collagen expression in keloid-derived fibroblasts by quercetin: a therapeutic potential use in the treatment and/or prevention of keloids. Br J Dermatol. 2003;148:544–52.
120. Baumann L, Spencer J. The effects of topical vitamin E on the cosmetic appearance of scars. Dermatol Surg. 1999;25:311–5.
121. Espana A, Solano T, Quintanilla E. Bleomycin in the treatment of keloids and hypertrophic scars by multiple needle punctures. Dermatol Surg. 2001;27:23–7.

# Chapter 11
# Skin Cancers in Skin of Color

**Brooke A. Jackson**

Skin cancer is the most common malignancy in the United States [1]. Although skin cancer is less common in patients with skin of color, it is associated with increased morbidity and mortality rates as compared to those in Caucasians [2, 3]. This statistical imbalance holds significant public health concern. Despite increased public awareness of skin cancer, many physicians do not immediately associate or recognize skin cancer in skin of color. While current skin cancer campaigns focus primarily on Caucasian patients in high-risk groups, little is known about sun-protective behaviors in patients with skin of color. Unlike melanoma, nonmelanoma skin cancers (NMSC) are not consistently reported to tumor registries, making collection of statistics for skin cancer in skin of color challenging. According to the 2000 census [4], 50% of the US population is projected to be nonwhite by the year 2050. This changing demographic, combined with the disparate mortality in patients of color, underscores the urgency for physicians to become familiar with skin cancer in their patients of color to better educate them on their risk factors, early detection, and prevention of this highly treatable disease.

## Histologic Differences in Skin of Color

While all skin, regardless of its color, contains the same number of pigment producing melanocytes, the melanosomes in skin of color are larger and more evenly dispersed throughout the entire epidermis compared to white skin [5]. These larger melanosomes allow dark skin to filter almost twice as much ultraviolet B (UVB) radiation than white skin [6], resulting in an estimated sun protection factor of 13.1

B.A. Jackson, M.D. (✉)
Founder and Medical Director, Skin Wellness Center of Chicago, SC, Chicago, IL, USA

Clinical Assistant professor, Department of Dermatology, Northwestern Medical School, Northwestern Memorial Hospital, Chicago, IL, USA
e-mail: bjacsonmd@mindspring.com

A.F. Alexis and V.H. Barbosa (eds.), *Skin of Color: A Practical Guide to Dermatologic Diagnosis and Treatment*, DOI 10.1007/978-0-387-84929-4_11,

**Table 11.1** Known risk factors of NMSC

| |
|---|
| Fitzpatrick skin type I–III |
| UV exposure including UV light treatment |
| Male gender |
| Organ transplant immunosuppression |
| Genetic disorders (XP) |
| Chemical exposure (arsenic, heavy metal) |
| HPV |
| Radiation exposure |

in black skin [7]. These unique histologic features of dark skin serve to protect it against actinic damage, making sun-induced skin cancers less prevalent. Despite this intrinsic photoprotection, the incidence of NMSC is increasing in skin of color [7], suggesting that UV exposure may play less of a role in the development of certain skin cancers in skin of color. Known risk factors for NMSC are listed in Table 11.1. [8]

## Ozone Layer

The ozone layer has decreased significantly over the past 20 years allowing increased penetration of UV radiation to the earth's surface [9]. While UV radiation is a known risk factor in the development of skin cancer in Caucasians [10] and Asians [11], its association with certain skin cancers in African Americans is less clear. UV radiation does play a causative role in the development of basal cell carcinoma (BCC) in African Americans evidenced by the predominately sun-exposed distribution of these tumors [6, 12]. However, squamous cell carcinoma (SCC), which occurs with equal frequency in sun-exposed and non-sun-exposed areas of the body in Caucasian patients, occurs 8.5 times more frequently in sun-protected skin in blacks, suggesting that UV radiation plays a less significant role in the development of SCC in blacks [13].

## Basal Cell Carcinoma

While the classically described basal cell carcinoma (BCC) of a pearly papule with central ulceration, rolled boarders, and surrounding telangiectasia may occur in skin of color, the presentation is more likely to be atypical in appearance [14]. In fact, pearly borders and telangiectasia, the hallmarks of diagnosis in Caucasians, may be difficult to appreciate in darkly complected patients. Pigmented BCCs occur more frequently in skin of color [15] while the morpheaform type is less common [16]. Although the majority of BCCs in skin of color are found in sun-exposed areas of the body, BCC is being seen with increasing frequency in non-sun-exposed sites [15].

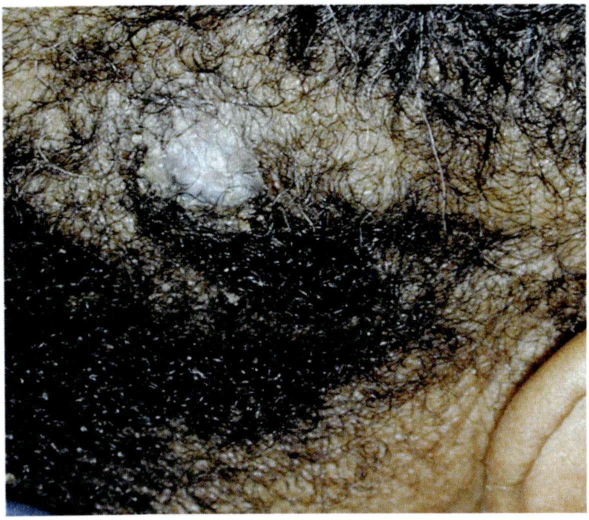

**Fig. 11.1** Nodular-pigmented basal cell carcinoma in elderly African American woman

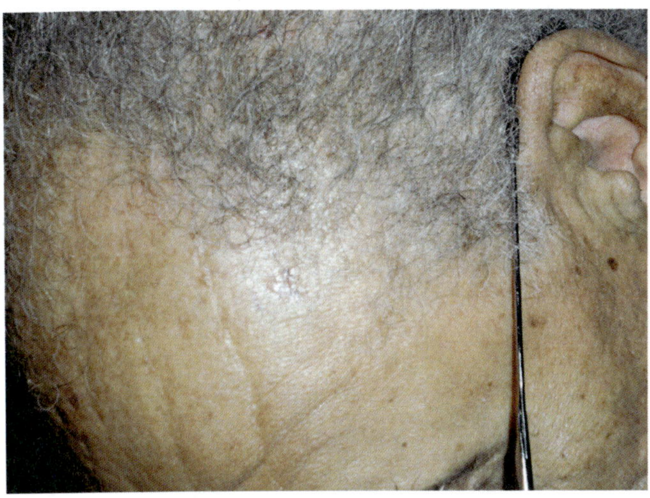

**Fig. 11.2** Basal cell carcinoma on frontal scalp of African American man

This divergence from the classical presentation of BCC in addition to the often atypical appearance in skin of color makes diagnosis challenging (Figs. 11.1 and 11.2). As with any patient, the physician should consider taking a biopsy of any suspicious or nonhealing lesion in a patient of color. The differential diagnosis of BCC in skin of color can be found in Table 11.2.

**Table 11.2** Differential diagnosis of BCC in skin of color

| |
|---|
| Trauma (curling iron burn) |
| Blue nevus |
| Sarcoid |
| Lupus erythematosus |
| Epidermal inclusion cyst |
| Melanoma |
| Nevus sebaceous |

## Squamous Cell Carcinoma

Squamous cell carcinoma (SCC) is the most common skin cancer in African Americans [17] and the second most common skin cancer in East Asians [11]. The precursor lesions to SCC, actinic keratoses, are not uncommon in Asians [18] yet tend not to occur in African Americans [19]. While SCC occurs with equal frequency on sun-exposed and non-sun-exposed skin in Caucasians, it is 8.5 times more likely to occur in non-sun-exposed areas (lower extremity, anogenital region) in African Americans (Fig. 11.3) suggesting the UV radiation plays a less significant role in the development of SCC in African Americans [20, 21]. Although Bowen's disease (SCC in situ) is less common in African Americans, it often occurs on the lower extremity presenting as a hyperkeratotic plaque (Fig. 11.4). Mortality rates for African Americans with SCC are as high as 29% [21, 22] and are particularly high with anogenital lesions. These alarmingly high rates may be related to delayed diagnosis of tumors in non-sun-exposed areas combined with potentially more biologically aggressive tumors [22]. Risk factors for SCC are listed in Table 11.3 [17]. Because of the increased mortality rate with African Americans, physicians should counsel their patients regarding their risks of SCC, evaluate new growths, and consider biopsy of any nonhealing, ulcerated, or chronically inflamed lesion regardless of sun exposure.

## Malignant Melanoma

Malignant melanoma is the deadliest form of skin cancer. It is estimated that in 2009, 8,650 deaths will be attributed to melanoma with one death each hour [23]. While malignant melanoma has received increased media attention due to high profile patients with melanoma (Senator John McCain, Maureen Regan, Sam Donaldson), the resultant public awareness messages have largely been aimed at high-risk Caucasian patients who burn easily. Few, if any skin cancer awareness and prevention messages are directed toward patients of color. Few know that the cause of death for reggae singer, Bob Marley, was acral lentiginous malignant melanoma at age 36 [24].

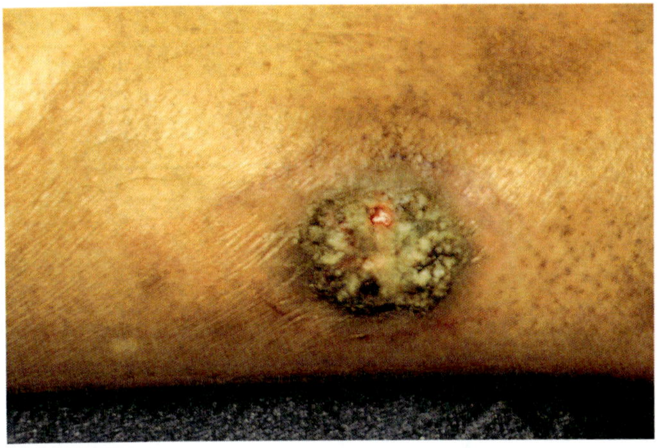

**Fig. 11.3** Invasive squamous cell carcinoma on lower extremity of African American woman with h/o childhood thermal burn

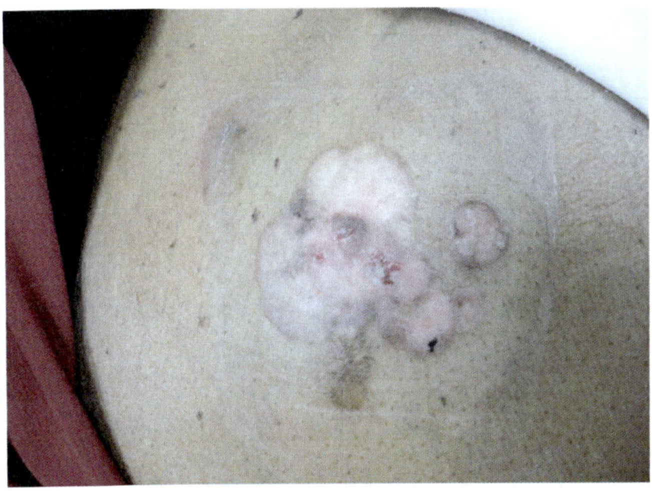

**Fig. 11.4** Bowen's disease (squamous cell carcinoma in situ) in African American woman on the right hip

**Table 11.3** Risk factors for SCC in skin of color

| | |
|---|---|
| Scars from burn or trauma | Hidradenitis suppurativa |
| DLE/LE | Granuloma annulare |
| Radiation sites | HPV |
| Immunosuppression | Albinism |
| Chemical exposure (tar, arsenic) | Cutaneous ulcers |

**Table 11.4** Differential diagnosis for MM in skin of color

| DDX for MM in skin of color | |
|---|---|
| Pigmented BCC | Tinea unguium |
| Seborrheic keratosis | Trauma (subungual hematoma) |
| Nevus | |
| Verruca | |

Although age-adjusted incidence rates (per 100,000) for melanoma are lower among blacks and Hispanics (1.0 and 4.3, respectively) compared to whites (20.8) [25], malignant melanomas in these groups are more likely to occur in sun-protected areas (acral and mucosal), to have delayed diagnosis, to metastasize, and therefore to have higher mortality than in whites [26, 27]. Because survival rates are directly correlated with Clark's level staging at diagnosis, early detection is critical for increased survival. Differential diagnosis for malignant melanoma in skin of color can be found in Table 11.4.

## Hypopigmented Mycosis Fungoides

Hypopigmented mycosis fungoides (HMF), a variant of cutaneous T cell lymphoma, occurs almost exclusively in younger persons of color and almost twice as frequently in African Americans than in Caucasians [28]. It presents as ill-defined hypopigmented patches and plaques, often in patients who have a preexisting history of eczema which may delay diagnosis [29] (Fig. 11.5). Consideration of serial biopsies should be given to any patient who is unresponsive to standard therapies for eczema or who has unexplained exacerbation of their disease. The differential diagnosis of HMF is found in Table 11.5.

## Treatment of Skin Cancers in Skin of Color

Treatment options for skin cancers in skin of color do not differ from those used in Caucasian patients (MOHS, wide local); however, because of the increased risk of keloid formation in persons of color [30, 31], caution must be taken to minimize tension on surgical wound closures. Patients should be counseled preoperatively regarding the possibility of keloid or hypertrophic scar formation both of which are responsive to intralesional Kenalog injection and pressure. Erythematous hypertrophic scars in lightly complected patients (skin type I–IV) may be treated successfully in one to three treatments with the 595-nm-pulsed dye laser. This author uses Cynosure 595 nm, 10-mm spot, 0.5-ms pulse duration, and 3–6 J. Atrophic scars respond well to the Affirm laser (1,440-nm YAG, Cynosure) using 10-mm spot, 2–4 J, double pass at 2–4-week intervals for 3–5 treatments. As the Affirm laser builds

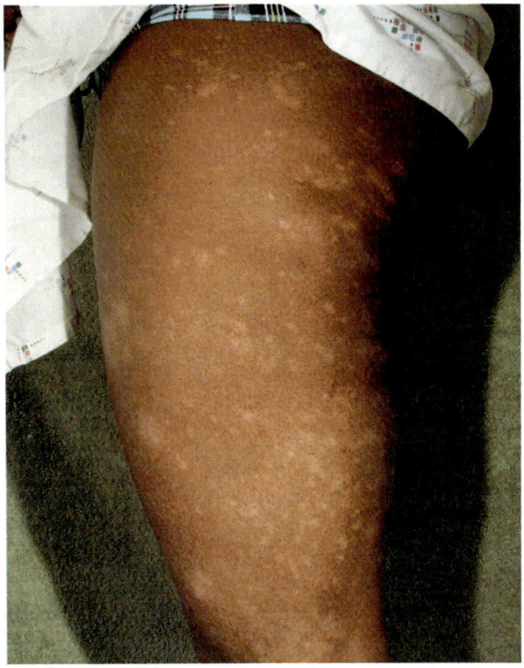

**Fig. 11.5** Patch-stage hypopigmented mycosis fungoides

**Table 11.5** Differential diagnosis for hypopigmented mycosis fungoides in skin of color

| | |
|---|---|
| Eczema | Post inflammatory hypopigmentation |
| Vitiligo | Sarcoid |
| Tinea versicolor | Contact dermatitis |

collagen, patients should be counseled that improvement is usually seen several months after the initiation of treatment.

When treating precancerous lesions, this author avoids the use of liquid nitrogen (or cryogen cooling with laser) in skin of color in favor of topical imiquimod or 5-FU in an effort to avoid post treatment hypopigmentation.

## Screening and Prevention

Skin cancer does occur in persons of color, although less commonly than in Caucasians [32]. Persons of color are more likely to die of their disease when compared to their Caucasian counterparts. This disparity is likely multifactorial and includes delayed diagnosis, potentially more biologically aggressive tumors, and lack of knowledge regarding risk factors for these tumors.

Current skin cancer awareness campaigns are aimed at Caucasians in high-risk groups. Because of this, patients with skin of color often have a false sense of security with regard to awareness of skin cancer risk and tend not to follow general guidelines of sun protection [30]. Patients of color who do not perceive themselves as being high risk for skin cancer are likely to ignore early warning signs. Physicians who do not associate skin cancer with their patients of color are less likely to consider it in a differential diagnosis, to perform a biopsy, or to counsel their patients on prevention, monitoring, and proper follow up, all of which are critical to early diagnosis. Public awareness skin cancer campaigns directed at persons of color should be considered, and physicians treating patients of color should consider skin cancer surveillance and counseling as they do with Caucasian patients.

## References

1. Centers for disease control and prevention. www.cdc.gov/cancer/skin/statistics. Accessed 18 Jan 2010.
2. Gloster Jr HM, Brodland DG. The epidemiology of skin cancer. Dermatol Surg. 1996;22:217–26.
3. Jemal A, Siegel R, Ward E, et al. Cancer statistics, 2006. CA Cancer J Clin. 2006;56:106–30.
4. US Census Bureau Population Division. Projections of the resident population by race, Hispanic origin, and nativity: middle series, 1999–2100. Washington, DC: US Census Bureau; 2000.
5. Montagna W. The architecture of black and white skin. J Am Acad Dermatol. 1991;24:29–37.
6. Halder RM, Bridgeman-Shah S. Skin cancer in African Americans. Cancer. 1995;75:667–73.
7. Halder RM, Ara CJ. Skin cancer and photoaging in ethnic skin. Dermatol Clin. 2003;21: 725–32.
8. American Cancer Society: Non melanoma skin cancer detailed guide. http://documents.cancer.org/118.00
9. Naruse K, Ueda M, Nagana T, Suzuki T. Prevalence of actinic keratoses in Japan. J Dermatol Sci. 1997;15:183–7.
10. Armstrong BK, Kricker A. The epidemiology of UV induced skin cancer. J Photochem Photobiol B. 2001;63:8–18.
11. Koh D, Wang H, et al. Basal cell carcinoma, squamous cell carcinoma and melanoma of the skin: analysis of the Singapore cancer registry data 1968–1997. Br J Dermatol. 2003;148:1161–6.
12. Halder RM, Bang KM. Skin cancer in blacks in the United States. Dermatol Clin. 1988;6:397–405.
13. Gloster HM, Neal K. Skin cancer in skin of color. J Am Acad Dermatol. 2006;55:741–60.
14. Chorun L, Norris JE, Gupta M. Basal cell carcinoma in blacks: a report of 15 cases. Ann Plast Surg. 1994;33:90–5.
15. Nadiminti U, Rakkhit T, Washington C. Morpheaform basal cell carcinoma in African Americans. Dermatol Surg. 2004;30:1550–2.
16. Lesher JL, d'Aubermont PC, Brown VM. Morpheaform basal cell carcinoma in a young black woman. J Dermatol Surg Oncol. 1988;14:2003.
17. Mora RG, Perniciaro C. Cancer of the skin in blacks: a review of 163 black patients with cutaneous squamous cell carcinoma. J Am Acad Dermatol. 1981;5:535–43.
18. Suzuki T, Ueda M, Naruse K, et al. Incidence of actinic keratosis of Japanese in Kasai city, Hyogo. J Dermatol Sci. 1997;16:74–8.
19. Hale EK, Jorizzo J, Nehal KS, et al. Current concepts in the management of actinic keratosis. J Drugs Dermatol. 2004;3((2 suppl)):S3–16.

20. Mora RG, Perniciaro C, Lee B. Cancer of the skin in blacks III: a review of nineteen black patients with Bowen's disease. J Am Acad Dermatol. 1984;11:557–62.
21. Sing B, Bhaya M, Shaha A, Har-El G, Lucente FE. Presentation, course and outcome of head and neck cancer in African Americans: a case controlled study. Laryngoscope. 1998;108:1159–63.
22. Mora RG. Surgical and aesthetic considerations of cancer of the skin in the black American. Am J Dermatol Surg Oncol. 1986;12:24–31.
23. American Cancer Society; Skin cancer facts. www.cancer.org. Accessed 6 Feb 2010.
24. Albreski D, Sloan SB. Melanoma of the feet: misdiagnosed and misunderstood. Clin Dermatol. 2009 Nov–Dec;27(6):556–63.
25. Cress RD, Holly EA. Incidence of cutaneous melanoma among non-Hispanic whites, Hispanics, Asians and Blacks: an analysis of California Cancer Registry data, 1988–1993. Cancer Causes Control. 1997;8:246–52.
26. Greenlee RT, Murray T, Bolden S, Wingo PA. Cancer statistics, 2000. CA Cancer J Clin. 2000;50(1):7–33.
27. Washington CV, Grimes PE. Incidence and prevention of skin cancer. Cosmet Dermatol. 2003;16:46–8.
28. Akaraphanth R, Douglass MC, Lim HW. Hypopigmented mycosis fungoides: treatment and a 6 1/2 year follow up of 9 patients. J Am Acad Dermatol. 2000;42:33–9.
29. Stone MC, Styles AR, Cockerell CJ. Hypopigmented mycosis fungoides: a report of 7 cases and review of the literature. Cutis. 2001;67:133–8.
30. LeFlore IC. Misconceptions regarding elective plastic surgery in the black patient. J Natl Med Assoc. 1980;72:947–8.
31. Arnold HL, Franer FH. Keloids; etiology and management by excision and intensive prophylactic radiation. Arch Dermatol. 1959;80:772.
32. Fleming ID, Barnawell JR, Burlison PE, et al. Skin cancer in black patients. Cancer. 1975;35:600–5.

# Chapter 12
# Overview of Cosmetic Concerns in Skin of Color

**Heather Woolery-Lloyd and Jenna N. Kammer**

Physicians are confronted with a myriad of cutaneous diseases affecting those with skin of color. Patients with skin of color, which include individuals of African, Asian, and Hispanic descent, have unique cosmetic concerns. Such patients often require special consideration when it comes to receiving cosmetic procedures. These patients are particularly vulnerable because any kind of significant trauma, whether it is from a laser or chemical peel, can cause long-lasting or permanent pigmentary changes. For the clinician, cosmetic procedures with patients of skin of color can be challenging because of this increased risk of hyperpigmentation and scarring. Due to enhanced technology and scientific advances, the demand to seek procedures to address these patients' cosmetic concerns has reached new heights. Patients with skin of color who request cosmetic procedures have various motivations and goals. They may want to attain even skin tone, remove unwanted hair, and/or reduce the signs of aging. This chapter will provide a systematic overview of the cosmetic concerns for those with skin of color by describing the practical approaches to treating pigmentary disorders, keloids, dermatosis papulosa nigra (DPN), unwanted hair, skin laxity, and photoaging in those with skin of color.

H. Woolery-Lloyd, M.D. (✉)
University of Miami Cosmetic Medicine and Research Institute,
4701 North Meridian Avenue, Suite, 7450, Miami Beach, FL 33140, USA
e-mail: Woolerylloyd@yahoo.com

J.N. Kammer, B.A.
Medical Student, Drexel University College of Medicine,
1425 Locust Street, Apt.24B, Philadelphia, PA 19102, USA
e-mail: jennakammer@gmail.com

A.F. Alexis and V.H. Barbosa (eds.), *Skin of Color: A Practical Guide to Dermatologic Diagnosis and Treatment*, DOI 10.1007/978-0-387-84929-4_12,

**Fig. 12.1** Hyperpigmentation after laser treatment

## Advantages and Disadvantages

Due to photoprotection from increased melanin, photoaging in dark-skinned individuals tends to be less severe and often occurs at a later age compared to light-skinned individuals. Grimes conducted a survey of age-matched white and black women, with a mean age of 43, regarding wrinkle self-assessments. Sixty-five percent of black women reported that their skin was not wrinkled compared to only 20% of white women reporting no wrinkles [1]. This reveals a marked distinction in perceived photoaging.

At the same time, there are other unique cosmetic concerns for those with skin of color. Inflammation or injury to the skin is almost immediately accompanied by alteration in pigmentation, namely, hyperpigmentation or hypopigmentation (Fig. 12.1). As follows, patients are most concerned with postinflammatory pigment changes. In a survey describing the cosmetic concerns in women of color (81 AA, 16 Hispanic, 3 Asian) with a mean age of 41, 86% of women reported hyperpigmentation or dark spots, and 80% stated blotchy or uneven skin [1].

## Hyperpigmentation

Hyperpigmentation is a common dermatologic condition in patients with skin of color. Treating hyperpigmentation can be a complicated and challenging process and, due to high recurrence rates, is often trying. A variety of topical agents are available to treat hyperpigmentation. These topical agents can interfere with the pigmentation process at several different levels. Commonly used agents to treat hyperpigmentation include tyrosinase inhibitors, melanosome-transfer inhibitors, and melanocyte-cytotoxic agents. Treatment can be greatly enhanced by using sunscreens, chemical peels, and microdermabrasion in conjunction with the topical agents, thus providing patients with a more comprehensive approach to treating hyperpigmentation.

When assessing facial hyperpigmentation, it is helpful to divide patients into two groups: localized and diffuse hyperpigmentation. Localized hyperpigmentation is characterized by well-demarcated brown patches on the face. This type of dyschromia is typically seen with acne and melasma. Diffuse or ill-defined hyperpigmentation can be more difficult to treat. Many patients with skin of color complain of "uneven skin tone." The cause of diffuse hyperpigmentation is unclear, but it is a common manifestation of aging and typically occurs in sun-exposed areas such as the face and dorsal hands.

### *Localized Hyperpigmentation*

Patients with localized hyperpigmentation due to conditions such as acne or melasma can apply hydroquinone topically to the affected areas nightly. A common side effect of using hydroquinone for treating dyschromia due to acne is the *halo* of hypopigmentation surrounding the dark macule due to bleaching of the surrounding normal skin. This is frequently observed when patients apply hydroquinone with their fingertips to small macules. Using of a cotton-tipped applicator is recommended to better localize treatment to the hyperpigmented areas and to prevent the hydroquinone halo. Additionally, applying a retinoid to the full face after the hydroquinone can also help to even the complexion.

For better results, a variation of Kligman's formula containing a topical hydroquinone combined with a retinoid and steroid can be used. Combination products that are currently available are very effective example Epiquin (fluocinolone acetonide 0.01%, hydroquinone 4%, tretinoin 0.05%) and EpiQuin® Micro (hydroquinone 4% with retinol); however, many patients with skin of color require formulations that are greater than 4% hydroquinone to achieve the greatest results. For these patients, a compounded product with concentrations of hydroquinone ranging from 6% to 10% may be useful for limited treatment durations (ideally 3 months or less) and in combination with a low-potency topical corticosteroid to prevent irritant contact dermatitis.

Hydroquinone used in combination with a retinoid and a steroid has a well-described mechanism of action and remains the gold standard for treating hyperpigmentation. Hydroquinone is a natural, plant-derived tyrosinase inhibitor and has been used in the United States to treat pigmentary disorders for several decades [2]. Despite its effectiveness, safety concerns have led to the ban of hydroquinone by regulatory agencies in parts of Europe and Asia as well as South Africa. In the United States, hydroquinone is currently available over the counter in 2% concentrations and by prescription in 4% concentrations. There is a continuing debate regarding whether or not the FDA will further regulate hydroquinone in the United States due to the reported mutagenic properties of hydroquinone when administered systemically in animals [3, 4]. However, no such effects have been reported in humans.

A rare side effect of hydroquinone is exogenous ochronosis. Exogenous ochronosis is paradoxical darkening of the skin. It usually begins with erythema followed by blue-black patches on the face where the hydroquinone was applied. In severe cases, blue-black macules can progress to papules and nodules on sun-exposed areas after long-term usage of hydroquinone [5]. It may be triggered from inhibition of homogentisic acid oxidase locally by hydroquinone. This rare side effect was common in South Africa where long-term hydroquinone use was widespread. In the United States, ochronosis is observed but is less common. It typically occurs with long-term continued use of hydroquinone over decades. The risk of ochronosis may be reduced with sunscreen since the pattern of ochronosis clinically is photodistributed. Due to the risk of ochronosis, long-term continued use of hydroquinone should be avoided. For patients with chronic conditions like melasma, hydroquinone should be switched to an alternative therapy such as azelaic acid after several months or once significant improvement is achieved.

More common side effects with hydroquinone include irritation and erythema. When prescribing hydroquinone, it is important to inform patients of this side effect and to recommend that patients discontinue the treatment if any significant redness or inflammation occurs. Irritation from hydroquinone is frequently due to the hydroquinone itself or to sodium metabisulfite, a common preservative in hydroquinone preparations [6]. Continuing hydroquinone regardless of irritation may lead to postinflammatory hyperpigmentation. Moreover, sunscreen is crucial in patients with hyperpigmentation to prevent recurrence, and this portion of the regimen should be equally stressed to the patient.

## *Diffuse Hyperpigmentation*

Diffuse and ill-defined hyperpigmentation can be challenging to treat. For this type of hyperpigmentation, the current authors recommend avoiding application of hydroquinone to the full face. When hydroquinone is applied to the full face, patients tend to develop an unnatural appearance where the skin on the face does not match the skin on the neck and the rest of the body. More subtle agents are more effective for this type of dyschromia. Azelaic acid daily combined with a retinoid at night is a simple and effective regimen.

Azelaic acid is a dicarboxylic acid, which has some antityrosinase effects in addition to its cytotoxic and antiproliferate effects [7]. Azelaic acid is available as a 15% gel which is approved for the treatment of rosacea and a 20% cream which is approved for the treatment of acne vulgaris. The use of azelaic acid for hyperpigmentation is off-label but has been documented in several published studies. Azelaic acid is typically well tolerated; however, stinging within the first few weeks is common. Therefore, patients should be informed of this potential side effect but assured that it usually resolves with time. The gel formulation is useful for those with oily skin, and the cream formulation is often preferable for those with dry skin.

## *Additional Therapies*

There are many alternative therapies for treating hyperpigmentation. Although none appears to reach the efficacy of hydroquinone, these alternatives can be used for patients that have hydroquinone sensitivities or during hydroquinone drug holidays. Mequinol, a 4-hydroxyanisole and derivative of hydroquinone, is a substrate of tyrosinase and acts as a competitive inhibitor of tyrosinase. In Europe, it is widely used in concentrations of 5–10%; in the United States, it is approved for the treatment of solar lentigines (Solagé, mequinol 2%/tretinoin 0.01%). Arbutin is a tyrosinase inhibitor, which can be extracted from bearberry (*Arctostaphylos uva-ursi*) and certain pear trees [8]. It is available in 1–3% formulations; however, there are not many controlled clinical studies available to support its efficacy.

Kojic acid is a fungal metabolite produced by Aspergillus, Acetobacter, and Penicillium. It is a well-known bleaching agent, which inactivates tyrosinase by chelation of copper. Garcia et al. compared 5% glycolic acid/2% hydroquinone gel with 5% glycolic acid/2% kojic acid gel for the treatment of melasma and found the two treatments to be equally effective [9]. However, kojic acid has a significant sensitizing potential, which should be taken into consideration when treating patients with sensitive skin [10].

Another tyrosinase inhibitor is aloesin, a glycosylated chromone derived from *Aloe vera*. Aloesin and a few chemically related chromones have been shown to contain a stronger inhibitory effect on tyrosinase than arbutin and kojic acid [11, 12]. In a study by Choi et al., aloesin and/or arbutin, administered four times a day for 15 days on pigmented human skin after UV radiation, showed a suppressed pigmentation by 34% for aloesin, 43.5% for arbutin, and 63.3% for aloesin and arbutin in combination [13].

Soy interferes with melanin transfer by inhibiting the protein-activated receptor 2 (PAR-2) pathway. PAR-2 is a G-protein-coupled receptor that regulates the ingestion of melanosomes by keratinocytes [14]. Two soy milk-derived proteins, namely, soybean trypsin inhibitor (STI) and the Bowman-Birk inhibitor (BBI) have been demonstrated to interfere with melanosome transfer by inhibiting the PAR-2 activation. The depigmenting activity of these agents and their ability to prevent ultraviolet-induced pigmentation suggests that inhibition of the PAR-2 pathway by soy milk may be used as a natural alternative to skin lightening [15]. A blinded controlled 12-week study evaluated the efficacy of a soy moisturizer containing STI and BBI on 65 women with moderate facial photodamage. A significant improvement in mottled pigmentation, blotchiness, dullness, fine lines, overall texture, and overall skin tone was demonstrated [16].

### Sunscreen

As mentioned previously, sunscreen is a crucial and fundamental component of the regimen when treating hyperpigmentation. Novel adjunctive therapies in treating

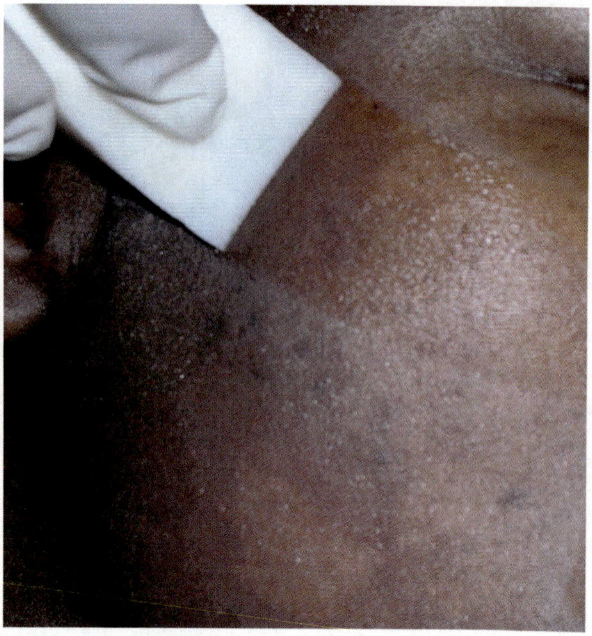

**Fig. 12.2** Salicylic acid peel of cheek

hyperpigmentation are oral photoprotectant. Polypodium leucotomos, a fern extract, (Heliocare®) is a commercially available oral photoprotectant. In clinical studies, Polypodium leucotomos was demonstrated to diminish sunburn cells after UVB exposure [17]. This oral therapy offers another sun protection option for patients with pigment disorders. A double blinded placebo-controlled pilot study with 21 subjects with melasma showed improvement with Polypodium leucotomos. The subjects were divided into two groups in which half received a placebo and half received Polypodium leucotomos (PL). The PL group demonstrated improvement in their melasma as measured by the patient assessments, investigator assessments and Mean Melasma Area and Severity Index (MASI) scores [18].

## Chemical Peels and Microdermabrasion

A more mechanistic approach to treating pigment disorders is the adjunctive use of chemical peels or microdermabrasion. These interventions work best in a series; typically, three to five monthly treatments are required to attain the greatest results. Absorption studies prove that these procedures not only remove superficial layers of the stratum corneum but also enhance penetration of topical therapies when treating hyperpigmentation [19, 20]. It is important to be aware of the prior use of a retinoid for it can cause a superficial peel to penetrate deeper than anticipated. Therefore, clinicians should consider discontinuing the use of retinoids, approximately 7–10 days prior to peels to reduce the risk of an adverse effect (Fig. 12.2).

## Keloids

Darker racial ethnic groups have unique wound healing characteristics that must be considered when performing cosmetic procedures. The main concern with surgical procedures in skin of color patients is the incidence of keloids and hypertrophic scars. Keloids and hypertrophic scars are most common in darker racial ethnic groups and are most prevalent in African-American, Hispanic, and Asian populations. Statistics on the incidence of keloids in specific populations vary greatly; however, an incidence of 5–16% has been reported in black and Hispanic populations [21]. Patients with keloids usually present in the second or third decade, and there is an equal risk among women and men. Keloids most commonly develop on earlobes (Fig. 12.3), shoulders, the upper back, and chest. Postsurgically, they appear to be most frequent in areas of highest tension. These scars consist of excessive dense fibrous tissue that extends beyond the borders of the original wound and do not regress spontaneously. Once excised, they tend to recur. Common symptoms include pruritus and tenderness at the site of the keloid. These symptoms are most severe in new scars and tend to diminish with time.

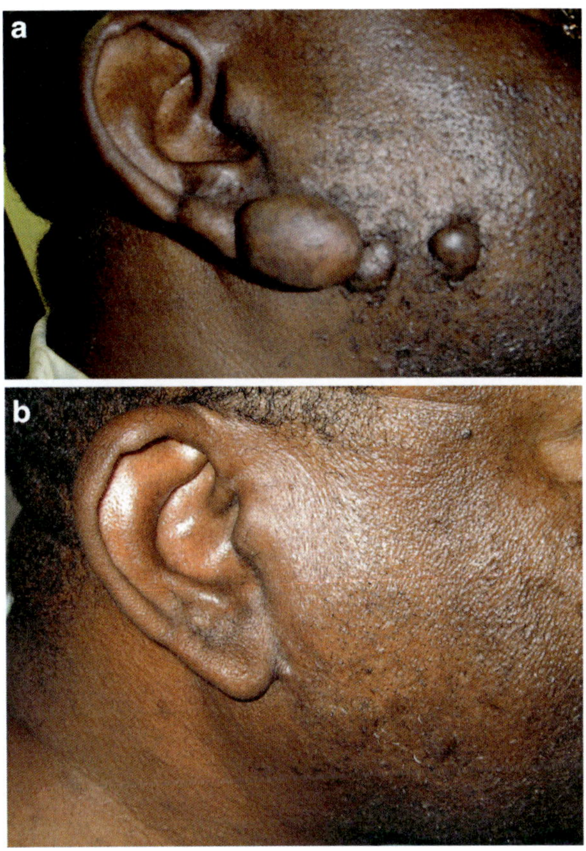


**Fig. 12.3** (**a**) Keloid jaw before. (**b**) After treatment

Prevention of recurrence is the biggest challenge with any keloid therapy. However, there are many treatment options for diminishing keloids. The standard therapies for keloids include intralesional corticosteroids, compression, laser therapy, and cryosurgery, yet still they do not provide optimal results. For example, cryotherapy can result in significant hypopigmentation. Surgical excision alone has a reported recurrence rate between 45% and 100% [22–25]. This high recurrence rate is decreased with the use of adjuvant therapy postexcision, such as intralesional corticosteroids, imiquimod 5% cream, and radiotherapy [26–28].

## Dermatosis Papulosa Nigra

Dermatosis papulosa nigra (DPN) is a benign epithelial tumor, common in darker racial ethnic groups. It is usually characterized by multiple, small, firm, hyperpigmented, asymptomatic papules on the face. DPN is a special topographic form of seborrheic keratosis. Lesions occur mainly on the malar area of the face and the forehead, although they also may be found on the neck, upper back, and chest. A small percentage of patients have similar lesions on the upper trunk. DPNs are one of the most common cosmetic concerns in those with skin of color. The treatment of choice in skin of color patients is hyfrecation. Treatment with hyfrecation on its lowest setting is important to avoid atrophic scars. Other treatment choices include cryotherapy and lasers; however, these should be avoided due to the significant risk of pigmentary changes [29]. Treatment should be superficial to minimize the risk of complications. Immediately after hyfrecation, the DPNs are slightly swollen with surrounding redness. Patients should be advised not to pick them, and the DPNs will typically fall off within 3–7 days following treatment. It is also important to perform cryotherapy with caution in skin of color due to the risk of pigmentary changes (Fig. 12.4).

## Unwanted Hair

Before the introduction of longer wavelengths and longer pulse durations, laser-assisted hair removal was largely limited to Fitzpatrick skin phototypes I–III with dark terminal hairs. Now, laser-assisted hair removal can be performed safely and efficaciously on darker skin types. The long-pulsed diode and Nd:YAG-wavelength-based laser systems are best suited to treat patients with darker skin types. By using conservative fluences, longer pulse durations, and multiple treatments, effective laser-assisted hair removal is possible for darker skin types. Topical eflornithine HCl 13.9% has been shown to be safe and effective in the management of unwanted facial hair in women [30]. It can be used in combination with laser hair removal and has been shown to be more effective when used for 6 months in conjunction with laser hair removal [31].

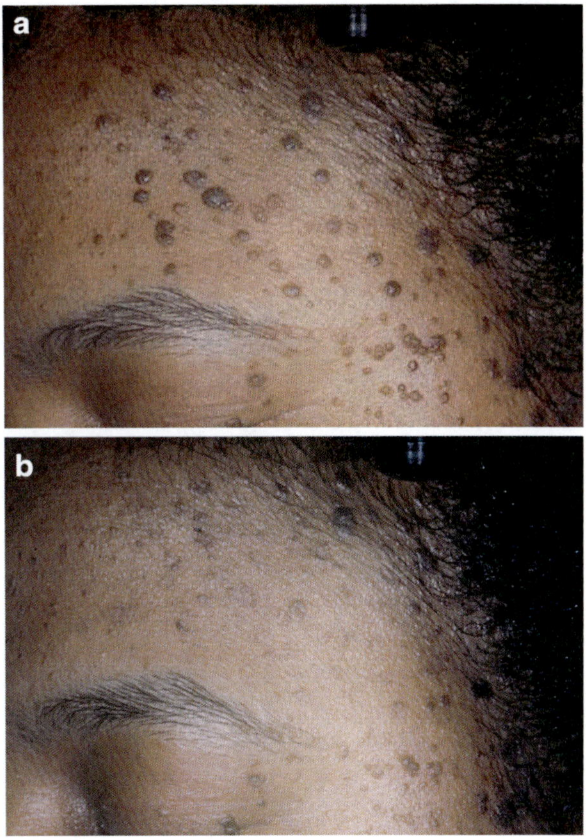

**Fig. 12.4** (**a**) Dermatosis papulosa nigra close-up before. (**b**) Dermatosis papulosa nigra close-up after

## *Diode Lasers*

The diode laser has been studied with great success in the treatment of darker-skinned patients. The 800-nm diode laser was examined with pulse widths of 30 ms and 100 ms. Adrian et al. reported that although both settings could be used safely, longer pulse widths (100 ms) allowed higher fluences to be utilized with fewer complications [32]. Another study used the 810-nm diode laser to treat eight patients with skin types V and VI. These patients were treated with a low fluence of 10mj/cm$^2$ and a pulse width of 30 ms. Transient blistering and pigment alterations were observed in some patients, despite the lower fluence utilization [33]. Overall, the diode laser offers an effective method for treating ethnic patients; however, complications remain problematic.

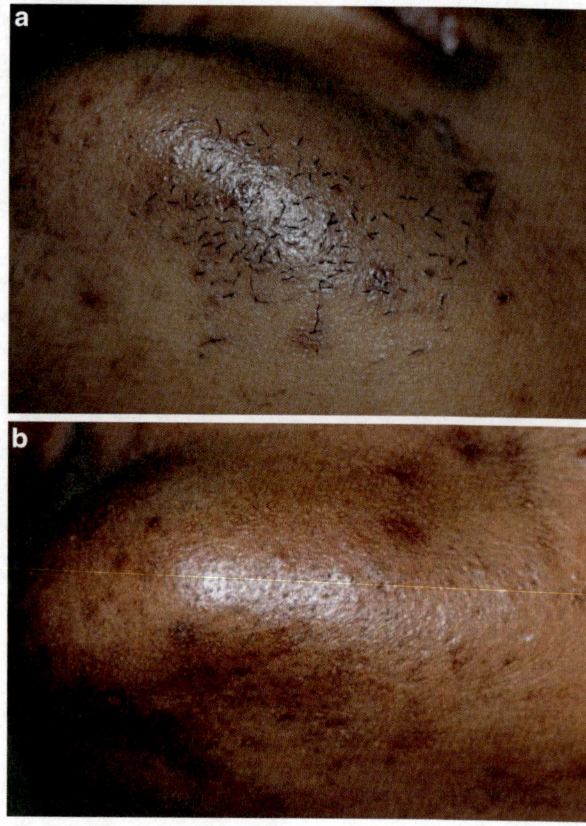


**Fig. 12.5** (**a**) Chin before laser hair removal (**b**) Chin after laser hair removal

## *Nd:YAG*

Due to the longer wavelength, the Nd:YAG system is the safest. Two factors contribute to the safety of the long-pulsed Nd:YAG in darker skin types. First, the longer wavelength of the Nd:YAG (1,064 nm) is located at the end of the absorption spectrum of melanin. This wavelength has the ability to achieve significant thermal injury in dark coarse hairs while not interfering with epidermal pigment. Second, the adjustable pulse width of the long-pulsed Nd:YAG laser allows the energy to be delivered over a longer period of time permitting the heat to dissipate, and thus allocating sufficient epidermal cooling. Darker racial ethnic groups typically have coarse, dark hair, and the Nd:YAG laser has proven to be effective at achieving permanent hair reduction after a series of treatments [34, 35] (Fig. 12.5).

Challenges arise with the long-pulsed Nd: YAG in darker skin types in patients who have dark skin but fine hair. This is generally seen in patients of Southeast Asian descent. With these patients, it is important to educate them on the limitations of laser hair removal. Patients must have realistic expectations and understand that lasers can offer an excellent hair management program but may not provide permanent long-term removal of fine hairs. Most patients who fall into this category still prefer lasers since irritation and dyschromia are frequently associated with shaving and waxing.

## Skin Laxity

Numerous patients with skin of color seek treatment to remedy skin laxity. An increase in skin laxity with advanced age is observed equally common among all races and ethnicities. Many older patients seek treatment to tighten the jowl and nasolabial fold areas, two areas which are well-known signs of aging. Many patients with skin of color seek nonsurgical interventions due to the significant risk of scarring. Devices that heat the dermis can be utilized to improve skin laxity. The idea behind noninvasive skin-tightening devices is to prevent epidermal injury with the desired injury occurring only at the site of maximal energy absorption in the dermis. This injury is speculated to create new collagen and elastic fibers and may contribute to immediate tightening due to denaturation and contraction of existing collagen fibers [36, 37]. There are different approaches to heating up the dermis to effect clinical skin tightening, including radiofrequency energy and infrared light. Both approaches are nonablative and do not require surgical incisions. Noninvasive skin tightening is especially useful in skin of color patients due to the significant risk of keloids and scarring that are associated with surgery in this population.

### *Radiofrequency*

Radiofrequency (RF) is an electromagnetic radiation in the frequency range of 3 kHz to 300 GHz. These devices induce dermal heating, denature collagen, and induce collagen remodeling [36]. Wound healing mechanisms promote wound contraction, which ultimately enhances the appearance of mild to moderate skin laxity. Since RF is not dependent on a specific chromophore interaction, epidermal melanin is not targeted, and treatment of all skin types is possible.

### *Infrared Tightening*

Infrared light can be used to volumetrically heat the dermis. It is designed to thermally induce collagen contraction, with ensuing collagen remodeling and neocollagen synthesis. The epidermis is protected by being cooled throughout the procedure. Chua et al. investigated the use of infrared light on 21 patients of skin types IV and V. The physician's assessments of photographs before and 6 months after treatment illustrated observable lifting of sagging skin folds in 86% of patients. The researchers concluded that the infrared light device is effective in treating mild

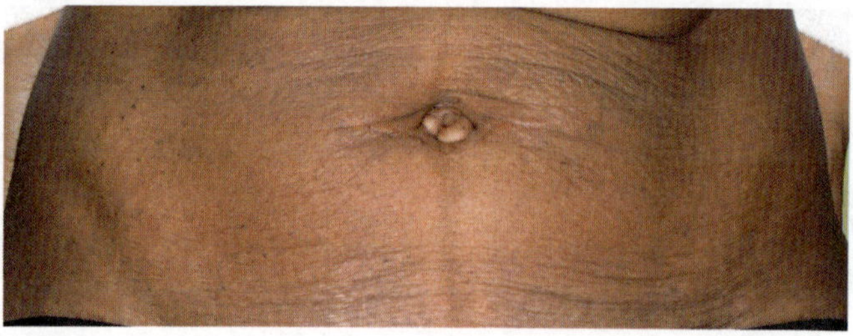

**Fig. 12.6** Postinfrared tightening

to moderate facial and neck skin laxity [38]. Infrared skin tightening has minimal downtime and is safe to use on all skin types, and multiple sessions are recommended for better results (Fig. 12.6).

## Photoaging in Skin of Color

Visible signs of aging are primarily a result of sun exposure. Studies have revealed that approximately five times as much ultraviolet light reaches the upper dermis of Caucasians compared to African Americans. This photoprotection is a result of having more melanin in dark skin [39]. Accordingly, fine and coarse lines are seen earlier in light than in dark skin. Despite the photoprotection presented by darker-skinned individuals, chronological aging is seen in darker racial ethnic groups [40]. In one study, older black subjects demonstrated flattening of the dermoepidermal junction when compared to younger subjects [41]. Additionally, there was elastic fiber degeneration, an increase in the superficial vascular plexus and a decrease in the number of melanocytes recorded with an increase in age in black patients. Thus, the number of overall cosmetic procedures is increasing in darker racial and ethnic groups, including the use of botulinum toxin type A and soft tissue augmentation.

### *Botulinum Toxin*

Botulinum toxin type A (BTX-A) can be used cosmetically to improve hyperkinetic facial rhytides, particularly of the upper one-third of the face. BTX-A treatment is the most common cosmetic procedure, with more than 2.7 million individuals receiving injections in 2007. Skin of color patients characterized almost 21% of all patients who received BTX-A, and the demand is increasing [42]. A recent study demonstrated that BTX-A is safe and effective in treating glabellar rhytides in African American women with skin types V and VI [43]. Despite the inherent differences in darker and lighter skin types, hyperfunctional facial muscles cause brow furrows and glabellar creases in all races [44].

The most commonly treated sites in African Americans patients include the forehead and glabellar areas. However, African American patients are less likely to seek treatment for crow's feet wrinkles as these rhytides are more dependent on photoaging. In a phase III clinical trial of the glabellar area, 21 out of 405 patients were African American. The study compared the overall efficacy of those 21 subjects to the remaining Caucasian subjects, and in the end there were no statistically significant differences in the efficacy or safety responses between the two groups [45].

In Asian patients, BTX-A has been shown to effectively recontour the upper and lower face. Some Asian patients desire a more open and wider eyelid. This can be achieved with the injection of 2 units of BTX-A into the lower lid to widen the eye slightly. In one study, 15 women had BTX-A injected into the orbicularis oculi muscle, and the results were more notable in the Asian eye. Two units of BTX-A injected into the lower eyelid's orbicularis oculi muscle improve infraorbital wrinkles, particularly when used in combination with BTX-A treatment of the lateral orbital area [46].

Another common concern in Asian women is a prominent mandibular angle and jaw fullness. Such patients usually present with hypertrophic masseter muscles causing jaw fullness. Intramuscular masseter injections with BTX-A can improve contours of the lower facial profile by reducing the bulkiness of masseteric muscles. Three-dimensional computed tomography evaluations demonstrated a statistically significant mean masseter reduction of about 30%, as well as the results lasting up to 6 months [47]. Treatment with BTX-A is a safe and effective alternative for contouring the lower facial profile in addition to its use for cosmetically improving rhytides in all racial and ethnic groups.

## *Soft Tissue Augmentation*

Soft tissue augmentation is another common noninvasive procedure sought by patients with skin of color. As a result, practitioners performing soft tissue augmentation must have proficient knowledge in the treatment of ethnic skin. In the young face, superficial and deep fat is distributed evenly, creating a homogenous topographical appearance. As the face begins to age, fat atrophy causes hills and valleys to develop, producing demarcations between the cosmetic components. Soft tissue augmentation attempts to restore an individual's face volume. Volume is primarily restored in areas of fat loss and atrophy [48]. Ethnic patients have a tendency toward midface aging with sagging of the malar fat pads toward the nasolabial folds, upper lid laxity, and jowl formation [49].

Based on the skin type, some soft tissue fillers will achieve better results than others. Collagen has an opaque white color which can be seen when injected superficially in skin of color patients. Hyaluronic acid and poly-L-lactic acid are transparent and thus are better choices for patients with skin of color. Calcium hydroxyl appetite is another beneficial choice for ethnic skin patients with deep rhytides.

Hyaluronic acid (HA) represents the most frequently used soft tissue augmentation filler and ranks second overall in surgical and nonsurgical cosmetic-performed procedures [42]. In a study of 60 patients injected with stabilized hyaluronic acid (Restylane ®), 40 patients were skin types I–III and 20 were skin types IV–VI. Of the skin types I–III, 2 of the 40 patients experienced temporary adverse events. Of the 20 patients with skin types IV–VI, no transient or permanent adverse events were observed. The investigators concluded that HA is a safe and effective treatment for darker skin types [50]. Since all the fillers mentioned offer a safe and effective treatment option for soft tissue augmentation, physicians should concentrate on the individual needs of the patient when choosing the appropriate filler.

## Conclusion

People with skin of color represent a significant growing group of patients seeking aesthetic procedures. Understanding the unique characteristics of skin of color is essential in cosmetic dermatology. The best way to approach cosmetic procedures in skin of color patients involves a thorough understanding and knowledge of the appropriate modalities available to treat their cosmetic concerns. Although effective cosmetic treatments in ethnic skin can be challenging, it is crucial that clinicians feel competent performing these treatments as the demand for cosmetic procedures will continue to soar worldwide.

## References


1. Grimes PE. Skin and hair cosmetic issues in women of color. Dermatol Clin. 2000;18(4): 659–65.
2. Penney KB, Smith CJ, Allen JC. Depigmenting action of hydroquinone depends on disruption of fundamental cell processes. J Invest Dermatol. 1984;82:308–10.
3. Bates B. Derms react to possible FDA ban of hydroquinone: cite poor scientific reasoning, ethnic bias. Skin Allergy News. 2007;38(1):20.
4. Nordlund JJ, Grimes PE, Ortonne JP. The safety of hydroquinone. J Eur Acad Dermatol Vener. 2006;20(7):781–7.
5. Lawrence N, Bligard CA, Reed R, et al. Exogenous ochronosis in the United States. J Am Acad Dermatol. 1988;18:1207–11.
6. Huang PY, Chu CY. Allergic contact dermatitis due to sodium metabisulfite in a bleaching cream. Contact Dermatitis. 2007;56(2):123–4.
7. Fitton A, Goa KL. Azelaic acid. A review of its pharmacological properties and therapeutic efficacy in acne and hyperpigmentary skin disorders. Drugs. 1991;41:780–98.
8. Grimes PE. Management of hyperpigmentation in darker racial ethnic groups. Semin Cutan Med Surg. 2009;28(2):77–85.
9. Garcia A, Fulton Jr JE. The combination of glycolic acid and hydroquinone or kojic acid for the treatment of melasma and related conditions. Dermatol Surg. 1996;22(5):443–7.
10. Nakagawa M, Kawai K, Kawai K. Contact allergy to kojic acid in skin care products. Contact Dermatitis. 1995;32(1):9–13.
11. Jones K, Hughes J, Hong M, et al. Modulation of melanogenesis by aloesin: a competitive inhibitor of tyrosinase. Pigment Cell Res. 2002;15(5):335–40.

12. Piao LZ, Park HR, Park YK, et al. Mushroom tyrosinase inhibition activity of some chromones. Chem Pharm Bull(Tokyo). 2002;50(3):309–11.
13. Choi S, Lee SK, Kim JE, et al. Aloesin inhibits hyperpigmentation induced by UV radiation. Clin Exp Dermatol. 2002;27(6):513–5.
14. Babiarz-Magee L, Chen N, Seiberg M, Lin CB. The expression and activation of protease-activated receptor-2 correlate with skin color. Pigment Cell Res. 2004;17(3):241–51.
15. Paine C, Sharlow E, Liebel F. An alternative approach to depigmentation by soybean extracts via inhibition of the PAR-2 pathway. J Invest Dermatol. 2001;116:585–95.
16. Wallo W, Nebus J, Leyden JJ. Efficacy of a soy moisturizer in photoaging: a double-blind, vehicle-controlled, 12-week study. J Drugs Dermatol. 2007;6(9):917–22.
17. Middelkamp-Hup MA, Pathak MA, Parrado C, Goukassian D, Rius-Díaz F, Mihm MC, Fitzpatrick TB, González S. Oral Polypodium leucotomos extract decreases ultraviolet-induced damage of human skin. J Am Acad Dermatol. 2004;51(6):910–8.
18. Woolery-Lloyd H, Martin L. A randomized double-blind placebo controlled study evaluating the effectiveness and tolerability of oral *Polypodium leucotomos* in patients with melasma J Am Acad of Dermatol. 2012;66(4(suppl 1)):AB21.
19. Lee WR, Shen SC, Kuo-Hsien W, Hu CH, Fang JY. Lasers and microdermabrasion enhance and control topical delivery of vitamin C. J Invest Dermatol. 2003;121(5):1118–25.
20. Rajan P, Grimes PE. Skin barrier changes induced by aluminum oxide and sodium chloride microdermabrasion. Dermatol Surg. 2002;28(5):390–3.
21. Berman B, Villa A. Imiquimod 5% cream for keloid management. Dermatol Surg. 2003;29: 1050–1.
22. Mathangi-Ramakrishnan K, Pothan-Thomas K, Cheyyur R. Study of 1,000 patients with keloidal scars in South India. Plast Reconstr Surg. 1974;53:276–80.
23. Cosman B, Wolff M. Correlation of keloid recurrence with completeness of local excision: a negative report. Plast Reconstr Surg. 1972;50:163–6.
24. Lawrence WT. In search of the optimal treatment of keloids: report of a series and a review of the literature. Ann Plast Surg. 1991;27:164–78.
25. Conway H, Gillette RW, Findley A. Differential diagnosis of keloids and hypertrophic scars by tissue culture techniques with notes on therapy of keloids by surgical excision and decadron. Plast Reconstr Surg. 1960;25:117–32.
26. Niessen FB, Spauwen PH, Schalkwijk J, Kon M. On the nature of hypertrophic scars and keloids: a review. Plast Reconstr Surg. 1999;104:1435–58.
27. Berman B, Kaufman J. Pilot study of the effect of postoperative imiquimod 5% cream on the recurrence rate of excised keloids. J Am Acad Dermatol. 2002;47(4):S209–11.
28. Tosa M, Ghazizadeh M, Shimizu H, et al. Global gene expression analysis of keloid fibroblasts in response to electron beam irradiation reveals the involvement of interleukin-6 pathway. J Invest Dermatol. 2005;124:704–13.
29. Lupo MP. Dermatosis papulosa nigra: treatment options. J Drugs Dermatol. 2007;6(1): 29–30.
30. Wolf Jr JE, Shander D, Huber F, Jackson J, Lin CS, Mathes BM, et al. Randomized, double-blind clinical evaluation of the efficacy and safety of topical eflornithine HCl 13.9% cream in the treatment of women with facial hair. Int J Dermatol. 2007;46(1):94–8.
31. Hamzavi I, Tan E, Shapiro J, Lui H. A randomized bilateral vehicle-controlled study of eflornithine cream combined with laser treatment versus laser treatment alone for facial hirsutism in women. J Am Acad Dermatol. 2007;57(1):54–9.
32. Adrian RM, Shay KP. 800 nanometer diode laser hair removal in African American patients: a clinical and histologic study. J Cutan Laser Ther. 2000;2(4):183–90.
33. Greppi I. Diode laser hair removal of the black patient. Lasers Surg Med. 2001;28(2):150–5.
34. Alster TS, Bryan H, Williams CM. Long-pulsed Nd:YAG laser-assisted hair removal in pigmented skin: a clinical and histological evaluation. Arch Dermatol. 2001;137(7):885–9.
35. Ross EV, Cooke LM, Timko AL, Overstreet KA, et al. Treatment of pseudofolliculitis barbae in skin types IV, V, and VI with a long-pulsed neodymium:yttrium aluminum garnet laser. J Am Acad Dermatol. 2002;47(2):263–7.

36. Zelickson BD, Kist D, Bernstein E, et al. Histological and ultrastructural evaluation of the effects of a radiofrequency based nonablative dermal remodeling device: a pilot study. Arch Dermatol. 2004;140(2):204–9.
37. Fitzpatrick R, Geronemeus R, Goldberg D, et al. Multicenter study of noninvasive radiofrequency for periorbital tissue tightening. Lasers Surg Med. 2003;33:232–42.
38. Chua SH, Ang P, Khoo LS, Goh CL. Nonablative infared skin tightening in Type IV to V Asian skin: a prospective clinical study. Dermatol Surg. 2007;33(2):146–51.
39. Kaidbey KH, Agin PP, Sayre RM, Kaidbey KH, Agin PP, Sayre RM, et al. Photoprotection by melanin – a comparison of black and Caucasian skin. J Am Acad Dermatol. 1979;1(3):249–60.
40. Woolery-Lloyd H. Skin of color. In: Baumann L, editor. Cosmetic dermatology. 2nd ed. New York: McGraw-Hill; 2009. p. 115.
41. Herzberg AJ, Dinehart SM. Chronologic aging in black skin. Am J Dermatopathol. 1989;11:319–28.
42. America Society for Aesthetic plastic surgery. Cosmetic surgery national data bank statistics. http://www.surgery.org/public/consumer/trends/cosmetic_procedures_in_2007. Accessed 5 July 2009.
43. Grimes PE, Shabazz D. A four-month randomized, double-blind evaluation of the efficacy of Botulinum Toxin type A for the treatment of glabellar lines in women with skin types V and VI. Dermatol Surg. 2009;35(3):429–36.
44. Jackson BA. Cosmetic considerations and nonlaser cosmetic procedures in ethnic skin. Dermatol Clin. 2003;21:703–12.
45. Hexsel DM, Hexsel CL, Brunetto LT. Botulinum toxin. In: Grimes PE, editor. Aesthetic and cosmetic surgery for darker skin types. Philadelphia: Lippincott Williams and Wilkins; 2007. p. 211–24.
46. Flynn TC, Carruthers JA, Carruthers JA. Botulinum A toxin treatment of the lower eyelid improves infraorbital rhytides and widens the eye. Dermatol Surg. 2001;27:703–8.
47. Yu CC, Chen PK, Chen YR. Botulinum toxin a for lower facial contouring: a prospective study. Aesthetic Plast Surg. 2007;31(5):445–51. discussion 452–453.
48. Brugges CM. Soft tissue augmentation in skin of color: market growth, available fillers, and successful techniques. J Drugs Dermatol. 2007;6:51–5.
49. Matory WE. Aging in people of color. In: Matory WE, editor. Ethnic considerations in facial aesthetic surgery. Philadelphia: Lippincott-Raven; 1998. p. 151–70.
50. Odunze M, Cohn A, Few JW. Restylane and people of color. Plast Reconstr Surg. 2007;120(7):2011–6.

# Chapter 13
# Laser Hair Removal for Darker Skin Types

**Eliot Battle**

Removing unwanted hair has been an accepted procedure since the beginning of civilized time. Prior to the onset of laser hair removal, popular procedures ranged from abrasion, threading, plucking, waxing, chemical depilatories, and shaving. These conventional procedures had different levels of effectiveness and were used mainly for hair growth delay and temporary hair removal. Permanent depilation became possible with the onset of electrolysis; however, the procedure was tedious and time consuming and led to a high incidence of postinflammatory hyperpigmentation and scarring in patients with curly hair and darker skin types (phototypes IV–VI).

Since its inception, laser hair removal has become an increasingly popular procedure to permanently reduce unwanted hair and has revolutionized the field of hair removal when it was introduced over a decade ago. It was originally recommended only for lighter skin patients (phototypes I–III) and contraindicated in patients with ethnically dark or sun-tanned skin. By combining longer wavelengths, longer pulse durations, and more efficient cooling devices, laser hair removal is no longer a treatment option only for lighter skin patients but available to all patients regardless of skin types, skin color, or ethnicity, including patients with darker skin types (phototypes IV–VI).

For lighter skin patients, whose hair is stereotypically straight and fine, it was viewed mostly as a time-saving cosmetic procedure. Previous conventional methods worked well but were considered by many to be mundane, tedious, and time consuming. In contrast, in patients with darker skin types (phototypes IV–VI), with curly and coarse hair, dermatologic conditions such as ingrown hair, pseudofolliculitis barbae, and hirsutism do not respond or improve with the previous conventional hair removal methods (threading, plucking, waxing, chemical depilatories,

E. Battle, M.D. (✉)
Department of Dermatology, Howard University Hospital,
5301 Wisconsin Avenue NW, Washington, DC 20015, USA
e-mail: eliotbattle@msn.com

A.F. Alexis and V.H. Barbosa (eds.), *Skin of Color: A Practical Guide to Dermatologic Diagnosis and Treatment*, DOI 10.1007/978-0-387-84929-4_13,

electrolysis, and shaving) and can even worsen the initial dermatologic condition, resulting in additional inflammatory papules, postinflammatory hyperpigmentation, and scarring.

This all changed when laser hair removal treatments became available for people with skin of color. For the first time there was an effective way to remove unwanted hair and, as important, improve the dermatologic conditions associated with coarse and curly hair in patients with darker skin types.

The backbone of cosmetic light-based laser therapy is the theory of selective photothermolysis. It is ironic that the most popular procedure in the field is based on a modified version of the theory. The theory of selective photothermolysis states that by using the appropriate wavelength, pulse duration, and fluence, thermal injury can be confined to the absorbing chromophore, protecting the surrounding tissue [1]. The target chromophore in laser hair removal is the melanin-rich hair shaft and bulb. Based on the original theory of selective photothermolysis to assure confinement of thermal damage to the selective target, the pulse duration should be shorter than or equal to the thermal relaxation time of the hair shaft. The thermal relaxation time of the hair shaft is estimated to be in the range of 10–100 ms [2]. But to achieve effective results with laser hair removal, thermal injury must go beyond the absorbing chromophore, the hair shaft, to destroy the surrounding tissue, which in this case is the surrounding hair follicle and stem cells.

Within the follicular unit, the laser targets are the melanocytic outer root sheath, shaft, and the matrix. In addition, stem cells are crucial for hair development and growth. In order to permanently inhibit hair growth, lasers must thermally destroy not only the entire hair follicle but also these progenitor cells. The *split fuse* hypothesis has identified two stem cell reservoirs in the human anagen hair follicle. The first is thought to be located in the proximal outer root sheath. These stem cells are amelanotic and may act as a melanocytic reservoir. It is suggested from this hypothesis that the second location is located in the distal outer root sheath [3]. By using the mouse model, this location of stem cells is identified within the bulge [4]. In the human hair follicle, the location of the bulge is thought to reside in the lower third of the follicle of the outer root sheath.

Therefore, to achieve permanent hair reduction with lasers, a modified theory of selective photothermolysis is used because the melanocytic chromophore, as well as the amelanotic hair follicle and stem cells, needs to be destroyed. To achieve this goal, longer pulse durations can be utilized to propagate heat to the entire hair follicle.

## Choosing Appropriate Laser Devices to Treat Darker Skin Types

To effectively treat unwanted hair, laser light must pass through the pigmented epidermis to treat the dermal hair target. The increased difficulty in performing laser hair removal on patients with skin of color is that the melanin in the epidermis competes as a chromophore for the laser light. The melanin within the pigmented epidermis absorbs the laser light and naturally converts it to heat. If enough heat is accumulated then it creates thermal damage which can cause epidermal blistering, dyspigmentation, and scarring. In addition to the increase potential for thermal injury, epidermal melanin absorption of laser light also decreases the amount of laser light that is able to reach its intended dermal chromophore and thus reducing its efficacy. However, utilizing longer wavelengths, longer pulse durations, and more efficient cooling devices, the laser surgeon can safely and effectively treat darker skin types.

By manipulating laser parameters, new generation laser hair removal devices can provide the safety necessary to effectively and safely treat darker skin types (phototypes IV–VI). The absorption spectrum of melanin is in the range of 250–1,200 nm. Melanin absorption decreases and there is a greater depth of penetration and less superficial chromophore absorption as wavelength increases thus making longer wavelengths safer in treating darker skin.

Longer pulse durations allow for more efficient cooling of the epidermis. The more slowly the light energy is deposited into the skin (longer pulse durations), the slower the pigmented epidermis absorbs the light and heats up, thus making cooling of the skin more efficient. It is easier and more efficient to remove heat from a slow-heating object then a fast-heating object. The main cause for laser-induced side effects is epidermal thermal damage when the epidermal temperature surpasses 45°C. If heat can be effectively removed from the epidermis by keeping it under 45°C, the risk of thermal-damage-induced epidermal side effects is minimal. Longer pulse durations are also safer for darker skin types based on the theory of thermokinetic selectivity. The theory states that smaller structures (e.g., epidermal melanin) will lose heat quicker than larger structures (dermal hair follicles). The quicker dissipation of heat of the epidermal melanocytes in comparison to the larger hair follicle serves as a protective mechanism for the epidermis [5].

In addition to longer wavelengths and pulse durations, inherent laser cooling devices are imperative to minimize thermal damage on the pigmented epidermis. Cooling devices cool the skin either by direct contact of a cooling plate or by non-contact cooling by emitting cooled spray, air, or gas. The use of excessive cooling, however, is not without risk on patients with darker skin types. Caution must be employed with overzealous cooling devices on pigmented skin. Excessive cooling, particularly cryogen-induced cooling and cold air cooling, can lead to blistering and dyspigmentation. Cryogen spray can reach temperatures as low as −26.2°C leading to both cooling-induced hypopigmentation and hyperpigmentation. Excessive cooling with cold air has also been reported; however, the exact mechanism in which cold air cooling is associated with dyspigmentation after laser treatment is unknown. However, in a study evaluating the incidence of continuous cold air cooling resulting in postinflammatory hyperpigmentation (PIH) after Q-switched Nd:YAG laser treatment of bilateral nevus of Ota, 62% of patients developed PIH on the cooled side and only 24% developed PIH on the uncooled side. The authors hypothesized that laser-irradiated melanocytes or keratinocytes may be more reactive to stimuli, such as cold temperature [6].

The available laser and light sources for photoepilation include the long-pulsed ruby (694 nm), long-pulsed alexandrite (755 nm), long-pulsed diode (810 nm), long-pulsed

Nd:YAG (1,064 nm), and noncoherent intense pulsed light (IPL; 590–1,200 nm) [7]. In terms of safely treating skin of color, the Food and Drug Administration (FDA) has approved two systems for photoepilation in darker skin types: the long-pulsed diode (810 nm) and Nd:YAG (1,064 nm) [8]. These two lasers have combined longer wavelengths, extended pulse durations, and active epidermal cooling to provide the greatest efficacy and safety in treating darker skin types (phototypes IV–VI). Of these options, the longer-wavelength Nd:YAG laser is the safest type to treat darker ethnic skin [9].

To improve the safety in treating darker skin types, the long-pulse diode laser system can utilize pulse durations of 100 ms or longer. In terms of treating very dark skin, phototype VI, with the long-pulsed diode laser, Battle and Hobbs [10] reported that very long pulse durations (>400 ms) and aggressive adjunctive skin cooling are required.

The Nd:YAG wavelength is inherently safer than the diode wavelength to treat darker skin types [9]. These systems are safer because the longer wavelength minimizes epidermal melanin absorption and maximizes wavelength penetration to the dermal hair follicular unit. Therefore, shorter, more effective pulse durations can be used more safely with the Nd:YAG lasers than with the diode lasers. When the Nd:YAG lasers are combined with aggressive skin cooling and pulse durations ≥30 ms, they can safely treat phototype VI skin [11]. As with the diode laser, longer pulse durations reduce the chance for epidermal thermal damage. Most of the FDA-approved Nd:YAG lasers incorporate efficient epidermal cooling devices as part of the system. With regard to overall hair reduction, however, the longer wavelength of the Nd:YAG is probably slightly less effective because of its reduced melanin absorption [12]. A study conducted by Galadari [11] showed a 35% reduction in hair at 12 months after 6 treatments with the Nd:YAG compared with a 40% reduction observed with the diode after a similar number of treatments and follow-up period. Because of the reduced pigment absorption with the longer Nd:YAG wavelengths, they are best used for patients with coarse dark hair.

## Choosing Appropriate Laser Parameters and Test Spots

Initiating treatments with appropriate conservative laser parameters (longer wavelengths, lower fluences, and longer pulse durations) are crucial when treating patients with darker skin types. Test spots are necessary in determining the appropriate laser parameters, particularly fluences and pulse duration. Test spots should be performed in the same or similar area to be treated in order to closely match the skin color, sun exposure, and hair density level. Test spot parameters should start with the safest parameters (lower fluences and longer pulse durations) and slowly progress to higher fluences and shorter pulse durations. To ensure safety one should wait a minimum of 48 h before performing a careful evaluation of epidermal tissue response to a laser test spot to determine the appropriate safe parameters. Patients with darker skin can have a 1–2-day delay in demonstrating cutaneous side effects.

A minimum of four overlapping test spots should be performed to simulate actual laser treatments. In high hair density areas, lower fluences should be used initially to decrease the risk of thermal damage caused by the pooling of heat from closely situated adjacent hairs. These high density areas occur most commonly on the beard area and upper back.

## Patient Selection

Because of the new generation of *color-blind* lasers, all phototypes can be safely treated with laser hair removal devices. There are very few contraindications for laser-assisted hair removal. Gold therapy or taking Saint John's wort are contraindications for laser hair removal, and patients should have been off those treatments for minimally 3 months prior to initiating laser hair removal treatments. Photosensitizing drugs activated by UVA wavelengths have often been considered contraindications; however, hair removal lasers are in the visible and near-infrared wavelength spectrum and therefore are generally thought to be safe to use on patients taking these medications.

People with a history of keloids or hypertrophic scarring should be treated cautiously, but new research and studies are showing promising results in treating keloids with lasers. Caution should be applied in treating patients with keloids to not use aggressive parameters to minimize any risk of dermal scarring.

It has been long held that patients taking Accutane (isotretinoin) is a contraindication for laser hair removal, and patients should be off the medication for at least 6 months prior to initiating treatments. There have been no studies showing that there is an increased incidence of laser-assisted hair removal side effects on patients that are on or have recently been on Accutane. Until new studies are published, practitioners should always err on the side of caution and have the patients wait 3–6 months after stopping Accutane prior to initiating laser hair removal treatments.

When indicated, prophylaxis antiviral medications are necessary for people with chronic or active herpetic infections, especially if they occur in the desired treatment area. Prophylaxis typically starts 1 day before continuing for a total of 5–7 days. Although there has been no evidence that pregnancy is a contraindication, it is widely practiced and recommended to not treat patients who are pregnant.

## Laser Hair Removal Consultation of Patients with Darker Skin Types

Appropriate management of the patient's expectations is critical when consulting the patient prior to laser-assisted hair removal. Patients should understand that multiple treatments are necessary to achieve permanent hair reduction. It usually takes a minimum of eight laser treatments (and often more) to reach the patient's desired hair reduction expectation. With each treatment, there is expected to be a decrease of between 10% and 20% in the hair count, color, and diameter of the hair. Patients with darker skin usually require more treatments than those with lighter skin because of the need to use more conservative parameters (longer wavelengths, lower fluences, and longer pulse durations) to ensure safety. How frequently one should treat is still controversial and is based on many factors, particularly the hair growth rate and the body region of the hair to be treated. It is generally agreed upon that more-frequent treatments are better than less-frequent ones because you want to treat again before the damaged hair has a chance to fully revitalize and strengthen. The treatments should usually be performed every 4–8 weeks, depending upon the body region. To maximize the amount of pigmented hair chromophore in the skin, the patient should not wax or pluck before or in between treatments. Shaving, bleaching, and using depilatory creams are preferable in between treatment methods.

Severe pain is another indicator that the parameters may be too aggressive. This is particularly helpful for patients who state that the pain is worse than their previous treatments. The discomfort that patients experience from laser hair removal is very subjective, but in general, it should be tolerable. There will be some level of discomfort during the procedure. This discomfort is described as feeling like the popping of small rubber bands, pin pricks or pinpoint heating. A topical anesthetic preparation (e.g., EMLA) and/or adjunct cooling (e.g., air cooling) help to decrease the pain during the procedure but are usually not required. After the treatment, there may be immediate perifollicular edema and mild erythema lasting from minutes to hours. However, this epidermal response is not always observed because of the more conservative parameters used on darker skin. Permanent hair reduction can still be achieved if this result is not seen. If these reactions last longer, this should serve as a warning of being close to the epidermal thermal damage threshold, and safer parameters may need to be used. Regardless of the patient's ethnicity or skin color, there should be no crusting, blistering, or scabbing posttreatment. In the event of any thermal damage–related cutaneous side effects, a topical antibiotic or corticosteroids should be applied and prescribed.

## Laser Treatment

The treatment area must be closely shaven or clipped prior to performing laser treatments to prevent the superficial hair from heating and causing superficial side effects, including blistering and discoloration. A gentle alcohol cleanse should be performed to make sure there is no residual makeup or anesthetic on the skin. A final wipe with water should be done to ensure that there is no residual alcohol remaining on the skin. Appropriate goggles must be worn by everyone in the room, including the patient and all observers. Treatment can begin once the appropriate parameters are determined. Laser pulses should overlap by 10–20%, depending on the type of laser system used.

In treating the upper lip and chin, the enamel of the teeth should be protected by overlaying the teeth with wet gauge. Facial hair is usually finer and lighter than the hair on the rest of the body, making it one of the most recalcitrant areas to treat. Therefore, more than the usual number of treatments may be required.

Although posttreatment cooling should not be required, immediate cooling (e.g., ice packs) can be used to reduce posttreatment discomfort, erythema, edema, and the risks of epidermal side effects. A mild topical corticosteroid can be used posttreatment if prolonged erythema, edema, or irritation takes place.

Caution should be applied when increasing the fluence since small increases can tip the scale beyond the patient's epidermal damage threshold, creating thermal damage. If the previous treatment has produced prolonged erythema, crusting, or any other form of epidermal side effects, a thorough history should be performed including asking them about recent sun exposure, new medications, new skin products, and their posttreatment regimen. More conservative parameters should be used to ensure treatment safety.

## Laser-Induced Side Effects

Combining conservative parameters with the long-pulse diode [13, 14] and Nd:YAG laser system will minimize the risk of any adverse events. When side effects occur, there needs to be immediate attention to minimize the risk for long-term or permanent side effects. Epidermal thermal damage can cause crusting, scabbing, blistering, pigmentary alterations, and scarring. The risk of infection is remote with laser-assisted hair removal, but a *folliculitis*-type reaction can take place and should be treated with antibiotics and/or corticosteroids. Although this risk is low, there is a possibility of herpetic infection for those with a history of chronic infections. Most side effects are transient in nature, and, if appropriate, wound care is exercised, then the chance for them to become permanent is greatly minimized.

## Hirsutism and Hypertrichosis

Excessive hair growth, whether from hirsutism or hypertrichosis, in women or men can create a major cosmetic and medical problem. In patients with darker skin types, there is a high incidence of epidermal side effects from conventional treatments, whether from shaving, plucking, electrolysis, or waxing. Laser hair removal treatments finally provide patients with darker skin and tightly curled hair a safe and successful therapeutic option. Pigmentary alterations and epidermal side effects affiliated with conventional methods of hair removal dramatically improve with each consecutive laser treatment. Patients are often as pleased with the improvement in their skin texture and decrease in their pigmentary disorders as they are with their permanent hair reduction.

## Pseudofolliculitis Barbae

Men and women with curly, tightly coiled coarse hair are often plagued with ingrown hairs, producing papules and pustules that easily lead to pigmentary disorders and scarring called pseudofolliculitis barbae (PFB). This is particularly seen in the beard area of men, or in the underarms or bikini area of women who shave. Like hirsutism, conventional methods of treatment are ineffective, leading to a high incidence of side effects. Laser-assisted hair removal is a successful treatment for pseudofolliculitis barbae (PFB). Temporarily or permanently reducing the hair from the PFB lesion dramatically improves the condition, leading to resolution of the papular and pustular condition and improvement in the skin's texture and associated postinflammatory hyperpigmentation [15, 16].

In treating the beard area of men, permanent hair removal of the entire beard is usually not the desired outcome. The beard stubble look is usually a more natural look in men and taking away their ability to grow a beard is not always an appropriate end result. The goal should be to improve both the papular and pigmentary disorder conditions to provide the patient with a cosmetically pleasing appearance. Most male patients who have beard PFB are most affected in the upper cheek or lower neck area. The practitioner's goal in treating this area should be to achieve permanent hair reduction in those select areas while keeping the majority of the beard intact. Safer parameters by using lower fluences and/or longer pulse durations can be used to minimize permanency and provide more of a hair delay management approach. In women who have PFB associated with excessive unwanted hair on the face, then permanent hair reduction of the entire face is usually the goal since excessive unwanted hair growth is usually as undesired as PFB.

## Acne Keloidalis Nuchae

Acne keloidalis nuchae (AKN) is most frequently seen in African-Americans. It is characterized by persistent follicular and perifollicular papules and plaques, which often lead to hyperpigmented scarring and keloidal thickening located on the occipital area of the scalp. AKNs are stubborn recalcitrant lesions and treatment with conventional methods is difficult with unpredictable and often marginal results. In early lesions, there is usually evidence of an entrapped hair, and laser-assisted hair removal is a somewhat helpful adjunctive therapy. Laser hair removal can be an effective treatment options for AKN. Lower fluences and longer pulse durations should be initially used to minimize permanent reduction of hair and provide more of a hair delay approach. For more chronic changes associated with long-standing acne keloidalis nuchae, such as scarring, foreign body reaction, and decreased hair growth, more aggressive laser hair removal parameters are necessary. The goal is to destroy the tufted-like hair that acts as a foreign body in hopes of decreasing further scarring. The clinical outcome in chronic cases is not as satisfactory.

## Paradoxical Hypertrichosis

Paradoxical hypertrichosis has been reported as a rare complication of laser hair removal [17, 18]. Published studies have reported these complications after alexandrite laser (755 nm) and IPL (590–1,200 nm) treatments [18, 19]. In the authors' experience, this complication is not dependent on a particular wavelength or light source and can occur with any wavelengths used with photoepilation, including the diode laser (810 nm) and Nd:YAG laser (1,064 nm). Studies suggest that patients with darker skin (phototypes IV–VI) may be at increased risk [17, 19], particularly patients of Mediterranean or Pacific Asian descent, but patients from most ethnic origins have been reported. With respect to location, paradoxical hypertrichosis may occur both within and beyond the treatment site [18].

## Conclusion

Everyone, regardless of skin color or ethnicity, can now be safely and effectively treated for unwanted hair with laser hair removal. The safest and most effective hair removal lasers to treat darker skin types are the long-pulsed diode and the long-pulsed Nd:YAG laser systems. Because of the longer wavelength, the long-pulsed Nd:YAG system is considered the safest. Conservative fluences and longer pulse durations are necessary in order to provide safe and effective treatments to patients with darker skin types.

## References

1. Anderson RR, Parish JA. Selective thermolysis: precise microsurgery by selective absorption of pulsed radiation. Science. 1983;220:524–7.
2. Van Gemert MJC, Welch AJ. Time constants in thermal laser medicine. Lasers Surg Med. 1989;9:405–21.
3. Commo S, Gaillardo O, Bernard BA. The human hair follicle contains two distinct K19 positive compartments in the outer root sheath: a unifying hypothesis for stem cell reservoir? Differentiation. 2000;66:157–64.
4. Cotsarelis G, Sun TT, Lavker RM. Label-retaining cells reside in the bulge area of pilosebaceous unit: implications for follicular stem cells, hair cycle, and skin carcinogenesis. Cell. 1990;61:1329–37.
5. Fuchs M. Thermokinetic selectivity – a new highly effective method for permanent hair removal: experience with LPIR Alexandrite laser. Derm Prakt Dermatologie. 1997;5:1.
6. Manuskiatti W, Elmpunth S, Wanitphakdeedecha R. Effect of cold air cooling on the incidence of postinflammatory hyperpigmentation after Q-switched Nd:YAG laser treatment of acquired bilateral nevus of Ota like macules. Arch Dermatol. 2007;143:1139–43.
7. Breadon JY, Barnes CA. Comparison of adverse events of laser and light-assisted hair removal systems in skin types IV–VI. J Drugs Dermatol. 2007;6:40–6.
8. Battle E, Suthamjariya K, Alora M, et al. Very long pulses (20–200 ms) diode laser for hair removal on all skin types (abstr). Lasers Surg Med. 2000;12:21–4.

9. Alster T, Bryan H, Williams CM. Long pulsed Nd:YAG laser assisted hair removal in pigmented skin. Arch Dermatol. 2001;137:885–9.
10. Battle Jr EF, Hobbs LM. Laser-assisted hair removal for darker skin types. Dermatol Ther. 2004;17:177–83.
11. Galadari I. Comparative evaluation of different hair removal lasers in skin types IV, V, and VI. Int J Dermatol. 2003;42:68–70.
12. Bouzari N, Tabatabai H, Abbasi Z, et al. Laser hair removal: comparison of long-pulsed Nd:YAG, long-pulsed alexandrite, and long-pulsed diode lasers. Dermatol Surg. 2004;30:498–502.
13. Greppi I. Diode laser hair removal of the black patient. Lasers Surg Med. 2002;28:150–5.
14. Adrian RM, Shay KP. 800 nm diode laser hair removal in African American patients: a clinical and histologic study. J Cutan Laser Ther. 2000;2:183–90.
15. Ross EV, Cooke LM, Timko AL, Overstreet K, Graham B, Barnette DJ. Treatment of pseudofolliculitis barbae in skin types IV, V, VI with a long pulsed Nd:YAG. J Am Acad Dermatol. 2002;47:263–70.
16. Ross EV, Cooke LM, Overstreet KA, Buttolph GD, Blair MA. Treatment of folliculitis barbae in very dark skin with Nd:YAG laser. J Natl Med Assoc. 2002;94:888–93.
17. Alajlan A, Shapiro J, Rivers JK, et al. Paradoxical hypertrichosis after laser epilation. J Am Acad Dermatol. 2005;53:85–8.
18. Radmanesh M. Paradoxical hypertrichosis and terminal hair change after intense pulsed light hair removal therapy. J Dermatol Treat. 2009;20:53–4.
19. Moreno-Arlas GA, Castelo-Branco C, Ferrando J. Side-effects after IPL photodepilation. Dermatol Surg. 2002;28:1131–4.

# Chapter 14
# Dermal Fillers in Ethnic Skin

**Cheryl M. Burgess**

## Growth of the Ethnic Patient Population

### *Growth of Cosmetic Products and Procedures in Ethnic Populations*

Growth in the ethnic patient population has been driven by growing diversity of skin types and shifting trends in US demographics. In addition, products and procedures that target the ethnic market are also bringing more ethnic patients into the clinic. Moreover, nearly one-third of ethnic patents indicated in a recent survey that they would consider having cosmetic surgery and many cosmetic surgeries are being performed in ethnic patients. According to recent surveys, 13 million cosmetic procedures were performed in 2010, an overall increase of 110% in minimally invasive procedures since 2000. However, of the total 13 million cosmetic procedures performed in 2010, 3.8 million (30%) procedures were performed in nonwhite racial or ethnic groups. Hispanics accounted for 11%; blacks accounted for 8%; Asians, 6%; and other nonwhites, 4%. This represents an increase of more than 50% among nonwhites since 2004 [1, 2]. Therefore, it is especially important for the dermatologist to incorporate safe and effective, ethnic-specific treatment procedures.

---

C.M. Burgess, M.D., F.A.A.D. (✉)
Department of Dermatology, Georgetown University Medical Center,
George Washington University, Center for Dermatology and Dermatologic Surgery,
2311 M Street, NW, Suite 504, Washington DC 20037, USA
e-mail: Cheryl.burgess@ctr4dermatology.com

A.F. Alexis and V.H. Barbosa (eds.), *Skin of Color: A Practical Guide to Dermatologic Diagnosis and Treatment*, DOI 10.1007/978-0-387-84929-4_14,

# Effects of Aging in Ethnic Skin

## *Morphology of Aging Face and Other Regions*

It has become widely acknowledged that volume loss in the skin, bone, and soft tissue contributes greatly to the resulting appearance of the aging face and various other regions of the hands, arms, neck, etc. In addition, experts recognize that the loss of craniofacial support from aging or disease exacerbates the effects of aging because of diminished surface area for the outer soft tissue to envelope. In fact, the individual and combined effects of fat atrophy, bone loss, changes in musculature, and changes in the skin itself are all factors that bring about the folding and sagging that is observed in the aging face. Changes in any of these components bring about individual and synergistic effects that result in the aging appearance of the face (Tables 14.1 and 14.2) [3].

Acknowledging the importance of the atrophy/hypertrophy model for aging skin, soft tissue, and hard tissue underscores the recent shift from treating wrinkles and gravitational sagging to a comprehensive approach that diagnoses and treats the aging face from "the inside out." Thus, it is vital that physicians understand the natural progression of changes in the aging face, the microstructural changes, and especially the macrostructural changes [3].

In the young face, superficial and deep fat is distributed evenly, creating a homogenous topographical appearance with smooth primary arcs and convexities. With age, the distribution of fat becomes altered by fat atrophy and hypertrophy, disturbing the contour of the face and producing hills and valleys with demarcations

**Table 14.1** Major age-related dermal changes in the human face

| | |
|---|---|
| Intrinsic aging of the skin | Causes histologic changes throughout the skin layers |
| | Flattening of the epidermal-dermal interface |
| | Loss of dermal papillae |
| | Reduction in dermal fibroblasts, mast cells, blood vessels, and elastic tissue |
| | Reduced type I and type III collagen production |
| | Lower epidermal turnover rate |
| | Reduced melanocyte activity |
| | Wound healing is impaired |
| Extrinsic aging of the skin | Histologic changes are distinct from those caused by intrinsic aging |
| | Photodamaged skin tissue is inflamed, characterized by elastosis, increased population of mast cells, histiocytes, and fibroblasts |
| | Reduced collagen and melanocyte activity, more pronounced in sun-exposed skin |
| | Wound healing is impaired, more pronounced in sun-exposed skin |

From [22], with permission

**Table 14.2** Major age-related structural changes

| | |
|---|---|
| Upper third of the face | Brow begins to droop |
| | Excess lid folds |
| | Deep horizontal and vertical rhytides develop on the forehead |
| Midface region | Soft tissue prominences near the cheeks recede, exposing the bony orbital rims |
| | Region between the lower lid and the cheek develops a hollow, with a deepening of the nasojugal fold |
| | Development of a palpebronasal groove |
| | Increased shadowing |
| Lower third of the face | Subcutaneous fat thins |
| | Malar fat pad descends and overlaps the cheek-lip groove, creating a prominent nasal fold |
| | Increased shadowing |
| Perioral region | Vertical rhytides develop above the vermilion border |
| | Lips become elongated and lose their fullness |
| | Excess skin and soft tissue accumulates near the draws and chin resulting in the development of jowls |

From [22], with permission

between the cosmetic units. Fat atrophy becomes clinically apparent in the temple and cheek and is followed by fat loss around the chin and mandibular areas. Features become concave, characterized by flat lips, sunken temple and cheek, scalloped mandible, and increased shadowing from hills and valleys. With aging, the gradual change from convex cosmetic units to concave regions brings about diminished reflection of light leading to a less radiant appearance. This may sometimes be reported by patients with darkly pigmented skin. With aging, the most significant change in appearance is the sagging of excess skin, which tends to drape inferiorly and diagonally from the temporal area toward the perioral region. This creates a central focus on the perioral and mandibular regions.

Fat atrophy is caused by decreased fat cell size, diminished fat cell function, impaired fat cell differentiation, and redistribution of fat cells. Fat hypertrophy occurs submentally, in the jowl, lateral nasolabial fold, lateral labiomental crease, and lateral malar areas. The accumulation of fat pulls the excessive skin downward under the force of gravity [4, 5]. Fat atrophy and hypertrophy are further compounded by bone loss due to aging. Changes in craniofacial skeleton volume occur as a natural process of aging but may be accelerated due to intrinsic or extrinsic factors. Morphologic modifications in the appearance of the head, face, and neck become more evident around 50 years of age in both genders, with greater bone loss in women, potentially from the effects of menopause. The aging of the craniofacial skeleton is thought to occur from changes in the relative dynamics of bone expansion and bone resorption. Significant volume changes are noted in the maxilla and mandible, resulting in sagging skin from diminished support for overlying soft tissue [3].

## Soft Tissue Augmentation in Ethnic Skin

### *Soft Tissue Fillers in Blacks*

While black patients may experience less frequency or severity of certain conditions, such as perioral rhytides or wrinkling, blacks experience a variety of other issues related to skin sagging and sinking, uneven complexion, loss of volume in skin laxity, and epidermal growths. Histologically, there is less thinning of collagen bundles and elastic tissue in this skin type. As a result, fillers that stimulate collagen production or skin tightening appear to be more effective in ethnic skin. Based on the particular ethnic skin type, some soft tissue fillers will achieve better results than others will.

#### Safety First

Because keloid scarring can occur in ethnic patients as a result of invasive procedures – for example, from full or partial facelifts – many patients and practitioners may be uncertain of what to expect from noninvasive procedures, such as soft tissue augmentation. Careful explanation can increase comfort levels in patients and cautionary measures will alleviate the occurrence of hyperpigmentation in ethnic patients. Clinician and patient education can lead to positive results for restoring a youthful facial appearance.

Soft tissue fillers are excellent for emphasizing cheeks and minimizing cheek festooning, filling accentuated tear troughs, and treating the prejowl sulcus and temples. Volumizing is accomplished in the infraorbital, upper cheek, and lateral cheek regions using cross-linked or larger-particle hyaluronic acid, calcium hydroxyapatite, or Poly-L-lactic acid (PLLA). Longevity of the effect varies with the type of substance. Temporary or less-permanent fillers provide immediate or delayed effects that last 9–18 months. For example, PLLA, which requires three sessions with 4 weeks or greater periods between treatments, produces a soft tissue augmentation that lasts between 18 months and 3 years. Around the eyes, laxity of the upper/lower eyelid skin may develop; therefore, volume enhancement of the subbrow region can be achieved by injecting the dermal filler just below the eyebrow hair for an instant brow lift.

### *Hyaluronic Acid*

Hyaluronic acid is a naturally occurring polysaccharide, a glycosaminoglycan that is a component of the "ground substance" or extracellular matrix of the dermis [6]. Hyaluronic acid was first used commercially in 1942 when Endre Balazs applied for a patent to use it as a substitute for egg white in bakery products. It plays an important role in giving volume to the skin, shape to the eyes, and elasticity to the joints. As we age, our cells lose their ability to produce hyaluronic acid, and the skin becomes drier, thinner, and looser, leading eventually to wrinkling, among other changes. Fillers containing hyaluronic acid are true fillers, in which the mechanism of augmentation is simply to fill space. Currently, there is one source of hyaluronic acid used for soft tissue augmentation: non-animal-stabilized hyaluronic acid (NASHA) produced from a bacterial biofermentation process (e.g., Restylane®, Medicis, Scottsdale, Arizona, USA; Juvederm®, Allergan, Irvine, California, USA; and Belotero®, Merz Aesthetics, San Mateo, California, USA, and Frankfurt, Germany). Hyaluronic acid is readily broken down in the dermis and eliminated via the lymphatics and the liver [7]. However, cross-linking with ester and ether linkages stabilizes the molecule for greater durability in dermal processes [8].

Bacterial-derived hyaluronic acid is available in different concentrations. Depending on the concentration, it can be injected into either the (1) reticular dermis and/or surface layer of the subcutis, or (2) papillary dermis. Various injection techniques apply and should not be overcorrected [9].

Viscoelastic hyaluronic acid is also available. Viscoelastic nonanimal hyaluronic acid gel (e.g., Juvederm®) is available in three different concentrations. It is intended for injection, based on concentration, into either (1) the superficial dermis, (2) the middermis, or (3) the mid- to deep dermis. It can be used in younger patients for shaping and volumizing, in addition to restoring lost lip structure in older patients. All hyaluronic acid fillers can be used in the body of the lips to reshape or enlarge the lips. However, collagen fillers are reserved for use in the vermillion border. Fillers containing hyaluronic acid are generally considered to last twice as long as fillers containing collagen [7]. Hyaluronic acid is cross-linked with ester and ether linkages to stabilize the molecule for dermal purposes. The amount of cross-linking of the molecule affects biocompatibility of hyaluronic acid; less cross-linking of the molecule achieves greater biocompatibility. Hyaluronic acid is indicated for the treatment of more superficial corrections, such as smoothing surfaces, as opposed to fillers used in deeper regions to create more supportive structure and foundation (Fig. 14.1). Theoretically, hyaluronic acid can be used to volumize. However, this application is considered cost prohibitive. Table 14.3 gives an overview of hyaluronic acid.

## Precautions for Enhancement with Hyaluronic Acid

Hyaluronic acid fillers are injected using prefilled syringes with 27-gauge or 30-gauge needles. These fillers can be used for the treatment of wrinkles, furrows, lip enhancement, lip plumping, and facial contouring and soft tissue augmentation. Hyaluronic acid fillers are placed in the middermis to avoid the Tyndall (blue discoloration) effect, which occurs when hyaluronic acid is injected too superficially. The use of hyaluronidase is to dissolve overcorrection and the Tyndall effect. Slower injection rates decrease the incidence of clinical bruising and postinflammatory hyperpigmentation in black patients [10]. Also, note that not all brown discoloration is a result of postinflammatory pigmentation; the discoloration could be hemosiderin deposition, which can occur

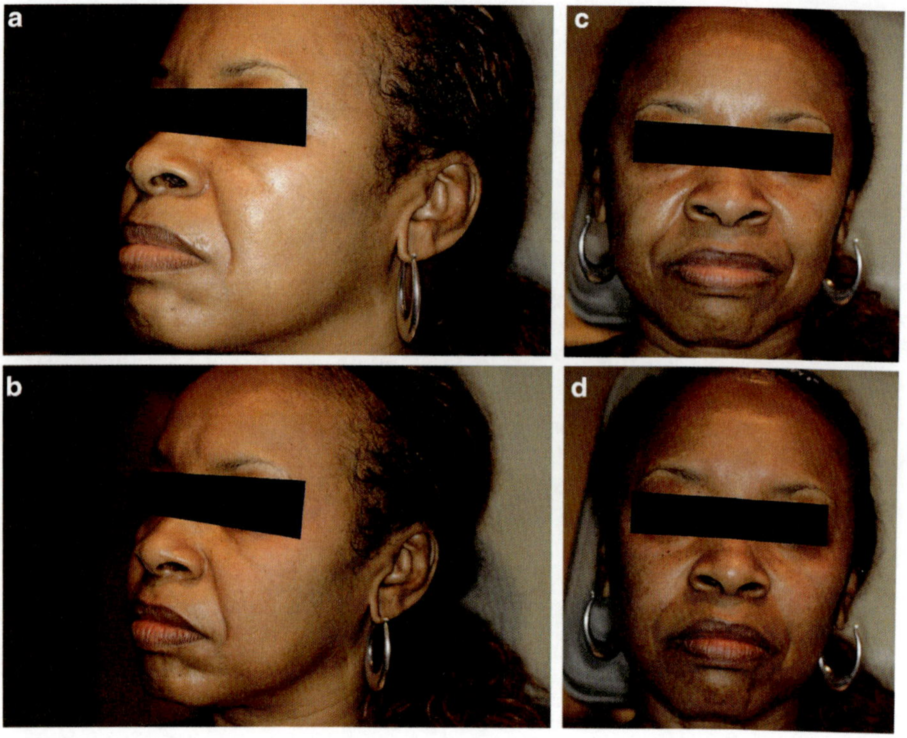

**Fig. 14.1** (**a**) *Before* 50+-year-old African American female with midfacial lipoatrophy. (**b**) *After* midface enhancement with hyaluronic acid filler. (**c**) *Before* photo of age-related midfacial lipoatrophy in 50+-year-old African American female. (**d**) *After* photo of age-related midfacial lipoatropy in 50+-year-old African American female enhanced with hyaluronic acid filler

**Table 14.3** Hyaluronic acid overview

| |
|---|
| **Hyaluronic acid derived from bacterial biofermentation process (e.g., Restylane, Perlane)** |
| Several preparations of nonanimal hyaluronic acid are derived from Streptococcus bacteria in a biofermentation process. Three forms differ in concentration, volume, and needle size and in recommended usage (Glogau 2004). Restylane contains hyaluronic acid particle size of 200 μm and 1% cross-linking. To stabilize the molecule, 20 mg/ml hyaluronic acid is cross-linked with ester and ether linkages. Some theorize that the less cross-linking of molecules, the more biocompatible the hyaluronic acid |
| *Granular consistency of hyaluronic acid* |
| **Viscoelastic, nonanimal hyaluronic acid gel derived from bacterial biofermentation (e.g., Juvederm)** |
| Another family of products containing a viscoelastic, nonanimal hyaluronic acid gel is available in three different concentrations (18 mg/ml and 30 mg/ml (Europe and Canada), 24 mg/ml (USA)) to address different correction needs. Hyaluronic acid gel is eventually absorbed into the body |
| *Smooth consistency of hyaluronic acid with gel mass sizing* |

**Table 14.4** Overview of stimulatory fillers: CaHa and PLLA

| |
|---|
| **Calcium hydroxyapatite (e.g., Radiesse)** |
| Synthetic calcium hydroxyapatite (CaHa) microspheres are identical in composition to the inorganic mineral portion of human bone and teeth. Augmentation develops over time as fibroblasts and collagen form over the gel matrix |
| **Poly-L-lactic acid (e.g., Sculptra, Sculptra Aesthetic)** |
| Poly-L-lactic acid is a biodegradable bioabsorbable synthetic polymer, which has been used for several decades in resorbable medical devices, such as sutures, surgical sealant meshes, screws, plates, and membranes for guided tissue regeneration. Augmentation takes place over time as the particles induced a local reaction characterized by increases in fibroblasts and new collagen production |

during bruising and can be confirmed through unresponsive hydroquinone bleaching. There is generally tissue swelling, so be cautious to avoid overcorrection, especially in the lips. Swelling typically dissipates in 3 days (Fig. 14.1).

## *Stimulatory Fillers: Calcium Hydroxyapatite and Poly-L-Lactic Acid*

As opposed to products that work solely by occupying space, the stimulatory fillers are a group of augmentation products that cause ongoing reactions that result in volumizing (Table 14.4). Two volumizing products are currently approved for use in the United States: calcium hydroxyapatite (e.g., Radiesse; Bioform Medical, Inc., San Mateo, California) and poly-L-lactic acid (e.g., Sculptra; Dermik Laboratories, Bridgewater, New Jersey).

Synthetic calcium hydroxyapatite (CaHa) microspheres are identical in composition to the inorganic mineral portion of human bone and teeth. As a result, the microspheres are nonimmunogenic, eliminating the need for allergy testing. The microspheres are gradually absorbed and set up a gel matrix that serves as a scaffold for fibroblast ingrowth and the production of new collagen. Augmentation slowly takes place and is semipermanent, lasting from 10–18 months, depending on injection depth, technique, and patient variability [11].

Calcium hydroxyapatite is approved by the FDA for the correction of fine lines and wrinkles around the nose and mouth, moderate to severe facial folds such as nasolabial folds and marionette lines, facial lipoatrophy due to the use of HIV antiviral drugs, oral/maxillofacial defects, vocal cord insufficiency, and radiographic tissue marking. Calcium hydroxyapatite is considerably viscous with the consistency of a thick paste and should be injected into the subdermal or intramuscular tissue. Do not inject CaHa into the vermillion border of the lip due to an increased incidence of submucosal nodule formation. Dilution is necessary for treating teardrops, finer wrinkles, whereas a thicker product is better for areas of volume loss, such as the cheek, nasolabial folds, and marionette lines. The CaHa preparation does not contain anesthesia, so topical or injectable anesthesia is necessary prior to use: lidocaine 1%, with or without epinephrine, as recommended [11].

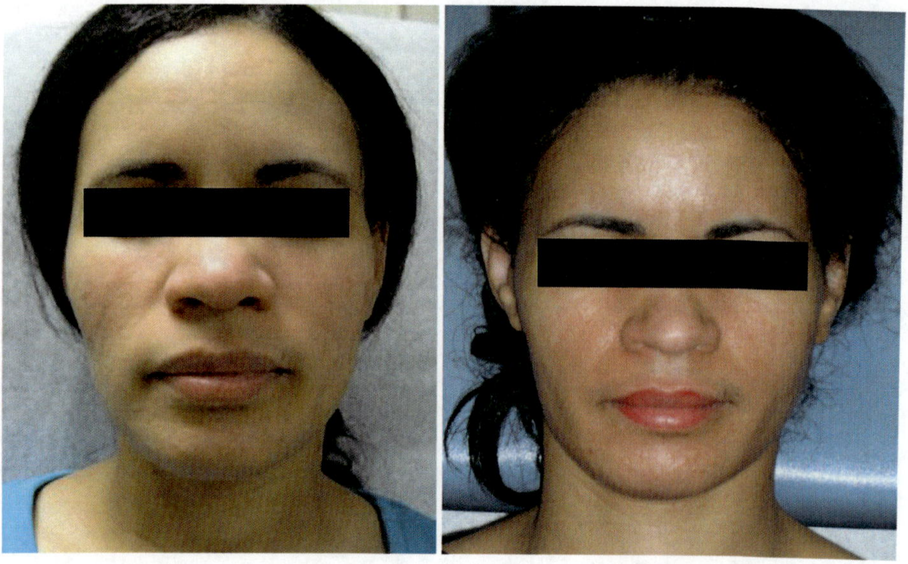

**Fig. 14.2** (**a**) *Before* PLLA volumization of the temporal and submalar regions in 30+ African American female. (**b**) 6 months *After* 2 sessions of PLLA volumization of the temporal and submalar regions in a 30+-year-old African American woman

Poly-L-lactic acid (PLLA; Sculptra® Aesthetic; Dermik, Bridgewater, NJ, USA) is an injectable medical device with approval by the US Food and Drug Administration (FDA) in 2009 for the treatment of shallow to deep nasolabial fold (smile lines) contour deficiencies and other facial wrinkles which are treated with the appropriate injection technique in healthy people; it is also approved for the treatment of facial lipoatrophy in patients with human immunodeficiency virus (HIV). Poly-L-lactic acid is a synthetic lactic acid polymer that is biodegradable, biocompatible, and immunologically inert. The safety of PLLA polymers has been demonstrated for many years through their use in a wide variety of therapeutic contexts, including use in vaccine vectors and medications; absorbable suture material (Ethicon® and Dexon®); screws, pins, and plates used in orthopedic surgery; and molded implants for craniofacial reconstruction. Poly-L-lactic acid was approved in Europe in November of 1999 and June of 2000 for cosmetic treatment of fine lines and wrinkles in immunocompetent individuals.

Poly-L-lactic acid is supplied as a dry monomer powder that can be stored at room temperature. It forms a poly-L-lactic acid hydrogel when mixed with bacteriostatic water. When injected into the deep dermis or dermal-subcutaneous plane, it causes an immediate physical improvement to the appearance (Figs. 14.2 and 14.3). The initial effect fades over the first week as the water is absorbed, causing a temporary return to at or near the pretreatment appearance. Over the following weeks, the PLLA microparticles induce the formation of collagen, leading to dermal thickening. It takes several months for treatment results to stabilize and for the full magnitude of

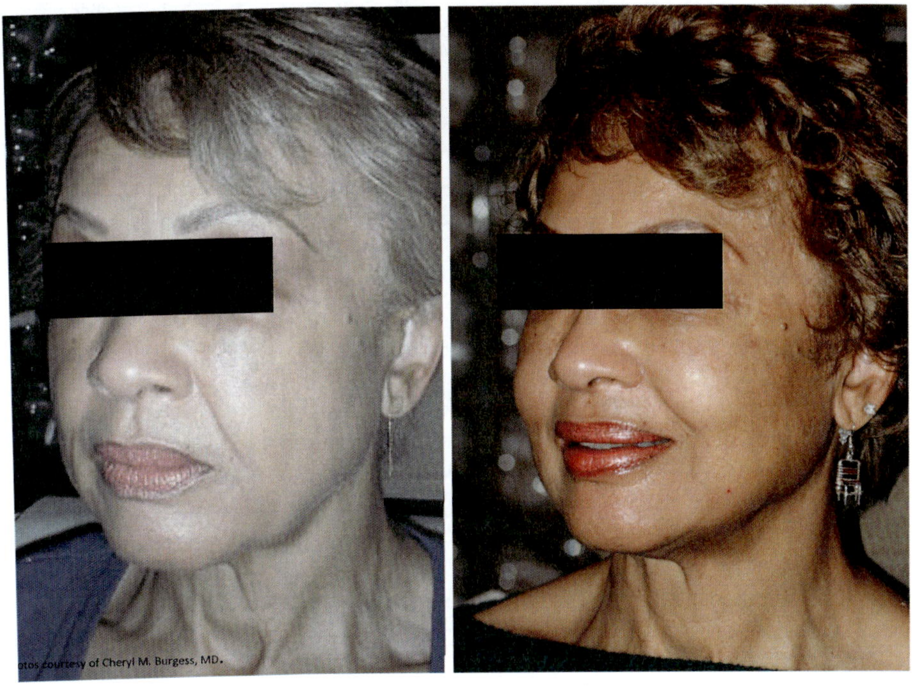


**Fig. 14.3** (**a**) *Before* photo of age-related lipoatropy of the face in 71-year-old African American female. (**b**) 6 months *After* 2 sessions of PLLA full face enhancement in 70+-year-old African American female

the facial augmentation to become apparent. The PLLA hydrogel is then slowly degraded into lactic acid microspheres and $CO_2$, thus leaving behind the crystals to stimulate a granulomatous reaction and dermal thickening [12].

## Safe and Effective Use of Poly-L-Lactic Acid

### *Avoiding Adverse Events Associated with Incorrect Use of Poly-L-Lactic Acid*

Studies have reported the development of granulomas and nodules after soft tissue augmentation using PLLA [13–15]. However, reports of adverse events can usually be traced back to poor technique involving injection preparation, incorrect location of injections, and use of a hasty treatment plan. It is crucial for dermatologists and plastic surgeons to recognize and acknowledge the distinct differences between PLLA and other soft tissue fillers. The characteristics that distinguish PLLA from traditional fillers are (1) the mechanism of action, (2) the treatment plan, (3) the preparation of the injection material, and (4) the injection technique [16]. Poly-L-lactic acid causes a gradual volume restoration that may take 3–6 months to develop. In addition, the rate of dermal thickening increases from the first to last injection. Since immediate correction is not the primary goal, as is the case in most traditional fillers, the use of PLLA requires a markedly different approach and treatment plan. Physicians should treat, wait, assess, and then decide how to proceed. Both patients and physicians need to observe great patience throughout the span of the treatment sessions. Unlike other cosmetic injectables, PLLA requires reconstitution before use. Although manufacturers recommend diluting in 3–5 mL of sterile water, 5–7 mL of sterile water is the customary reconstitution volume in the United States. In fact, some studies have reported that adverse effects, such as granulomas and nodules, have resulted because PLLA is difficult to dissolve completely [14]. However, Dreschnack notes that failure to allow sufficient time for reconstitution is probably the most common clinical error made by clinicians. Dermik laboratories recommend a 2-h period of stabilization and dissolution of the microparticles after reconstitution [15]. What is most critical for successful outcomes is that physicians receive sufficient training before attempting to inject PLLA. This training should include distinctions in injection technique. For example, as opposed to treating a specific line, the strategy of PLLA treatment is to return volume to a facial area. In addition, PLLA is injected into the dermal-subcutaneous plane, unlike collagen or hyaluronic acids. Finally, it is important that PLLA injection be accompanied by massage of the treatment area and continued by the patient posttreatment [16].

Poly-L-lactic acid has been used effectively in both the younger and older patients. However, in the older or aging patient, the thickness of the dermis plane is diminished, leading to a greater likelihood for bruising that results from increased fragility of blood vessels. In these patients, it is recommended that clinicians allow 8 weeks between treatment sessions, as opposed to the regular 4 weeks or greater waiting period. For clinicians, the learning curve is longer in these patients, due to the concerns associated with treating patients with a thin dermis plane [17]. Experts recommend that physicians acquire sufficient knowledge and training before attempting procedures and performing less-ambitious corrections before injecting around the orbits or into the perioral region [18].

## *Age-Related Lipoatrophy and Facial Enhancement*

### Safety and Efficacy History

A recent study by Hanke and Redbord found PLLA to be safe and efficacious for the satisfactory treatment of lipoatrophy in HIV and lipoatrophy of aging. In their study, 65 patients (27 HIV positive; 38 HIV negative) were treated with PLLA for facial lipoatrophy from August 2004 to August 2006. Nearly all patients reported that they were very satisfied with the PLLA treatments (93% of HIV-positive patients; 89.5% of HIV-negative patients). PLLA can be used to treat cosmetic patients with a lipoatrophy severity of grade 2 to grade 5 (Table 14.5).

**Table 14.5** Facial lipoatrophy grading scale to assess the degree of lipoatrophy in all patients

| | |
|---|---|
| **Grade 0** | No facial lipoatrophy |
| **Grade 1** | Mild flattening or shadowing of one or more facial regions<br>No prominent bony landmarks<br>No visibility of underlying musculature |
| **Grade 2** | Intermediate point between grade 1 and grade 3 |
| **Grade 3** | Moderate concavity of one or more facial regions<br>Prominence of bony landmarks<br>May have visibility of underlying musculature |
| **Grade 4** | Intermediate point between grade 3 and grade 5 |
| **Grade 5** | Severe indentation of one or more facial regions<br>Severe prominence of bony landmarks<br>Clear visibility of underlying musculature |

Adapted from [23], with permission

Experts recommend reconstituting in a minimum of 5 ml of sterile water to allow for light-to-moderate plunger pressure and to help distribute the product evenly [18]. In highly mobile areas, such as around the eye and around the lip, it is recommended to reconstitute PLLA in 6–8 ml. However, it is not recommended to use large dilutions in large areas or in nonmobile areas [19].

### Treatment Plan and Injection Technique

Several treatments, administered 4 or more weeks apart, are required to achieve maximum benefit; the exact number depends on the severity of the lipoatrophy. Mild cases may require 2–3 treatment sessions; moderate cases approximately 3–4 treatment sessions; and severe lipoatrophy could require 4–6 treatment sessions [12]. Injection technique is outlined in Table 14.6.

## *Lip Rejuvenation*

In the 1990s, the desire among white women for full, voluptuous lips began to stimulate the market for collagen injections used to enhance the appearance of lips. Over the years, the desire for full lips has gained widespread popularity and fueled the demand for lip augmentation. By contrast, full lips have historically been viewed as an unattractive feature by most black women. However, changes in self-perception are motivating more black women to emphasize the beauty of their lips. As a result, many of these women are now choosing procedures to rebuild an aging lip [20, 21].

Whereas the typical goal of lip augmentation in white women is to increase the lip size beyond the original volume, black women generally seek augmentation to only restore the size of the lip to the original volume and appearance. Although the intrinsic aging process causes similar effects to the lips of black and white patients, some

**Table 14.6** Poly-L-lactic acid injection steps

| |
|---|
| Obtain preoperative photographs |
| Prior to injection, in the areas of correction, thoroughly cleanse the skin |
| The treatment areas are anesthetized with topical lidocaine, nerve blocks, or 1% lidocaine with or without 1:100,000 epinephrine infused into the reconstituted vial of PLLA |
| Areas of concavity are outlined with a wax marking pencil or eyeliner pencil |
| For the enhancement of the under-eye area, prevent the development of subcutaneous nodules in the thin skin of the orbital rim, by injecting under the orbicularis oculi musculature |
| If at the time of injection, the PLLA suspension is not fully reconstituted, vigorously shake and then warm the suspension to 92–96°C (197.6–204.8°F) by submerging the suspension in hot water. This causes the covalent bonding to occur more rapidly. In more sophisticated laboratories, use a laboratory vortex mixer prior to the procedure and during the procedure to prevent settling of the suspension |
| The PLLA suspension is injected into the dermal-subcutaneous juncture with a 25-gauge 1/2–1½-inch needle. Move the needle in a fan-like sweep in the horizontal plane, while injecting the PLLA with a retrograde technique. Place the needle adjacent to the first location in the same horizontal plane and repeat the injection using a fanning motion so that the fans overlap and cross to create a lattice of PLLA deposits |
| Vigorous massage and manual sculpting was performed by the physician and/or nurse on patients with and without HIV for 5 min to treatment areas to distribute the material evenly. To minimize bruising and swelling, patients were given instructions to apply ice packs to the injected areas for 15 min of every hour over the next 12–24 h |

subtle differences are important to note. Whereas in white women lip aging usually occurs relatively early in life, these effects typically occur later in black women. In white women, supravermilion rhytides develop above and below the vermilion borders because of thinning of the dermis, volume loss, loss of vermillion border, and the overactivity of the periorbicularis oris musculature.

The lips of white women appear thin, long, flat, and wrinkled, with down-turned corners of the mouth that appear sad or angry looking. However, for black women, rhytides occur predominantly in the body of the lip below the vermilion border, in response to loss of volume of the upper lip. In addition, the lower lip usually maintains the same appearance; however, it sometimes becomes flat and more visible. Unlike white women, collagen enhancement of the vermillion border is rarely performed, and therefore, the primary treatment consists of rolling the lip up using injections of hyaluronic acid. If there is overactivity of the periorbicularis oris musculature, botulinum toxin A is the preferred method to relax muscles perioral rhytides [8] (Fig. 14.4).

## *Foot Corrections: Treatment of Metatarsal Fat Pad Wasting*

As we age, the fat pads of the feet thin and undergo lipoatrophy, causing discomfort with standing and ambulation (Fig. 14.5). Poly-L-lactic acid has been used effectively in restoring volume to areas of metatarsal fat pad wasting in the foot. Before treating the fat pad area, apply topical anesthetic cream for 45 min or perform an intradermal

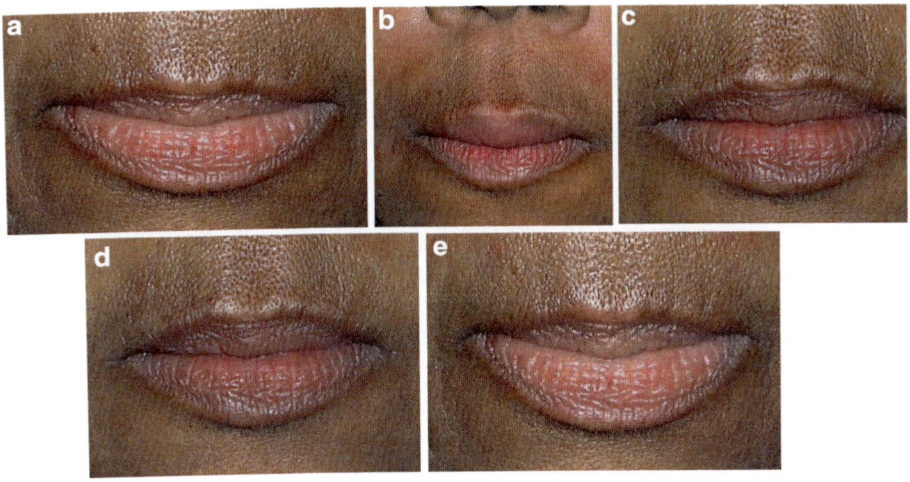

**Fig. 14.4** (**a**) *Before*: Aged upper lip in 70+-year-old African American female. (**b**) Several days following hyaluronic acid filler enhancement of the upper lip. (**c**) 1 month *After* hyaluronic acid filler enhancement of the upper lip in 70+-year-old African American woman

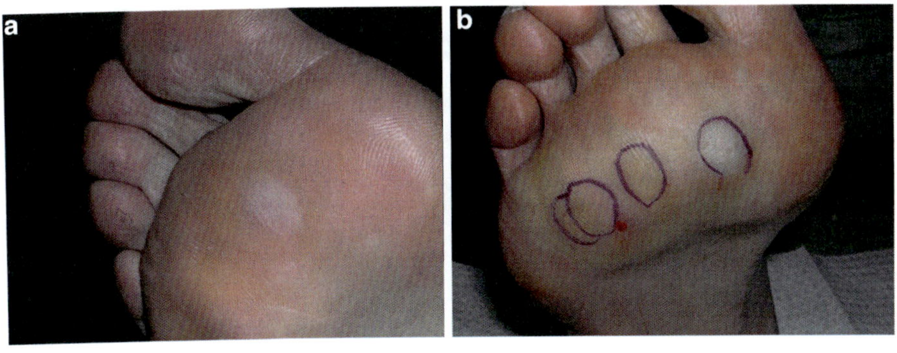

**Fig. 14.5** (**a**) Lipoatrophy of the foot pad in a male athlete. (**b**) PLLA injections into the metatarsal spaces of the foot pad

injection of 1% lidocaine to minimize pain on injection. The process of injecting PLLA at the base of the metatarsal joint stimulates fibroblastic enhancement of dermal collagen and subsequent thickening of the foot pad. Augmentation slowly takes place and may require several injection sessions. Unlike with facial rejuvenation, the reconstitution volume of PLLA dilution is with 3–4 cc of sterile water.

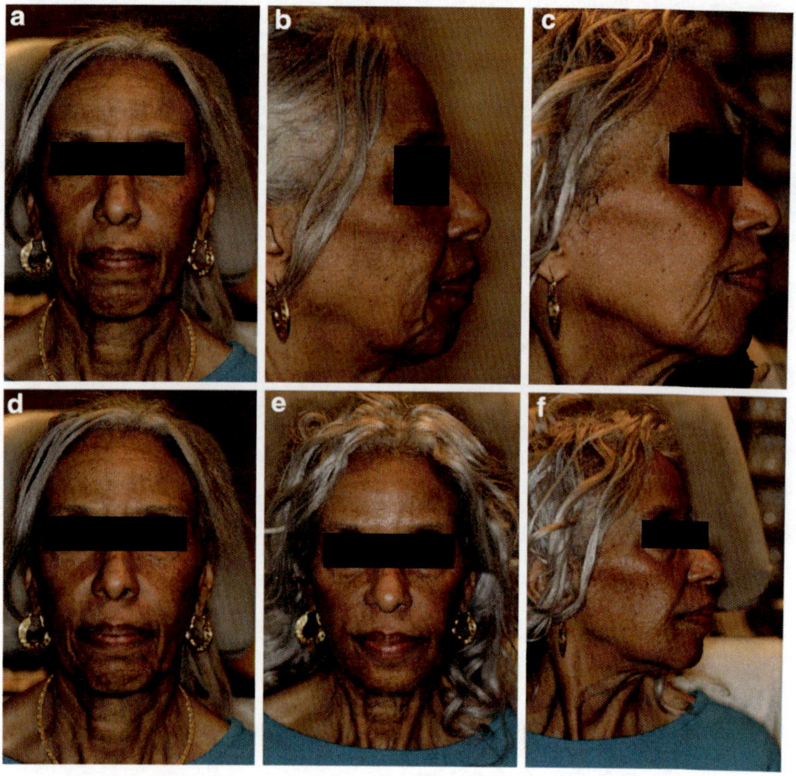


**Fig. 14.6** (**a**) *Before* (frontal view) lower face rhytides in 70+-year-old African American female. (**b**) *Before* (lateral view) lower face rhytides in 70+-year-old African American female. (**c**) Botulinum toxin type A injected in the depressor anguli oris and mentalis in 70+-year-old African American female. (**d**) (Frontal view) *After* botulinum toxin type A injected in the depressor anguli oris and mentalis regions with hyaluronic filler enhancement of the lower face in 70+-year-old African American female. (**e**) (Lateral view) *After* botulinum toxin type A injected in the depressor anguli oris and mentalis regions with hyaluronic filler enhancement of the lower face in 70+-year-old African American woman

## *Combination Treatment: Botulinum Toxin Type A with Dermal Filler*

Facial shaping can be accomplished by injecting with botulinum toxin type A in combination with dermal fillers. The botulinum toxin is injected first to minimize or alleviate folds and creases so that less correction is needed during the subsequent injection of dermal filler. After injection with the neurotoxin, allow 2 weeks for the full effect to develop and then perform the dermal filler injections (Fig. 14.6).

The formation of crease lines and rhytides is a natural component of the aging process that can lead to deep furrows and frown/scowl lines. Such furrows and frown/scowl lines are referred to as dynamic rhytides because they arise when we laugh, frown, or smile. Dynamic rhytides are caused by the repeated forces generated by hyperkinetic muscles including the frontalis (responsible for forehead furrows), corrugator supercilii (involved in frown/scowl lines), orbicularis oculi (crow's feet), and procerus and depressor supercilii (also involved in frown/scowl lines) [21]. Although botulinum toxin has FDA approval for treatment of the glabellar region of the face, it is often used off-label for relaxation of the upper and lower hyperkinetic muscles. However, in ethnic skin, there is very little need to treat crow's feet, which rarely develops as seen in Caucasian patients.

## Summary

In recent years, people with pigmented skin have become an increasingly important market force for the cosmetics industry. In addition, it is predicted that people with darkly pigmented skin will eventually comprise a majority of the domestic and international population during the twenty-first century. Not surprisingly, people with skin of color are increasingly seeking out products and procedures to fight the effects of aging, including increased use of nonsurgical cosmetic procedures. In some cases, skin of color patients may be skeptical about the safety of certain cosmetic procedures. Because keloid scarring can complicate invasive procedures such as full or partial facelifts in patients with skin of color, many patients and practitioners are uncertain of what to expect from noninvasive procedures, such as soft tissue augmentation. Fortunately, careful technique can minimize the risk of hyperpigmentation in darkly pigmented skin and lead to positive results for restoring a youthful facial appearance. Clinicians must also be aware of the different manifestations of fat atrophy and hypertrophy that are experienced by patients with skin of color. As with patients of all skin types, a comprehensive approach to assessment and treatment of the face is paramount. A variety of injectable fillers and volume stimulators exist that can be used alone or in combination. These fillers differ in composition, mechanism of action, longevity, and price. It is critical that clinicians receive specialized training for specific soft tissue fillers before attempting to treat patients. With proper training and technique, clinicians can provide successful outcomes with little risk of adverse events to patients with skin of color.

## References

1. American Society for Aesthetic Surgery: Cosmetic surgery National Data Bank statistics. Available at: www.surgery.org/download/2005stats.pdf (2005). Accessed 24 Aug 2006.
2. American Society for Aesthetic Surgery: Cosmetic surgery National Data Bank statistics. Available at: www.surgery.org/download/2008stats.pdf (2008). Accessed 20 July 2009.

3. Vleggaar D, Fitzgerald R. Dermatological implications of skeletal aging: a focus on supraperiosteal volumization for perioral rejuvenation. J Drugs Dermatol. 2008;7(3):209–20.
4. Donofrio LM. Fat distribution: a morphologic study of the aging face. Dermatol Surg. 2000;26(12):1107–12.
5. Alster T, Jorizzo J, Hanke W, Weinkle S, Werschler P. The aging face: more than skin deep CME. Available at: http://www.medscape.org/viewprogram/3401
6. Lupton JR, Alster TS. Cutaneous hypersensitivity reaction to injectable hyaluronic acid gel. Dermatol Surg. 2000;26(2):135–7.
7. Klein AW, Elson ML. The history of substances for soft tissue augmentation. Dermatol Surg. 2000;26(12):1096–105.
8. Burgess C. Soft tissue augmentation. In: Burgess C, editor. Cosmetic dermatology. Heidelberg: Springer; 2005. p. 93–110.
9. Lowe NJ, et al. Hyaluronic acid skin fillers: adverse reactions and skin testing. J Am Acad Dermatol. 2001;45(6):930–3.
10. Taylor SC, Burgess CM, Callender VD. Safety of nonanimal stabilized hyaluronic acid dermal fillers in patients with skin of color: a randomized, evaluator-blinded comparative trial. Dermatol Surg. 2009;35 Suppl 2:1653–60.
11. Hamilton T. Skin augmentation and correction: the new generation of dermal fillers-a dermatologist's experience. Clin Dermatol. 2009;27:13–22.
12. DAAI. Legal and regulatory issues regarding new-Fill. Resources DAAI, Inc; 2001.
13. Beljaards RC, de Roos KP, Bruins FG. NewFill for skin augmentation: a new filler or failure? Dermatol Surg. 2005;31(7 Pt 1):772–6.
14. Saylan Z. Facial fillers and their complications. Aesthet Surg J. 2003;23:221–4.
15. Dreschnack P, Farber G. Complications of Sculptra for cosmetic skin contour enhancements. Am J Cosmet Dermatol. 2007;24(3):143–5.
16. Werschler W, Bondar G, Esch P. Six simple steps to Sculptra success: expert advice for incorporating this new filler agent into your practice. Skin and Aging. 2005;13(1):56–64.
17. Burgess C, Lowe N. Letter to the editor: regarding "NewFill" for skin augmentation: a new filler or failure? Dermatol Surg. 2006;32:1530–2. author reply 1530–2.
18. Vleggaar D, Bauer U. Facial enhancement and the European experience with Sculptra (poly-l-lactic acid). J Drugs Dermatol. 2004;3(5):542–7.
19. Anonymous. Questions and answers: ASCDAS 3rd annual meeting. New options in the recognition and treatment of lipoatrophy with volume restoration. Cosmet Dermatol. 2005;18(3):235–9.
20. Burgess CM. Soft tissue augmentation in skin of color: market growth, available fillers, and successful techniques. J Drugs Dermatol. 2007;6(1):51–5.
21. Carruthers A, Kiene K, Carruthers J. Botulinum A exotoxin use in clinical dermatology. J Am Acad Dermatol. 1996;34(5 Pt 1):788–97.
22. Sadick NS, Karcher C, Palmisano L. Cosmetic dermatology of the aging face. Clin Dermatol. 2009;27:3–12.
23. Ascher B, Coleman S, Alster T, et al. Full scope of effect of facial lipoatrophy: a framework of disease understanding. Dermatol Surg. 2006;32(8):1058–69.

# Chapter 15
# Botulinum Toxin A

**Elena Jones and Carlos A. Charles**

There is a trend toward greater use of cosmetic procedures by ethnic minorities. The greatest level of increased interest is among Latino and African American patients, with Latino patients leading all minority groups in the number of cosmetic procedures performed in 2008. African American and Asian American patients closely trail Latino patients, comprising 8% and 7% of all of the cosmetic procedures performed in 2008. The most commonly requested surgical procedures are nose reshaping, breast reduction, and liposuction, whereas botulinum toxin A, facial fillers, and chemical peels are the most commonly requested minimally invasive procedures.

Botulinum toxin A (BtxA) continues to be the most popular cosmetic procedure in the United States. More than five million procedures were performed in 2008. In the United States, there are two botulinum A toxins approved by the Food and Drug Administration for the treatment of moderate to severe glabellar lines. This chapter will review both of these toxins, commercially known as *Botox* and *Dysport*, and their use in the improvement of facial aesthetics in ethnic minorities (Tables 15.1 and 15.2).

Botulinum toxins are derived from various strains of the bacterium *Clostridium botulinum.* There are seven serotypes of botulinum neurotoxin: A, B, C1, D, E, F, and G. These neurotoxins produce chemodenervation and atrophy of skeletal muscle by blocking acetylcholine release from the presynaptic neuron at the neuromuscular junction. Consequently, this results in a reversible flaccid paralysis of the muscles. Botulinum toxin A can be used to smooth hyperdynamic lines of the glabella, forehead, crow's feet, as well as perioral and platysmal lines. In addition, due to its ability

E. Jones, M.D. (✉)
Department of Dermatology, St. Luke's – Roosevelt Hospital,
108 East 86th Street, Suite IN, New York, NY 10028, USA
e-mail: elenajonesmd@gmail.com

C.A. Charles, M.D., F.A.A.D.
Department of Dermatology, Weill Medical College of Cornell University,
New York Presbyterian Hospital/Cornell, 1300 York Avenue, New York, NY 10065, USA

A.F. Alexis and V.H. Barbosa (eds.), *Skin of Color: A Practical Guide to Dermatologic Diagnosis and Treatment*, DOI 10.1007/978-0-387-84929-4_15,

**Table 15.1** Comparison of botulinum A toxins

| | Botox | Dysport |
|---|---|---|
| | Botulinum toxin A (*Clostridium botulinum* toxin type A hemoagglutinin complex) | Abobotulinum toxin A (*Clostridium botulinum* toxin type A hemoagglutinin complex) |
| *Vial sizes* | 50 u,100 u | 300 u |
| *Composition* | 500 ug (0.5 mg) | 125 ug (0.125 mg) |
| | Human serum albumin/0.9-mg sodium chloride | Human serum albumin/2.5-mg lactose |
| *Molecular weight of neurotoxin* | 150 kDa | 150 kDa |
| *Total protein content* | ~5 ng | ~3 ng |
| *Storage* | 2–8°C for 36 months (Postreconstitution: 2–8°C, use within 4 h) | 2–8°C until vial expiration (Postreconstitution: 2–8°C, use within 4 h) |
| *Label preparation* | Dilute 100 u with 2.5-ml *PRESERVATIVE FREE SALINE,* use within 4 h on single patient | Dilute with 1.5 or 2.5-ml *PRESERVATIVE FREE SALINE, use within 4 h on single patient* |
| *Most common OFF-LABEL preparation* | Dilute 100u with 1–3 ml of *PRESERVED SALINE,* use within 7–10 days, More than one patient per vial (preserved saline, less painful) | Dilute with 1–3 ml of *PRESERVED SALINE, use within 7 = 10 days, more than one patient per vial* |
| *Units* | 1 Botox unit | 2–3 Dysport units |
| *Onset of effect* | 1–7 days | 2–4 days |
| *Duration of effect* | ~90 days | 88–114 days |

**Table 15.2** Botox and Dysport vial dilutions

| | Botox 100 u/vial | Dysport 300 u/vial |
|---|---|---|
| Saline diluent volume (ml) | Units/0.1 ml | Units/0.1 ml |
| 1 | 10 units/0.1 ml | 30 units/0.1 ml |
| 1.5 | 6.7 u | 20 u |
| 2.0 | 5.0 u | 15 u |
| 2.5 | 4.0 u | 12 u |
| 3.0 | 3.3 u | 10 u |
| 4.0 | 2.5 u | 7.5 u |
| 5.0 | 2.0 u | 6.0 u |

to block acetylcholine release from autonomic nerve endings innervating glandular tissue or smooth muscle, BtxA is increasingly being used for axillary hyperhidrosis.

Treatment sites and BtxA doses must be individualized to the patient. Patients 30–50 years of age are the most responsive to BtxA. Muscle mass, muscle action, gender of the patient, and the patient's preference for degree of muscle relaxation all play a significant role in the aesthetic goal. All patients, regardless of skin color, respond to botulinum toxin injections in the same manner.

The aging process and the unique facial features of ethnic minorities help to indicate the BtxA injection sites that are more relevant to this population.

Darker skin types age slower than fairer skin types. The aging African American face is similar to the aging Latino and Asian face in that there are fewer rhytides than the aging Caucasian face. The glabella, brow ptosis, upper eyelid laxity, and marionette lines are areas of the aging African American face that benefit from BtxA. Crow's feet and marionette and platysmal lines may be visible earlier in the aging Asian or Latino face. Rarely is perioral BtxA needed in darker skin types. Yet, with an increase in the mixed ancestral lines within ethnic minorities and their growing interest and comfort in obtaining cosmetic procedures, BtxA will be increasingly used to treat more varied facial lines in ethnic skin.

## History

The clinical use of botulinum toxin originated from the application of the physiologic effects of the disease process known as botulinum. This disease was first described in 1817 by Justinus Kerner [1] and is characterized by muscle paralysis caused by the intake of poisoned food. In the late 1800s, Emile Pierre Van Ermengen isolated an anaerobic bacteria from contaminated food and injected the toxin of this bacteria in animals, demonstrating a specific disease in laboratory animals [2]. He reported this anaerobic Gram-positive bacillus to be the cause of botulinum and thus penned the name *Bacillus botulinus*. As the anaerobic nature of this organism was discovered, the name was appropriately amended to *Clostridium botulinum* [3]. *Clostridium botulinum* produces the most potent neurotoxin known in nature, botulinum toxin. Seven different serotypes of botulinum neurotoxins have been described: A, B, C1, D, E, F, and G; BT types A, B, and E are most commonly responsible for causing botulinum in humans.

The cosmetic applications of BT type A began in the latter half of the 1980s. Carruthers and Carruthers noted an improvement in the glabellar lines after the injections of BT for the treatment of blepharospasm [4]. Initially, BT was only applied for the clinical treatment of the upper third of the face; however, as the cosmetic use was further explored, the mid- and lower face as well as the neck were treated. Over time, other important clinical applications have been developed including the treatment of hyperhidrosis [5] and gingival smile [6].

## Commercially Available Botulinum Toxins

Seven neurotoxin serotypes have been purified and identified. They have been designated as BT types A to G. The serotype A has been shown to have the most potent physiologic effects. Currently, both serotypes A and B are commercially available and indicated for therapeutic use. Only serotype A is currently used for cosmetic purposes. However, serotype B has shown some efficacy in the treatment of patients resistant to serotype A on other clinical applications such as for the treatment of cervical dystonia [7].

Botulinum toxin type A is available in several commercial preparations that are indicated for cosmetic application in several countries: OnabotulinumtoxinA (Botox®, Allergan Inc., Irvine California, USA), AbobotulinumtoxinA (Dysport®, Ipsen Limited, Paris, France; Medicis, Scottsdale, Arizona, USA), and incobotulinumtoxinA (Xeomin®, Merz Aesthetics, San Mateo, CA, USA). All of these products produce similar effects in the human musculature and sweat glands, with individual characteristics regarding strength, onset of action, and duration of action.

Botulinum toxin type B is commercially available as Myobloc/NeuroBloc (Elan Pharmaceuticals Inc., South San Francisco California, USA). Myobloc was approved by the FDA in 2000 for the treatment of cervical dystonia [8] and has been investigated in patients who developed antibodies to type A [9]. Additionally, studies have demonstrated the safety and efficacy of BT type B for the treatment of axillary hyperhidrosis [10]. Little data exists evaluating the treatment of facial wrinkles with BT type B.

## Mechanism of Action

Botulinum toxin type A prevents the release of acetylcholine (Ach) from the presynaptic neuron of the neuromuscular junction of striated muscles. This action produces a chemical denervation resulting in reversible paralysis of the muscle via three important steps [11]. In the first step known as binding, the toxin binds to a receptor at the surface of the cell membrane of the presynaptic neuron. In the second step, internalization, the toxin is internalized within the neuron. The third and final step is blockage in which the release of Ach-containing vesicles is blocked by the interaction of the toxin with intracellular proteins that are responsible for vesicle release. Muscular strength is mitigated by the toxin beginning 6–36 h after injection of BT depending on the dose, and these effects are clinically apparent approximately 3–7 days after treatment. Clinical evidence of the BT treatment lasts for 3–6 months, at which time the formation of new neuromuscular junction occurs allowing for proper muscular function [12].

## Pre- and Postoperative Botulinum Toxin A Care

1. Obtain a complete medical history.
2. If possible, stop medications that may cause prolonged bruising 7 days prior to injections (e.g., anticoagulants, NSAIDS, analgesics).
3. Obtain photographs at rest and at maximal contraction before and 7–14 days after the injections.
4. Cool area with ice pack pre- and postprocedure or apply topical anesthetic cream 30 min to 1 h before procedure to minimize pain.
5. Patient should not massage treated area.
6. Prepare patient for transient redness, swelling, or bruising at injection sites.

## Contraindications to Botulinum Toxin A

1. Patients with myasthenia gravis, amyotrophic lateral sclerosis, and Lambert-Eaton disease
2. Drug interactions with aminoglycoside antibiotics, calcium channel blockers, cyclosporine, and cholinesterase inhibitors
3. Pregnant/lactating women: pregnancy category C
4. Patients known to be allergic to any ingredient of the formulation, i.e., BtxA, lactose, human albumin, and saline
5. Patients who are psychologically unstable, overly anxious, or have unrealistic expectations

## Injection Technique

1. Sit patient upright.
2. Clean area to be treated with 70% alcohol.
3. Examine facial musculature at rest and at maximal contraction.
4. Mark areas to be treated with marking pen (Fig. 15.1).

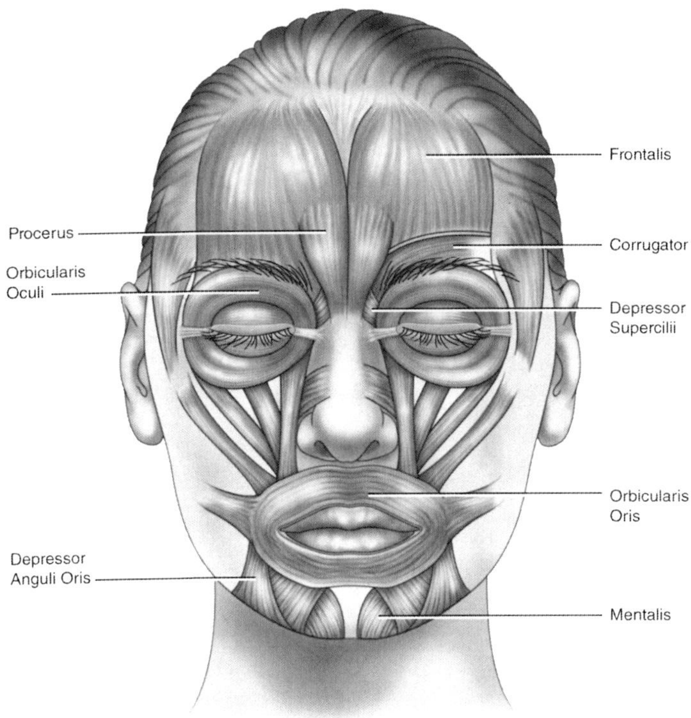


**Fig. 15.1** Botulinum treatment sites

5. Use 1-ml syringe with 30-gauge needle or BD ultrafine II short needle 0.3-cc syringe.
6. Inject slowly either IM, SQ, or ID.

## Guidelines for Treatment

### *Glabellar Lines*

Glabellar lines are caused by the combined action of three muscles: *corrugator supercilii* (causes vertical lines), *procerus* (causes horizontal lines), and *depressor supercilii* (draws the medial eyebrows down).

- Inject into corrugator and procerus.
- *Procerus*: 1 injection point in center of *procerus.*
- Dose range: 2–4 units of Botox or 5–20 units of Dysport.
- *Corrugator*: 1 injection point 0.5–1 cm above the medial orbital rim on each side AND 1 lateral injection point 1 cm above the orbital rim (Fig. 15.2).
- Dose range: 16–18 units of Botox or 40–60 units of Dysport.

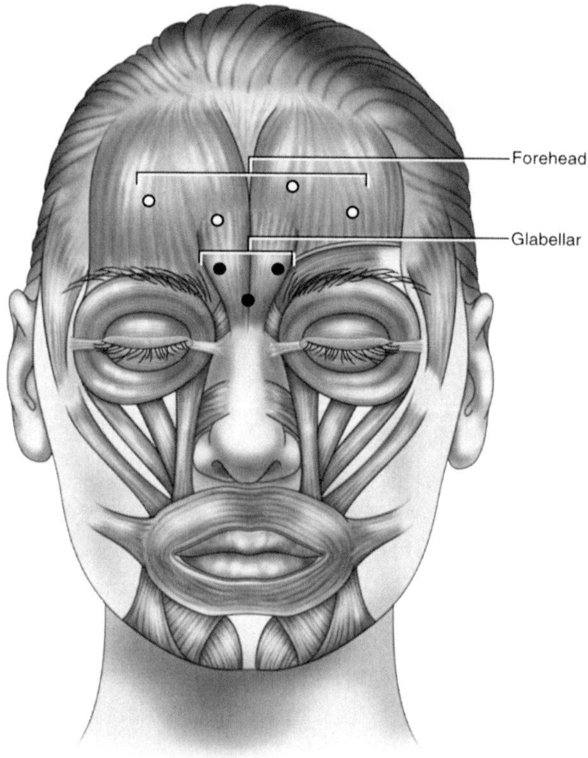


**Fig. 15.2** Injection points for treatment of glabellar lines and forehead lines

## Forehead Lines

- Depends on current brow position, gender, age, and patient preference.
- Muscles that impact brow position are the *frontalis*, *corrugator*, *procerus*, and *orbicularis oculi*.
- Inject in horizontal orientation in *frontalis* muscle.
- Four to eight injection points depending on brow (Fig. 15.2).
- Dose range: 10–20 units Botox or 25–60 units Dysport.

## Lateral Brow Lift

- Inject superior and lateral aspect of *orbicularis oculi*, 1 injection per side, approximately 0.5 cm above orbital rim.
- Dose range: 4 units Botox per side or 8–12 units Dysport per side.
- Inject into glabellar midline (Fig. 15.2).
- Dose range: 7–10 units Botox or 20–30 units Dysport.

## Crow's Feet

- The *orbicularis oculi* muscle has three components: orbital, palpebral, and lacrimal.
- The size, shape, and distribution of each component vary among patients.
- Inject via three SQ or ID sites into the lateral canthus approximately 1 cm from orbital rim (Fig. 15.3).
- Dose range: 8–20 units Botox per side or 16–60 units Dysport.

## Bunny Lines

- Inject into each side of *nasalis* muscle (keep injection out of trough and medial to *levator labii superioris alaequae nasi* to avoid lip ptosis) (Fig. 15.3).
- Dose range: 5–10 units Botox or 10–30 units Dysport.

## Marionette Lines

- Caused by the contraction of the *depressor anguli oris (DAO)* which causes the downward angulation of mouth (ask patient to pull down corners of mouth to identify DAO).

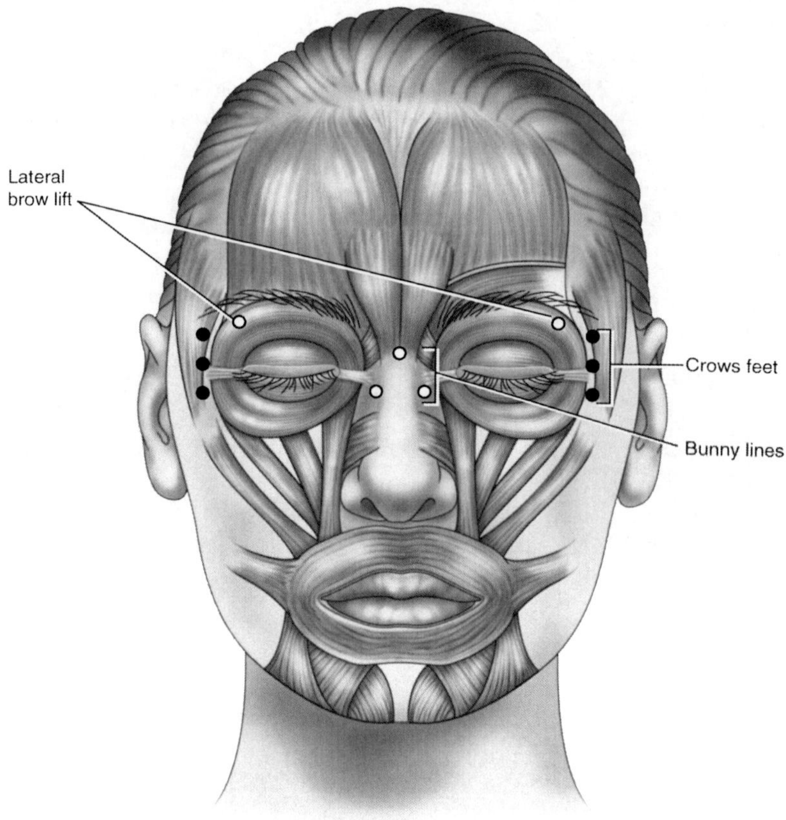


**Fig. 15.3** Injection points for lateral brow lift, crow's feet, and bunny lines

- One injection point into the posterior aspect of each *depressor anguli oris* (Fig. 15.4).
- Inject at least 1 cm lateral to the oral commissure.
- Dose range: 3–8 units Botox or 6–20 units Dysport.

## *Chin Lines*

- Caused by the contraction of the *mentalis* muscle
- One injection superficially in the center of the chin or 2 lateral superficial injections approximately 0.5–1 cm above the chin (keep injection 1 cm from the lower lip because it can affect ability to eat, speak, or move mouth) (Fig. 15.4)
- Dose range: 3–10 units Botox or 6–25 units Dysport

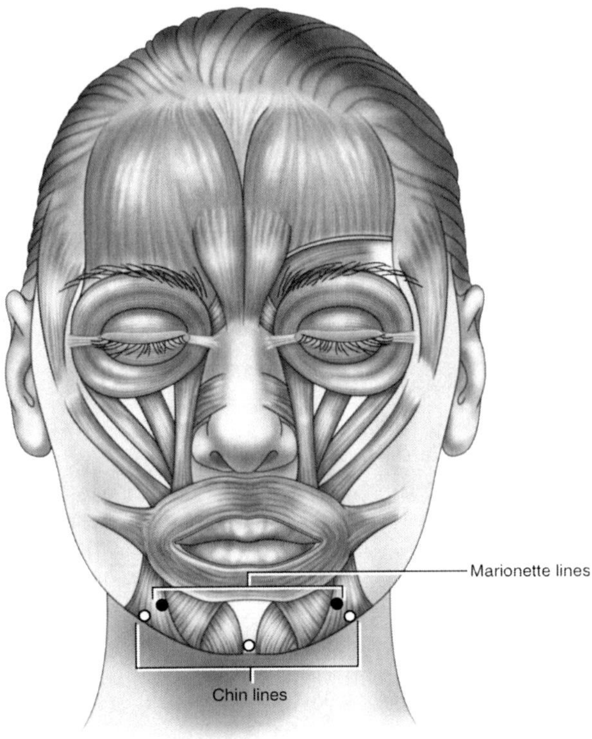


**Fig. 15.4** Injection points for treatment of marionette lines and chin lines

## *Axillary Hyperhidrosis*

- Dilute with 5 ml of preserved saline.
- Perform Minor's starch-iodine test to accurately define the affected area.
- Inject superficially 1.5–2 cm apart and 1 cm from edge of affected area.
- Inject every 4–12 months.
- Dose range: 50–150 units of Botox divided among 10–20 injection sites (no equivalent studies on Dysport in this region).

## *Eyelid Ptosis*

- Alpha-adrenergic agonist ophthalmic drops: Iopidine 0.5% (Apraclonidine, Alcon) and Neo-synephrine 2.5% (Phenylephrine HCl).
- Use 1–2 drops three times daily until ptosis resolves.

## Side Effects and Complications

The cosmetic use of BT is associated with a low incidence of side effects or complications. However, most of the toxin-related complications are secondary to injection in incorrect sites. Further complications are characterized by excessive weakness of the injected muscles. This phenomenon is usually secondary to the use of excessively high doses, incorrect equivalence between the available toxins, or diffusion of the toxin into beyond the injection site. Complications can also be secondary to inappropriate selection of patients.

Mild pain, paresthesia, and/or bruising at the injection site may occur at the time of treatment or shortly thereafter. Bruising tends to occur more commonly with the treatment of the lateral orbital area because of the superficial blood vessels and thin skin characteristic of the periorbital sites [13]. Other common postprocedural symptoms include headache and mild nausea [14].

Concern for postprocedural postinflammatory hyperpigmentation or hypopigmentation in dark-skinned patients is always present; however, previous studies have shown minimal need for concern. A small study of 26 African American patients treated repeatedly with periocular BT type A injections found no evidence of posttreatment depigmentation [15].

Brow ptosis is commonly described as the main side effect resulting from treatment of the frontal and glabellar wrinkles. This phenomenon is rare and is likely secondary to improper technique [16]. Complications related to treatment of the glabellar and periorbital areas also include blepharoptosis and diplopia. These are caused by weakness of the upper eyelid levator muscle as well as the action of BT in the extraocular muscles [17]. Drooping of the lower eyelid may occur when treating the lateral orbital area. This can often lead to corneal exposure, dry eye, and superficial punctate keratitis [18].

Treating the mid- and lower face can also lead to unwanted side effects. The most common complications are secondary to undesired paralysis of the muscles related to the lips and mouth. This can lead to an asymmetric smile and incompetence of the function of the mouth sphincter, which cause difficulty in swallowing, speaking, whistling, smoking, and/or playing wind instruments. Additionally, patients experiencing these unwanted effects can display involuntary biting of the lips, difficulty moving the lips for lipstick application, and involuntary loss of saliva when speaking [19]. Treatment of the neck muscles can lead to excessive weakness of the platysmal bands resulting in difficulty swallowing and lifting the head as well as neck discomfort [20].

## Conclusion

This brief chapter presents an overview of the use of botulinum toxin for the treatment of dynamic wrinkles in patients with darker skin types. It is well established that darker racial ethnic groups age more slowly than fair-skinned counterparts.

However, dynamic wrinkles do play a role in the aging process regardless of skin type. Through the appropriate application of botulinum toxin, these effects can be greatly mitigated thereby greatly enhancing the cosmetic appearance of patients. Physicians must be educated on several important factors when performing BT injections. These include the proper injection techniques and the knowledge of the possible complications as well as their prevention and treatment. Careful screening of patients must be performed prior to treatment to exclude those patients with preexisting contraindications. Additionally, proper patient selection with special attention to facial characteristics, skin color, and patient's expectations will help to assure good outcomes when treating with botulinum toxin.

## References

1. Erbguth FJ. Historical notes on botulinum, *Clostridium botulinum*, botulinum toxin, and the idea of the therapeutic use of the toxin. Mov Disord. 2004;19:S2–6.
2. Cherington M. Clinical spectrum of botulinum. Muscle Nerve. 1998;21:701–10.
3. Bengston IA. Studies on organisms concerned as causative factors in botulinum. Hyg Lab Bull. 1924;136:101.
4. Carruthers JD, Carruthers A. Treatment of glabellar frown lines with C. botulinum-A exotoxin. J Dermatol Surg Oncol. 1992;18:17–21.
5. Glogau RG. Botulinum A neurotoxin for axillary hyperhidrosis: no sweat Botox. Dermatol Surg. 1998;24:817–9.
6. Curruthers A, Carruthers J. Botulinum toxin type A. J Am Acad Dermatol. 2005;53:284–90.
7. Lew MF, Brashear A, Factor S. The safety and efficacy of botulinum toxin type B in the treatment of patients with cervical dystonia: summary of three controlled clinical trials. Neurology. 2000;55 Suppl 5:S29–35.
8. Schwetz BA. First drug for cervical dystonia. JAMA. 2001;285:724.
9. Brin MF, Lew MF, Adler CH, et al. Safety and efficacy of Neurobloc (botulinum toxin type B) in type A-resistant cervical dystonia. Neurology. 1999;7:1431–8.
10. Baumann L, Slezinger A, Halem M, et al. Pilot study of the safety and efficacy of Myobloc (botulinum toxin type B) for the treatment of axillary hyperhidrosis. Int J Dermatol. 2005;44:418–24.
11. Carruthers A, Carruthers J, Kiena K. Botulinum A exotoxin use in clinical dermatology. J Am Acad Dermatol. 1996;34:788–95.
12. Tsui JKC. Botulinum toxin as a therapeutic agent. Pharmacol Ther. 1996;72:13–24.
13. Frankel AS. Botox rejuvenation for the periorbital region. Facial Plast Surg. 1999;15:255–62.
14. Klein AW. Complications and adverse reactions with the use of botulinum toxin. Semin Cutan Med Surg. 2001;20:109–20.
15. Roehm PC, Perry JD, Girkin CA, et al. Prevalence of periocular depigmentation after repeated botulinum toxin A injections in African American patients. J Neuroophthalmol. 1999;19:7–9.
16. Klein AW. Complications, adverse reactions, and insights with the use of botulinum toxin. Dermatol Surg. 2003;29:549–56.
17. Wollina U, Konrad H. Managing adverse events associated with botulinum toxin A: a focus on cosmetic procedures. Am J Clin Dermatol. 2005;6:141–50.
18. Carruthers A, Carruthers JA. Botulinum toxin in the treatment of glabellar frown lines and other facial wrinkles. In: Jankivic J, Hallet M, editors. Therapy with botulinum toxin. New York: Marcel Decker Inc; 1994. p. 577–95.
19. Klein AW. Contraindications and complications with the use of botulinum toxin. Clin Dermatol. 2004;22:66–75.
20. Atamoros FP. Botulinum toxin in the lower third of the face. Clin Dermatol. 2003;21:505–12.

# Chapter 16
# Chemical Peels and Microdermabrasion in Skin of Color

**Fran E. Cook-Bolden, Jocelyne Papacharalambous, and Tanasha Sylvester**

The desire to reverse the aging process has generated great interest throughout history. Ancient texts document the practice of applying various substances to the skin in an attempt to rejuvenate the appearance. More recently, numerous factors have contributed to the rise in popularity of skin resurfacing procedures, including excess ultraviolet exposure, smoking, the aging baby boomer cohort, and our youth-centric culture. The result is a boom in the desire to allay the aging process, prolong youth, and enhance beauty. Resurfacing procedures have long provided a foundation to achieve these goals.

At the same time, skin of color has provided challenges in the area of rejuvenation, especially in the area of skin resurfacing. These challenges occur largely due to melanocyte and fibroblast reactivity in response to injury or inflammation, which leads to an increased risk of dyschromias and keloids following resurfacing procedures in darker skin types.

Two resurfacing treatments, microdermabrasion and chemical peels, have a long history of success in restoring youth and reversing physical signs of aging. Variations of these resurfacing treatment methods have also been successfully performed on all skin types. Although both microdermabrasion and chemical peel treatments are generally safe and beneficial in pigmented skin, both can yield inconsistent results and have potentially severe complications when performed on the wrong subject in the wrong hands.

F.E. Cook-Bolden, M.D. (✉)
Department of Dermatology, The College of Physicians and Surgeons of Columbia University, 150 East 58th Street, 3rd Floor Annex, New York, NY 10155, USA
e-mail: admin.skinspecialtygroup@gmail.com

J. Papacharalambous, M.D. • T. Sylvester, M.D.
Skin Specialty Group, 150 East 58th Street, 3rd Floor Annex, New York, NY 10155, USA
e-mail: admin.skinspecialtygroup@gmail.com; admin.skinspecialtygroup@gmail.com

A.F. Alexis and V.H. Barbosa (eds.), *Skin of Color: A Practical Guide to Dermatologic Diagnosis and Treatment*, DOI 10.1007/978-0-387-84929-4_16,

## Microdermabrasion

Microdermabrasion is a noninvasive procedure in which the superficial layer is gently abraded. It has been described as a form of polishing of the skin or as a process of mechanical exfoliation and is popular in day spas, medical spas, and physicians' practices. Dermabrasion, often compared to microdermabrasion, is a much more intensive and deeper-penetrating procedure that is performed solely by physicians. This procedure can be performed on skin of color with great caution, only by a skilled experienced physician with expertise in performing in pigmented skin.

Microdermabrasion stimulates the production of collagen in the skin and also is an excellent alternative for people with skin that is sensitive to or unable to tolerate chemical peels [1, 2]. The goal of treatment is to stimulate healthy epidermal tissue growth, improve skin tone, and improve elasticity of the skin. It can be performed on any area of the body, although the face is the most popular location. When performed properly, it is a safe, efficacious, and efficient cosmetic procedure with little or no downtime. This treatment can be especially useful in skin of color, in which it has been used to address a variety of dermatologic concerns, including dullness, postinflammatory hyperpigmentation, fine lines and wrinkles, mild acne scarring, acne vulgaris, and pseudofolliculitis barbae. It has also been used to exfoliate plugged pores and reduce the appearance of enlarged pores [1] by stimulating collagen production.

### *Procedure*

During microdermabrasion, abrasive crystals are propelled onto the skin within a controlled, closed vacuum suction system that gently sprays the crystals through a tube from a handpiece onto the patient's skin, leading to exfoliation of the stratum corneum. The device mixes the gentle abrasion of the crystals with suction to remove the dead or damaged outer layers of the skin. The skin debris and particles are sucked back into the tube and then into a waste canister for proper disposal. The goal of the crystals is to polish and/or exfoliate, while the suction stimulates blood flow and collagen production. Most treatments last approximately 15–30 min and do not require anesthesia.

There are many different devices using different types of crystals and suction pressure systems. The four most common crystals used are aluminum oxide, sodium bicarbonate, sodium chloride, and magnesium oxide.

Aluminum oxide is a naturally occurring compound found on earth in a variety of colors. The crystals used in microdermabrasion are often white but can also be brown. They are available in large quantities and are a popular choice for the procedure due to their hard, rough texture, antibacterial properties and because they are inexpensive. Second to diamonds, they are one of the hardest known materials. This makes them well suited for the procedure because they can be blasted without fragmenting. They are light in weight which allows them to be blasted through the device without much air pressure, and their rough edges make them useful for exfoliating the top layer of skin. The crystals should be 99.4% pure and between 100 and 120 μm. Larger crystals tend to be too harsh, especially when used on skin of color. Sodium bicarbonate crystals are an alternative to aluminum oxide crystals. They are organic in nature, hence environmentally friendly and water soluble which allows them to be easily washed off if any crystals remain on the skin after the procedure. They possess antiseptic properties, have a neutral pH, and are generally soothing and nonirritating.

Microdermabrasion with aluminum oxide and sodium bicarbonate crystals each have their advantages. Aluminum oxide crystals are harder which makes them more suitable for deeper conditions such as acne scars. Although rare, there have been complaints of itchy eyes and throat, headaches, and accidental inhalation causing temporary respiratory problems. Although the use of sodium bicarbonate, sodium chloride, and magnesium oxide crystals avoid respiratory issues, professional microdermabrasion systems are designed to be closed circuit; hence, the crystals should never be let out in the air. Sodium bicarbonate crystals are very light and take very little air pressure to deliver to the skin, resulting in decreased redness or soreness after the procedure.

There are systems that do not use crystals; hence, there are no disposables to replace. They use a sandpaper- or diamond-tipped handpiece that mechanically abrades the skin. Other units use positive instead of negative pressure systems [2].

The technology was first performed in Italy in 1985 by Marini and Lo Brutto and introduced to the United States in 1996 [3]. Marini and Lo Brutto employed a closed-circuit negative pressure system that used microcrystals to abrade the skin [2]. Dr. Arnoldo Canella, a colleague of Marini and Lo Brutto, demonstrated that the instrumentation operates at three potential levels.

- *Level 1* corresponds to a superficial epidermal abrasion. The handpiece is passed across the skin in one to two passes to achieve a cosmetic cleaning of the skin. This method is usually performed on the whole cosmetic unit.
- *Level 2* is achieved when a higher vacuum pressure and additional passes are used to approach the level of the papillary dermis. Here, one can see minute pinpoint bleeding. This level is usually used for improving fine wrinkles, superficial scars, and striae.
- *Level 3* reaches the papillary dermis and can potentially remove the entire epidermis, reaching the reticular dermis in some areas [3]. This level is used to improve striae, as well as wrinkles around the lips.

Deeper levels of microdermabrasion are associated with a higher incidence of adverse events in darker skin types and should be performed with caution. Given the considerable risk for hyperpigmentation, hypopigmentation, and scarring [4], Level 3 microdermabrasion should be avoided in skin of color. When performed by a skilled and experienced dermatologist or a certified and well-trained skin care professional, risks are often minimal (Table 16.1). Furthermore, it has been suggested

**Table 16.1** Microdermabrasion

| Candidates for microdermabrasion | Contraindication to performing microdermabrasion | Complications [17] | Benefits |
|---|---|---|---|
| Posttraumatic scarring | Active rosacea | Urticarial reaction | New collagen deposition in the dermis |
| | Facial rejuvenation procedures in the past 3–6 months such as Botox injection or collagen implants | Transient skin dryness | Improved texture |
| Grade 1 acne (open and closed comedones) | | Transient increased sensitivity | Enhanced skin hydration |
| Facial wrinkles prior to aging ("soften and feather out") | | | Improved epidermal barrier |
| | | Transient erythema | Convenience "lunchtime facial" |
| | Fragile capillaries | Petechiae or purpura | It is a safe and highly effective way to restore a clear, youthful glow to the skin |
| Sun damage (uneven texture and skin tone) | Vascular lesions | Worsening of telangiectasia or erythema | |
| | Widespread acne | | |
| | Herpetic lesions (herpes) | | Improve oily or dull skin, enlarged pores, clogged pores, fine lines, mild acne scars, and complexion problems |
| Pigmentary disorders (melasma-macular hyperpigmentation of the face) | | Corneal trauma | |
| | Warts | Reactivation of herpes simplex infection | |
| | Open sores | | |
| | Skin lesions | | |
| Normal aging of facial and body skin | Anyone who takes anticoagulants | | |
| | Eczema | | |
| | Dermatitis | | |
| Dormant superficial acneform scars | Psoriasis | | |
| | Lupus | | |
| | Erythematosus | | |
| Seborrheic keratosis | Diabetes mellitus | | |

that complications can be minimized or avoided by removing the following from one's skin care routine 5–7 days prior to microdermabrasion [5]:

- Chemical depilatories and other chemical processes
- Electrolysis/waxing
- Loofah sponges/facial brushes
- Facial scrubs and masks
- Alpha hydroxy acids, e.g., glycolic acid and lactic acid
- Beta hydroxy acids, e.g., salicylic acid
- Topical retinoids and retinols

For most skin disorders, it is shown that a minimum of five to six treatments is recommended for the best results with a 2-week interval between each procedure [6]. This 2-week interval is very important for recovery of the skin barrier function that is compromised by the microdermabrasion treatment. Some can see a temporary effect on the skin tone immediately. Depending on the condition and its severity such as acne scarring, more treatments may be required. After the procedure, the patient may experience some erythema, or redness, which resolves within minutes but can last for 2–4 h after treatment. The patient may also experience a sunburn-like sensation which can be soothed by a protective barrier and healing cream. A sensitive-skin sunscreen should also be used due to increased photosensitivity even in pigmented skin.

## *Benefits*

The benefits of microdermabrasion have been supported by several scientific and histological studies. It has been postulated by some that repetitive intraepidermal injury causes gradual improvement in damaged skin by stimulating fibroblast proliferation and collagen production [3]. This leads to new collagen deposition in the dermis. The skin is ultimately smoother with few blemishes and new collagen deposition [7]. Modification in epidermal barrier function, such as transepidermal water loss, hydration, pH, and sebum production, may be responsible for the improved texture and overall appearance of the skin following microdermabrasion [7, 8]. A split study was performed where half the face was treated with aluminum oxide microdermabrasion and the other half with sodium chloride microdermabrasion in eight patients, three of whom were African American and two were Hispanic. After three passes, transepidermal water loss (TEWL), stratum corneum hydration, skin pH, and sebum production were measured. The study concluded that microdermabrasion enhanced skin hydration and improved epidermal barrier [7].

More recently, another a study provided the first evidence of changes in the lipid barrier following microdermabrasion treatments. The study investigated the changes in lipid levels in the stratum corneum subsequent to microdermabrasion and noted changes in ceramide levels [8]. A statistically significant increase in the ceramide level was observed after two microdermabrasion treatments.

## Chemical Peels

Egyptians were among the first to use chemicals as exfoliating agents (alabaster, animal oils, and salt) for aesthetics purposes [9]. Next, the Romans and Greeks used pumice, myrrh, frankincense, mustard, and sulfur for lightening of the skin and to improve wrinkles. Fox, Hebra, and Unna described chemical peeling in Europe [2], and in 1882, Unna continued his experience by using peeling agents such as resorcinol, phenol, trichloroacetic acid (TCA), and salicylic acid. Chemical peeling of facial skin has become an integral part of the armamentarium for resurfacing aging, sun-damaged, and diseased skin. It is an alternative to microdermabrasion and dermabrasion to improve the appearance of photodamaged and wrinkled facial skin and other skin conditions.

Chemical peeling or chemical exfoliation is a form of skin resurfacing in which chemical agents are applied to the skin surface to produce epidermal and/or dermal injury and exfoliation. The main goal is generation of a new epidermis, while stimulating dermal collagen remodeling. Chemical peeling agents are classified as superficial, medium-depth, or deep chemical peels. More recently, very superficial has been added as an additional classification (Table 16.2). Each peeling strength has different efficacies, outcomes, and safety precautions.

- *Very superficial peels* include low-strength glycolic acid, lactic acid, and salicylic acid.
- *Superficial peels* include higher-strength glycolic acid, salicylic acid, Jessner's solution, tretinoin, and TCA in concentrations of 10–30%. They target the stratum corneum to the papillary dermis, (Table 16.3) [1].
- *Medium-depth peels* refer to a peeling agent or a combination of agents that penetrate the epidermis and papillary dermis and may extend to the upper reticular dermis. They include TCA in concentration of 35–50%, solid $CO_2$ and TCA, combined glycolic acids 70%/TCA 35%, and Jessner's/TCA 35%.
- *Deep peels* penetrate to the midreticular dermis and utilize occluded or unoccluded Baker-Gordon phenol formula.

Very superficial, and superficial-depth peels can be safely performed on all Fitzpatrick skin types including skin types IV–VI (Table 16.4) [10]. Medium-depth peels can be performed safely on darker skin types, but caution is advised due to the

**Table 16.2** Types of peels

| Depths | Solutions | Techniques | Treatment options |
|---|---|---|---|
| Very superficial | AHAs/BHAs | | |
| | Glycolic | | |
| | Salicylic | Gauze | Acne |
| Superficial | Lactic acid | Cotton-tipped swab | Acne scars |
| Medium | Trichloroacetic acid | Sponge wedge | Photodamage |
| Deep | Jessner's | | Pigmentation |
| | Phenol | | Not to be used in Fitzpatrick skin types IV–VI |

**Table 16.3** Superficial chemical peels

| Candidates for chemical peel | Glycolic acid | | |
|---|---|---|---|
| | Indication | Contraindication | Complications |
| Person in good physical health | Rosacea | History of allergy to the peeling solution, neutralizing agent, diluting agent, or any of their components | Hyperpigmentation |
| | Dyschromias, including melasma and postinflammatory hyperpigmentation from acne or burns in skin types IV to VI | Relative contraindications<br>Prior cosmetic surgery<br>Extensive exposure to sun<br>Smoking<br>Poor general physical or mental health<br>History of herpetic lesions | Hypopigmentation |
| Psychologically stable<br>Who understand the procedure<br>Who do not smoke<br>Wanting to look younger and more refreshed<br>Unhappy with the appearance of wrinkles or brown spots, especially around the mouth or eyes | Pseudofolliculitis barbae<br>Photodamage<br>Improving skin texture | Prior cosmetic surgery<br>Extensive exposure to sun | Scarring |
| | **Salicylic acid** | | |
| | Indication | Contraindication | Complications |
| | Acne vulgaris (inflammatory and noninflammatory lesions) | Salicylate hypersensitivity/allergy | Crusting |
| | Acne rosacea<br>Melasma<br>Postinflammatory hyperpigmentations<br>Freckles<br>Lentigines<br>Mild to moderate photodamage<br>Texturally rough skin | Pregnancy<br>Isotretinoin therapy within 3–6 months of peeling | Prolonged erythema<br>Dryness<br>Intense exfoliation<br>Hyperpigmentation<br>Salicylism or salicylic acid toxicity |

(continued)

**Table 16.3** (continued)

| | Indication | Contraindication | Complications |
|---|---|---|---|
| | **Jessner's solution** | | |
| | Indication | Contraindication | Complications |
| | | Absolute contraindication<br>Allergy to resorcinol, salicylic acid, or lactic acid<br>Relative contraindications<br>Active inflammation<br>Dermatitis or infection of the area to be treated<br>Isotretinoin therapy within 6 months of peeling<br>Delayed or abnormal wound healing<br>Pregnancy | Allergy to resorcinol<br><br>Resorcinol toxicity |
| | **Trichloroacetic acid** | | |
| | Indication | Contraindication | Complications |
| | Sun damage<br>Dilated skin pores<br>Superficial scars<br>Wrinkles and fine lines<br>Keratosis<br>Melasma | Salicylate hypersensitivity/allergy<br>Unrealistic patient expectations<br>Active inflammation/dermatitis of the area to be peeled<br>Acute viral infection<br>Pregnancy<br>Isotretinoin therapy within 3–6 months of peeling<br>History of poor or delayed wound healing | Erythema and increased desquamation in some patients |
| | **Tretinoin** | | |
| | Indication | Contraindication | Complications |
| | Fine lines<br>Wrinkles and fine lines<br>Dyschromia of photoaging<br>Acne | Hypersensitivity to retinoids | |

**Table 16.4** Chemical peel indications in skin types I–III versus skin types IV–VI

| Skin types I–III | Skin types IV–VI |
|---|---|
| Fine wrinkles, rhytides | Postinflammatory hyperpigmentation |
| Solar keratoses | Melasma |
| Photodamage | Acne vulgaris |
| Melasma | Oily skin |
| Postinflammatory hyperpigmentation | Textural changes |
| Acne vulgaris | Acne scarring |
| Rosacea | Fine wrinkles |
| Superficial scarring | |

risk of dyspigmentation. The risks of deep chemical peels outweigh the advantages and therefore are not recommended in darker-skinned patients [11]. Whether it is a salicylic, glycolic, lactic, or a trichloroacetic acid (TCA) or stronger agent, the lowest strength and time interval should always be used initially to assess the response of the skin and then adjusted accordingly. Although important with all procedures, when considering a stronger peel, such as TCA, patient selection and ability to comply with treatment is extremely important due to a greater epidermal response with such peels.

## *Benefits*

Darker skin has significant photoprotection because of the increased content of epidermal melanin. While clinical photodamage, sun spots, actinic keratosis, and skin malignancies are less common problems in darker skin types, patients with skin of color are plagued with dyschromias [2]. Despite major concerns with hyperpigmentation/hypopigmentation, scarring, and postinflammatory changes, recent studies have shown that peeling procedures, specifically superficial peels, are most often successful in persons with darker skin tones (Table 16.5). It is important to keep in mind that peel indications differ between light and darker skin (Table 16.4). Grimes compared the histological variations induced by a variety of chemical peels in 17 patients with skin types IV, V, and VI. Peeling agents used included glycolic acid 70%, salicylic acid 30%, Jessner's solution, and 25% and 30% TCA [2]. Peels were applied to areas in the back and postauricular sites and biopsies were performed at 24 h. Results included glycolic acid-inducing stratum corneum necrosis, while salicylic acid and Jessner's peels caused mild lymphohistiocytic dermal infiltrates. Twenty-five percent and 30% TCA caused the most severe damage, inducing epidermal necrosis and papillary dermal lymphocytic infiltrates with resistant postinflammatory hyperpigmentation. The study proposed that glycolic, salicylic acid, and Jessner's peels produce less postpeeling complications as compared to 25% and 30% superficial TCA peels as expected.

Not only should special issues be raised when considering chemical peels in darker skin types, peel preparation also depends upon the condition being treated.

**Table 16.5** Studies evaluating chemical peeling in skin of color

| Author, year | Skin type/ ethnicity/gender | Diagnosis | Topical therapy | Type of peel | Response | Adverse events |
|---|---|---|---|---|---|---|
| Burns et al. 1997 | 19 IV–VI African Americans | PIL | T 0.05% cream + 2% HQ/10% GA | GA 50%<br>GA 68% | Decreased HASI by 0 % in peel group vs 42% in controls | Erythema, superficial desquamation, and vesiculation |
| Lim 1997 | 10 Asian women | Melasma, fine wrinkles Acne | 20% HQ and 10% HQ | GA 20–70% | NSS | 20% Redness burns and transient PIH |
| Wang 1997 | 40 Asians | Acne | 15% GA | GA 35%<br>GA 50% | Significant resolution in acne | 5.6% PIH, HSV flare, and mild skin irritation |
| Grimes 1999 | 25 V–VI African American and Hispanic women and men | Acne, PIH, Melasma, oily skin, enlarged pores, and rough texture | 4% HQ | SA 20%<br>SA 30 | 88% Moderate to significant improvement | 15% Temporary crusting hypopigmentation, dryness, and hyperpigmentation |
| Javaheri 2001 | 25 Indian women and men | Melasma | Sunscreen SPF 15, 10% GA, and oral acyclovir | GA 50% | 46.7% Epidermal, 27.8% mixed, and 0% dermal | Hyperpigmentation |
| Al-Waiz 2002 | 15 Dark-skinned women and men | Acne scars | RA cream in three patients | Jessner's solution + TCA 35% | 6.6% Significant<br>53.3% Moderate<br>26.6% Mild<br>6.6% Minimal<br>6.6% No response | 73.4% Transient PIH |

| | | | | | | |
|---|---|---|---|---|---|---|
| Sarkar 2002 | 40 Indian patients | Melasma | HQ 5% + T 0.05% + HC 1% cream | GA peel in 20 patients | Decreased MASI in all patients, faster in peel group | Erythema, superficial desquamation, HSV, vesiculation, and PIH |
| Lee 2003 | 35 Korean patients | Acne vulgaris | N/A | 30% Salicylic acid peels | Decreased in inflammatory and noninflammatory lesion counts | Tolerable |
| Khunger 2004 | 10 Indian women | Melasma | N/A | Split-faced study: 1% tretinoin peel vs 70% GA | Significant decrease MASI; no difference between right vs left sides | Minimal |
| Kadhim et al. 2005 | 12 Dark-skinned women and men | Periorbital wrinkles (fine/medium sized) | N/A | Jessner's solution + TCA 35% | 33% Marked<br>25% Moderate<br>25% Mild<br>8% Minimal<br>8% No response | Mild |

*PIH* postinflammatory hyperpigmentation, *T* tretinoin, *HQ* hydroquinone, *GA* glycolic acid, *SPF* sun protection factor
*MASI* Melasma Area Severity Index, *HSV* herpes simplex virus, *NSS* not statistically significant

Different regimens have been suggested when dealing with photodamage, melasma, hyperpigmentation, acne vulgaris, as well as other conditions. A detailed history and physical examination should be performed in patients before any type of chemical peeling. Photographs should be taken at baseline and subsequent visits, including full-face frontal and lateral views. In lighter skin types, the use of topical retinoids is often allowed for 2–6 weeks before peeling in order to thin the stratum corneum and enhance epidermal turnover. They also enhance the penetration and depth of chemical peeling. Because those with darker skin types are more predisposed to postinflammatory hyperpigmentation and scarring, the following guidelines have been implemented to minimize and prevent postpeel complications in those with darker skin. While optimal effects are shown with the use of retinoids when dealing with photodamage in Fitzpatrick skin types I to III, it has been suggested that they should be discontinued 1–2 weeks before peeling or stopped completely when treating conditions such as melasma and postinflammatory hyperpigmentation in darker skin. Others suggest discontinuing these agents a minimum of 3–5 days before the procedure depending on the depth of the peeling agent. Topical alpha hydroxyl acids or polyhydroxy acid formulas can also prep the skin and tend to be less aggressive in postpeel complications. Darker skin can also be prepped with hydroquinone 4% or a higher-percent-compounded formula for 2–4 weeks to reduce epidermal melanin. Regardless of the prepeel regimen used, broad-spectrum sunscreens (UVA and UVB) should be applied by the patient consistently.

## *Superficial Chemical Peels*

### Alpha Hydroxy Acids

Alpha hydroxy acids have been excellent in improving the skin surface by thinning the stratum corneum, promoting epidermolysis, dispersing basal layer melanin, and increasing collagen synthesis within the dermis [2]. They have been among the best-known superficial peeling agents since the early 1800s. Glycolic acid is most commonly used today, although there are commercially available peels containing lactic acid, mandelic acid, and recently pyruvic acid. Their strengths range from 20% to 70%, and they can treat a variety of defects ranging from the epidermis to the papillary dermis. Their effects depend on the pH, strength, and time of application. Glycolic acid peeling agents include buffered, partially neutralized, and esterified formulations. It has been shown that unbuffered formulations with low pH induce the greatest epidermal and dermal damage.

Glycolic acid peels, can be used on all Fitzpatrick skin types. It is most commonly used for dyschromias including melasma and postinflammatory hyperpigmentation from acne, burns, or other inflammatory disorders in skin types IV to VI [12, 13] (Table 16.3). It is usually performed in a series of 6–8 peels, with each peel spaced 2 or 3 weeks apart.

Indications

- Acne vulgaris (inflammatory and noninflammatory lesions)
- Melasma
- Postinflammatory hyperpigmentations
- Freckles
- Lentigines
- Mild to moderate photodamage
- Texturally rough skin

Absolute Contraindications

- History of allergy to the peeling solution, neutralizing agent, diluting agent, or any of the peel components
- Active infection in peeling area

Relative Contraindications

- Prior cosmetic surgery
- Extensive exposure to sun
- Smoking
- Poor general physical or mental health
- History of herpetic lesions

Complications

Generally, glycolic acid peels are well tolerated in darker skin. Erosions that can resolve with residual hyperpigmentation, hypopigmentation, and rarely scarring can occur.

Studies have been conducted to evaluate whether glycolic acid peels would augment improvement in darker skin when combined with topical regimens such as tretinoin or topical steroids. Sarkar et al. [14] assessed the efficacy of a series of glycolic acid peels combined with a topical bleaching agent compared to the use of the bleaching agent alone in darker skin patients with melasma. They compared the efficacy of serial glycolic acid peels (three 30% glycolic peels and three 40% glycolic peels) in combination with a modified Kligman bleaching formulation consisting of hydroquinone 5%, hydrocortisone acetate 1%, and tretinoin 0.05%, versus the bleaching agent alone. Forty women were included in each group, and each group showed improvement. The group that utilized the series of glycolic acid peels with the bleaching agent displayed the most improvement.

Technique for Applying Glycolic Acid Peels

- The area can be cleansed with 70% isopropyl alcohol, acetone, or other prep solution using cotton balls, 2 × 2 in. gauze, or sponges.
- The orbicular angles, nasolabial folds, and lips should be protected with white petrolatum.
- The eyes should be covered with moistened gauze.
- If working on the eyelids, a protective ointment such as petrolatum should be applied at the lid margin to protect the eyes.
- The peeling agent can be applied with cotton balls, sable brush, 3 × 3 in. gauze, or sponge.
- The response of the skin should be monitored visually while remaining alert to mild discomfort, burning, and temporary mild darkening of the skin, which are common during the procedure.
- Skin contact with glycolic acid should take place for 2–6 min (Note: 4 min is an appropriate duration for most patients with skin of color).
- Glycolic acid peels are neutralized with 10% sodium bicarbonate solution or copious water.

## Beta Hydroxy Acid

Salicylic acid is the only beta hydroxy acid commonly used in chemical peels and other skin care preparations. Many formulations of salicylic acid have been used in superficial chemical peels including 50% ointment formulations and 10%, 20%, and 30% ethanol formulations [15]. The 20% and 30% salicylic acid in ethanol formulations are the most commonly used. Beginning with the 20% concentration for the first salicylic acid peel is recommended. The concentration can be increased with subsequent peels depending on the patient's sensitivity and response [16]. Peels are typically spaced 2–4 weeks apart.

Indications

- Same as glycolic peels
- Acne rosacea
- Oily skin

Contraindications

Even though salicylic peels are well tolerated in all skin types, contraindications include salicylate hypersensitivity/allergy, pregnancy, or isotretinoin therapy within 3–6 months of peeling (Table 16.3).

### Complications

Side effects of salicylic acid peeling are mild and transient and include the following:

- Crusting
- Prolonged erythema
- Dryness
- Intense exfoliation
- Hyperpigmentation
- Salicylism or salicylic acid toxicity

In a series of 25 patients comprising 20 African Americans and five Hispanics, 16% experienced mild side effects [17]. One patient experienced temporary crusting and hypopigmentation that cleared in 7 days. Three patients had transient dryness and hyperpigmentation that resolved in 7–14 days. In a series of 35 Korean patients, 8.8% had prolonged erythema that lasted more than 2 days [18]. Dryness occurred in 32.3%, responding to frequent applications of moisturizers. Intense exfoliation occurred in 17.6%, clearing in 7–10 days. Crusting was noted in 11.7%. There were no cases of persistent postinflammatory hyperpigmentation or scarring. Salicylism is characterized by rapid breathing, tinnitus, hearing loss, dizziness, abdominal cramps, and central nervous system reactions. Grimes has peeled more than 1,000 patients with the current 20% and 30% marketed ethanol formulations and has observed no cases of salicylism [17]. We have had a similar experience, confirming that although salicylism can occur, it is rare.

### Technique for Peeling or Applying Salicylic Acid Peels

- A standard peel-tray setup is utilized, similar to the glycolic peel.
- A total of 2–3 coats can be applied to the face, first applying to the lateral face, including the forehead, chin, and perioral area. The initial peel can be performed by applying one coat to assess patient response and sensitivity.
- Application is then applied to the center of the face, including the medial cheeks.
- Although the peel is considered self-neutralizing, it is usually left on for 3–5 min (some patients may experience mild burning, in which a portable handheld fan can be used).
- A white precipitate begins to form around 30 s to 1 min and should not be confused with whitening of the skin. Frosting represents crystallization of the salicylic acid, and most patients will experience crusting and peeling following the procedure.
- Some suggest that it is best to have minimal frosting when treating conditions except in the case of photodamage, especially with the initial treatment.
- After 3–5 min, the patient is instructed to rinse and apply a bland moisturizer.
- A combination of bland cleansers and moisturizers are continued for 48 h. After that time, patients can resume their typical skin care regimen as tolerated.

## Jessner's Solution

Jessner's solution is a superficial peeling agent that contains a mixture of salicylic acid, resorcinol, and lactic acid in 45% ethanol that has been used for many years to treat hyperkeratotic epidermal lesions. It typically has effects to the depth of the papillary dermis. Each component has specific effects. Not only is salicylic acid a lipophilic compound that removes intercellular lipids that are linked to the cornified envelope surrounding epithelial cells, it also enhances the effects of other compounds [19]. Resorcinol disrupts the hydrogen bonds in keratin [20]. Lactic acid causes corneocyte detachment and desquamation of the stratum corneum [21]. Jessner's solution has an outstanding safety profile and can be used in all skin types. It has considerable efficacy with minimal "downtime" and augments the penetration of TCA. As disadvantages, there may be some instability with exposure to light and air, and some darker-skinned patients may experience increased exfoliation with Jessner's peeling.

### Contraindications

Jessner's peels are generally well tolerated in Fitzpatrick skin types IV to VI with few contraindications; however, there is scant published information on its use in this group of patients.

### Complications

In rare cases, allergic reactions to resorcinol are reported [22, 23]. There are concerns regarding resorcinol toxicity, including thyroid dysfunction; however, a recent toxicological review on the risk of resorcinol-inducing thyroid abnormalities did not support an association [22]. In addition, no known case reports of salicylism from Jessner's formulation have been reported.

### Technique for Applying Jessner's Peels

- The skin is usually degreased with alcohol, followed by a mild acetone scrub.
- After cleaning, Jessner's solution is applied to the face with a sable brush, cotton-tipped applicators, cotton balls, or 2 × 2 in. gauze sponges.
- Typically, the forehead, nose and chin are treated first, working from the lateral to medial areas, followed by application to the cheeks. Alternatively, the cheeks can be treated first.
- For superficial peeling, two coats are usually applied. Additional coats increase the depth of peeling.
- Neutralization or dilution with Jessner's solution is not indicated.

- After application of product, some visible precipitate may appear on the skin surface. This should be distinguished from true frosting, which correlates with the depth of peeling.
- Extent of erythema and desquamation following a Jessner's peel correlates with extent of and type of prepeel prepping, number of coats of product applied, and level or degree of frosting during the procedure [24].
- Postpeel care is the same as salicylic acid.

## Trichloroacetic Acid

Although TCA peels are considered the gold standard by which other peels are measured, it has the greatest benefit in Fitzpatrick skin types I through III. Darker skin is more prone to postpeel complications. A superficial peel is usually achieved in concentrations of 10–15% (up to 30%). TCA peels have a small window of safety when compared to glycolic acid, Jessner's solution, and salicylic acid in skin types IV–VI, and the incidence of TCA induced hyperpigmentation is significantly more common in skin types V and VI. Therefore, it is not used as a first-choice agent and is usually chosen when patients are resistant to glycolic acid, salicylic acid, or Jessner's peels. Low-strength TCA can be used in combination with salicylic acid 20% and 30% for superficial peeling. The mixture produces added efficacy compared with salicylic acid peels or TCA 10% peels, at the same time minimizing complications reported with higher concentrations of TCA or glycolic acid, especially in darker skin.

### Indications

- Sun damage
- Prominent pores
- Superficial scars
- Wrinkles and fine lines
- Keratosis
- Melasma
- Same conditions as glycolic peels in cases of resistance

### Contraindications

There are few contraindications to combination salicylic acid/TCA peeling. The combination regimen is tolerated in all Fitzpatrick skin types. Contraindications include the following:

- Salicylate hypersensitivity
- Unrealistic patient expectations
- Active inflammation/dermatitis of the area to be peeled

- Acute infection
- Pregnancy
- Isotretinoin therapy within 6 months of peeling
- History of poor or delayed wound healing

Complications

Side effects are usually low; however, there is erythema and increased desquamation in some patients that can last longer than usual with the combination mixture than observed with salicylic acid peels or TCA 10% alone (Table 16.3).

Technique for Applying Combination TCA/Salicylic Acid Peels

- After thorough cleansing of the face with alcohol and acetone, up to three coats of salicylic acid (20% or 30%) are applied to the entire face with a 2 × 2 in. wedge sponge, 2 × 2 in. gauze sponge, or cotton-tipped applicator for 3–5 min.
- Typically, the forehead and chin are treated first, applying the peel from lateral to medial areas, followed by application to the cheeks (this may be reversed).
- Most patients experience some mild burning and sting during the procedure; others may experience sensation of peel-related facial anesthesia.
- Portable handheld fanning during the procedure substantially mitigates the sensation of burning and stinging.
- A white precipitate begins to form at 30 s to 1 min following peel application.
- After 3–5 min, the face is thoroughly rinsed with tap water to remove salicylic acid crystals.
- The face is gently blotted to remove excess water.
- When treating hyperpigmentation, TCA 10% or 15% is then applied to the areas of hyperpigmentation with a cotton-tipped swab for 2–3 min, producing minimal or no frosting [2].
- The face is again rinsed with tap water.
- If treating photodamage, acne, or texturally rough skin, TCA is applied to the entire face.
- This protocol usually involves a regimen of two or three combination peels performed at 2–4 week intervals.

## Tretinoin

Tretinoin 1% is also used as a chemical peeling agent. Many studies have shown its efficacy in improvement of fine lines, wrinkles, and dyschromia of photoaging. In histological studies, it increases epidermal thickness, increases granular cell layer thickness, decreases melanin content, and improves the density of the stratum corneum [2]. A split-face study was performed in ten Indian women with melasma.

**Table 16.6** Classification of medium-depth and deep chemical peeling agents

| |
|---|
| Medium depth |
| TCA 35–50% |
| Glycolic acid 70% applied for 3–30 min |
| Combinations |
| CO2 snow + 35% TCA |
| Jessner's + 35% TCA |
| Glycolic acid 70% + 35% TCA |
| Deep |
| Phenol 88% |

One percent tretinoin was applied to half of the face, while 70% glycolic acid was applied to the opposite side. Treatments were performed weekly and a modified MASI (Melasma Area and Severity Index) score was taken as well as photographs at each visit. A reduction was noted on both sides of the face at 6 and 12 weeks. There were similar responses between the tretinoin-peeled side and the glycolic-treated areas. The indications, contraindications, and application technique are most similar to those of salicylic acid peels.

## *Medium-Depth Chemical Peels*

Medium-depth peels cause destruction from the epidermis extending to the papillary dermis. It could also extend to the upper reticular dermis [14]. A simplified classification based on the depth of the wound created by the chemical peeling agent is provided by Rubin (Table 16.6). According to his classification, medium-depth peels include glycolic acid 70%, TCA 35–50%, and combination of 35% TCA, with CO2 snow, Jessner's solution, 70% glycolic acid, or unoccluded 88% phenol. Instead of using solo agents, recent movement is to combine two less potent peels and reduce the risks by first penetrating the epidermis with a superficial peeling agent.

### Indications

Generally, medium-depth peels are not often used in darker skin due to greater risk of postinflammatory hyperpigmentation. They are primarily used by trained dermatologists in skin types of I and II who suffer from conditions such as actinic elastosis, actinic keratosis, fine wrinkles, postinflammatory hyperpigmentation, and hard to treat melasma that has not responded to other treatments (Tables 16.7 [15] and 16.8).

Each experienced dermatologist has a standardized peeling process in the way he or she primes, cleans, and degreases the patient's skin. As previously noted, the

**Table 16.7** Indications for medium-depth and deep-chemical peelings

| |
|---|
| *Medium depth* |
| Actinic keratoses |
| Moderate photoaging skin: Glogau II |
| Pigmentary dyschromias (lentigines blotchy hyperpigmentation, postinflammatory hyperpigmentation, and melasma) |
| Fine to medium rhytides |
| Superficial acne scars |
| Blending photoaging skin with laser resurfacing and deep chemical peeling |
| *Deep* |
| Photoaging skin (severe) |
| Acne scars |
| Perioral wrinkles |

**Table 16.8** Medium-depth chemical peels

| Candidates for chemical peel | Indication | Contraindication | Complications |
|---|---|---|---|
| Person in good physical health | Actinic elastosis | Active herpes simplex | Hyperpigmentation |
| | Actinic keratosis | Warts | Hypopigmentation |
| Psychologically stable | Fine facial wrinkles | History of keloidal scarring | Scarring |
| Who understand the procedure | Postinflammatory hyperpigmentation | Unreliable patient | |
| Who do not smoke | Hard to treat melasma that has not responded to other treatments | Any type of recent facial surgical procedures | |
| Wanting to look younger and more refreshed | | Pregnancy or lactating | |
| Unhappy with the appearance of wrinkles or brown spots, especially around the mouth or eyes | | Autoimmune diseases | |
| | | Collagen disease | |
| | | Atopics | |
| | | Eczema | |

factors that affect the depth of the peel include the concentration, number of coats applied, technique, skin type, and anatomic location, as well as duration. It is very important to obtain a detailed history before the peeling procedure, including medication history, occupation, social history, and history of sun exposure. A cutaneous examination is obtained while taking note of the texture and tone of the skin. Realistic expectations should be explained to the patient.

## Contraindications

- Active herpes simplex
- Warts
- History of keloidal scarring
- Unreliable patient
- Any type of recent facial surgical procedures
- Pregnancy or lactating
- Autoimmune diseases
- Collagen disease
- Atopics
- Other types of eczema

## Trichloroacetic Acid

TCA (35–50%) is also considered to be a gold standard due to its low cost, long history of use, and stability [15]. It does not require a lengthy consultation (the consultation should be thorough) and has few medical contraindications, no systemic toxicity, and the pain is less severe as compared to phenol peels. TCA peels usually causes dermal inflammation, necrosis, and sloughing as it precipitates epidermal proteins. This can be noticed visually by white frosting on the skin that correlates with depth of the peel. Because of increased risk of scarring, hyperpigmentation, or hypopigmentation in darker skin types, strengths of 50% or greater are not recommended.

## Technique for Applying Medium-Depth Peels

Combination Jessner's/TCA 35%:

- The procedure begins by applying Jessner's solution with a cotton-tip applicator or gauze pads to the affected areas of the face.
- Within 2–3 min, an erythematous response with frosting is noted.
- Another application of Jessner's solution can be applied; however, solid frosting should be avoided.
- The peel should be applied starting from the least sensitive areas of the skin to the most sensitive areas.
- After the frost is noted, 35% TCA is applied in the same manner and a frosting is noted within 2–4 min which denotes an upper reticular dermis peel [2].

- The patient may feel a burning sensation, and gauze with cool saline is applied soon afterward for 5–10 min.
- In the postpeel period, the patient should soak the area treated with bland moisturizers for the first 24 h.
- After 48 h, the patient can wash their face with a mild soap and water.
- In the first week, a topical antibiotic ointment can be applied twice daily.
- There have been some dermatologists who use a topical steroid antibiotic ointment twice daily in darker skin types [16].
- After 2 weeks, a bleaching agent may be applied to the face area. During this time, the patient should be aware to avoid the sun for at least 10–14 days and be directed to use sunscreen.
- Erythema, edema, and desquamation can be severe in the first 3–4 days.

### Glycolic Acid

Glycolic acid can be used at varying concentrations, but the higher the concentration, the more the depth of the peel increases. When used in concentrations of 70 %, glycolic acid is useful as a medium-depth peel. It has been noted that 70% glycolic acid peels were well tolerated in those with darker skin types and the postinflammatory hyperpigmentation and hypopigmentation were minimal.

When used by trained and experienced dermatologists in darker skin types, the free nonneutralized glycolic acid works better than the partially neutralized glycolic acid [4]. Good results are noted when the peel contains a lower pH of the acid and higher concentration of the free glycolic acid. It is usually neutralized with water or 10–15% sodium bicarbonate

Coleman and Futrell demonstrated the use of 70% glycolic acid and 35% TCA as a medium-depth peel to have similar results as compared to Jessner's solution and 35% TCA peel [25]. Phenol 88% is rarely used in darker skin types due to side effects of hypopigmentation. Cardiac and renal toxicity are other limitations.

Technique for Applying 70% Glycolic Acid and 35% TCA

- Seventy percent glycolic acid is first applied with cotton-tipped applicators.
- Washed off with tap water.
- After 2 min, 35% TCA is applied with 2 × 2 in. gauze pads.

## *Deep Chemical Peels*

Deep chemical peels can improve the texture, quality, and appearance of the skin. It can evoke changes in the deeper reticular dermis by causing necrosis of the skin and can induce production of collagen and ground substance. The risks associated with deep chemical peels in skin of color generally outweigh the benefits and therefore should be avoided in this patient population.

## Conclusion

Many patients have turned to nonsurgical procedures when other measures have not given them their desired results. Treatments like microdermabrasion and chemical peels usually require little to no recovery time and are appropriate for patients with darker skin types. Ethnic skin treatments should follow the same recommended guidelines as Caucasian patients, but treatment strengths and times should be decreased and other adjustments made as required (e.g., adjustments in prepeel regimens and preparation). Whether the chemical peel uses salicylic, glycolic, lactic, TCA, or a combination of the above or many other ingredients and chemicals, the lowest strength and time interval should always be part of the initial protocol. With a stronger peel, such as TCA, as with all procedures, patient condition, skin type, sensitivity, and ability to comply with treatment is extremely important due to a greater epidermal response. Ultimately, the success of any peel is crucially dependent on the physician's understanding of the chemical and biological processes, as well as of indications, potential clinical effectiveness, and side effects of the procedures, along with patient selection, education, and compliance before and after the procedure.

## References

1. www.mayoclinic/health/acne-treatments. Accessed 20 Apr 2010.
2. Susan Taylor's Brownskin.net. http://www.brownskin.net/microdermabrasion.html. Accessed 10 Sept 2006.
3. Grimes P. Aesthetics and cosmetic surgery for darker skin types. 1st ed. Philadelphia: Lippincott Williams &Wilkins; 2007. p. 147–54.
4. Shim E, Barnette D, Hughes K, et al. Microdermabrasion: a clinical and histopathic study. Dermatol Surg. 2001;27:524–30.
5. Saraf V. Chemical rejuvenation of the face and nonfacial areas in Asian skin. 1st ed. Mumbai: Saraf Vinay; 2003.
6. Ottmar Stubler. Microdermabrasion: a protocol for treatment. Les Nouvelles Esthetiques. http://www.docstoc.com/docs/2980377/Microdermabrasion-A-Protocol-For-Treatment. Accessed 10 Sept 2009.
7. Rajan P, Grimes PE. Skin barrier changes induced by aluminum oxide and sodium chloride microdermabrasion. Dermatology. 2002;28:390–3.
8. Jackson BA. Cosmetic considerations and nonlaser cosmetic procedures in ethnic skin. Dermatol Clin. 2003;21:703–12.
9. Lew BL, Cho Y, Lee MH. Effect of serial microdermabrasion of the ceramide level in the stratum corneum. Dermatol Surg. 2006;32:376–9.
10. Brody HJ, Monheit GD, Resnick SS, et al. A history of chemical peeling. Dermatol Surg. 2000;26:405–9.

11. Callender Valerie D, Young Cherie M. Cosmetic procedures in skin of color: chemical peels, microdermabrasion, hair transplantation, augmentation, and sclerotherapy. In: Kelly Paul A, Taylor Susan C, editors. Dermatology for skin of color. Philadelphia: Lippincott Williams & Wilkins; 2008. p. 513–9.
12. Savant SS. Superficial and medium depth chemical peeling. In: Savant SS, editor. Textbook of dermatosurgery and cosmetology. 2nd ed. Mumbai: ASCAD; 2005. p. 177–95.
13. Farber GA. Prolonged erythema after chemical peel. Dermatol Surg. 1998;24:934–5.
14. Rendon MI, Gaviria JI. Review of skin-lightening agents. Dermatol Surg. 2005;31:886–9.
15. Brody H. Variations and comparisons in medium depth chemical peeling. J Dermatol Surg Oncol. 1989;15:953.
16. Moheit GD. Medium depth chemical peels. Dermatol Clin. 2001;19:413–25. vii.
17. Al-Waiz M, Al-Sharqi AI. Medium depth chemical peels in the treatment of acne scars in dark-skinned individuals. Dermatol Surg. 2002;28:383–7.
18. Grimes PE. The safety and efficacy of salicylic acid chemical peels in darker racial-ethnic groups. Dermatol Surg. 1999;25:18–22.
19. Lee HS, Kim IH. Salicylic acid peels for the treatment of acne vulgaris in Asian patients. Dermatol Surg. 2003;29:1196–9.
20. Lazo ND, Meine JG, Downing DT. Lipids are covalently attached to rigid corneocyte protein envelope existing predominantly as beta-sheets: a solid state nuclear magnetic resonance study. J Invest Dermatol. 1995;105:296–300.
21. Robin MG. Jessner's peels. In: Rubin MG, editor. Manual of chemical peels: superficial and medium depth. Philadelphia: JB Lippincott; 1995. p. 9–88.
22. Van Scott EJ, Yu RJ. Hyperkeratinization, corneocyte cohesion, and alpha hydroxyl acids. J Am Acad Dermatol. 1984;11:867–79.
23. Lynch BS, Delzell ES, Bechtel DH. Toxicology review and risk assessment of resorcinol: thyroid effects. Regul Toxicol Pharmacol. 2002;36:198–210.
24. Barbaud A, Modiano P, Cocciale M, et al. The topical application of resorcinol can provoke a systemic allergic reaction. Br J Dermatol. 1996;135:1014–5.
25. Griffiths WAD, Wilkinson JD. Topical therapy. In: Rook A, Wilkinson DS, Ebling FJ, editors. Textbook of dermatology. Oxford: Blackwell Science; 1998. p. 3538–9.

## Further Reading

26. Monheit GD, Kayal JD. Chemical peeling. In: Nouri K, Leal Khouri S, editors. Techniques in dermatologic surgery. 1st ed. Mosby: St. Louis; 2004. p. 233–44.
27. Rubin MG. What are skin peels? In: Winters SR, James M, Caputo GR, editors. Manual of chemical peels: superficial and medium depth. 1st ed. Philadelphia: JB Lippincott; 1995. p. 17–25.
28. Stagnone GJ, Orgel MG, Stagnone JJ. Cardiovascular effects of topical 50% trichloroacetic acid and Baker's phenol solution. J Dermatol Surg Oncol. 1987;13:999–1002.
29. Beeson WH. The importance of cardiac monitoring in superficial and deep chemical peeling. J Dermatol Surg Oncol. 1987;13:949–50.

# Chapter 17
# Cultural Considerations in People of African Descent

**Victoria H. Barbosa**

The demographics of the United States and those of the world are continuously evolving. Many doctors find that their patients come from an ever increasing diversity of racial and ethnic backgrounds. No physician evaluates and manages disease in a vacuum; the racial background of the patient and cultural context within which he or she exists may influence many aspects of the interaction between the two. The terminology chosen to communicate effectively with patients, the diseases on the physician's differential, and medications selected for management of a condition may vary according to the patient's ethnicity. For instance, when communicating with an African American woman, one might choose to ask about her *flesh moles* rather than her dermatosis papulosa nigra. Or a dermatologist might steer clear of 10% benzoyl peroxide in an African American acne patient whose skin is prone to postinflammatory hyperpigmentation due to concerns of irritation. It is incumbent upon the provider to be knowledgeable about both the medical and relevant cultural aspects of his or her patients so that he or she has the ability to provide quality care. This chapter addresses the cultural considerations in treating patients of African descent.

The conversation about race and ethnicity is complicated. There is discussion and debate in natural and social scientific communities about the validity of race, the meaning of ethnicity, and the significance of each. Terms keep changing and are sometimes confusing. And for some, it is just plain uncomfortable to talk about at all, and avoidance can seem easier than risking saying the wrong thing or inadvertently offending an entire group of people. That being said, most patients are not involved in anthropological or biological debates, and their race and/or culture are important to them. These factors may impact their perceptions of disease, utilization of health services, and disease outcomes. So understanding the cultural context in which the patient and his or her disease exist is paramount.

V.H. Barbosa, M.D., M.P.H., M.B.A (✉)
Department of Dermatology, Millennium Park Dermatology,
30 N Michigan Avenue Suite 1429, Chicago, IL 60602, USA
e-mail: vbarbosa@millenniumparkdermatology.com

A.F. Alexis and V.H. Barbosa (eds.), *Skin of Color: A Practical Guide to Dermatologic Diagnosis and Treatment*, DOI 10.1007/978-0-387-84929-4_17,

## Who Are People of African Descent?

The world's population is approaching seven billion people [1]. With 800 million sub-Saharan Africans and another 140 million people of African descent living on other continents, Blacks make up 14% of the world's population [2]. Speaking literally, anyone who is a citizen of one of Africa's 57 countries is African, regardless of their racial background [3]. And again, speaking literally, since all populations of people can be traced back to Africa, then everyone on the planet is "of African descent." The term is most commonly used as a proxy to indicate race rather than continent of origin, since the term "negro" has fallen out of favor and "Black" has decreased in popularity. The term generally refers to people whose ancestors are from sub-Saharan Africa. The seven countries that make up Northern Africa include Algeria, Egypt, Libya, Morocco, Sudan, Tunisia, and Western Sahara. These countries are more heavily influenced racially, religiously, socially, and culturally by the Middle East, Europe, and Asia given their physical proximity and the barrier created to the rest of Africa by the Sahara Desert [4]. Sub-Saharan Africa is comprised of 50 countries where the populations are predominantly people with brown skin and curly hair, the phenotype originally given the racial classification Negroid.

Millions of Africans were transported from Africa during the slave trade, more migrated voluntarily in the centuries that followed. This fact gives rise to the concept of the African diaspora, people of African descent living outside Africa. Many of these people are of mixed race, and each country has its own way of categorizing their mixed race inhabitants. While exact numbers are difficult to find, there are approximately 23 million people of African descent in the Caribbean, 111.5 million in South America, 44 million in North America, and 7 million in Europe [5]. People of African descent make up 14% of the world population and 12.9% of the United States population [5, 6].

It goes without saying that many people of African descent are of mixed race, and racial and ethnic heritage is not always apparent. Patients should be afforded the opportunity to self-identify their racial and ethnic background rather than the provider making assumptions based upon physical attributes. This information should be gathered routinely on new paper intake forms or during the taking of the medical history.

## Health Services Utilization

As we contemplate cultural considerations for treating African-Americans medical needs, many issues come to mind. Issues in health services like access to care, barriers to treatment, perceptions of the medical system, and trust in physicians and willingness to participate in clinical research have all been explored in the medical literature in general, but specific studies pertaining to dermatological care are lacking. There is virtually no literature published in scientific journals exploring African American treatment-seeking or health-seeking behaviors for dermatological conditions. There is, however, a plethora of research on the subject for medical care in general as well as for other fields, particularly for primary care and psychiatric services.

Recent studies both in the United States and Europe document common reasons that people of African descent visit the dermatologist. In a study by Alexis et al., the five most common diagnosis codes listed for African-Americans visiting a dermatology practice were acne, dyschromia, contact dermatitis and other eczema, alopecia, and seborrheic dermatitis. Interestingly, dyschromia and alopecia were not among the top ten diagnoses of Caucasian patients. The top five diagnoses for Caucasians were acne, lesion of uncertain behavior on the trunk, benign neoplasm on the trunk, contact dermatitis and other eczema, and psoriasis [7]. Similar patterns have been noted among people of African descent elsewhere in the world. For instance, a study of 1,000 patients in Jamaica noted the four most common diagnoses to be acne, seborrheic eczema, pigmentary disorders, and atopic eczema [8]. In a study of Africans and Afro-Caribbeans in Paris, adults were noted to be diagnosed with acne, dyschromia, alopecia, and eczema. [9]

## Common Misconceptions Among African Americans

In the African-American community, knowledge about hair and skin and their care and treatments for problems comes from many sources. Information is commonly passed from mother to daughter and among the female relatives and friends. Information is also sought from sources like the Internet, beauty magazines, and hairdressers. Unfortunately not all information is correct, and there are many beauty myths that are accepted as fact. The dermatologist treating an African-American patient should be aware of common misconceptions so that they can be dispelled during the office consultation.

In order to explore commonly held beauty myths among African Americans, a Google search was performed using the terms "African American Beauty Myths," "African American Skin Myths," and "African American Hair Myths." The top ten posts from beauty blogs, magazine and radio websites, and other online resources were analyzed for common themes. Commercial websites selling cosmetic products and containing press releases were excluded. The top five myths for skin and hair are presented here, along with strategies for dispelling the myths.

## Skin Myths

The top five myths regarding African American skin are listed in Table 17.1. It is not surprising that three of the top five myths relate directly or indirectly to sun exposure and protection. African Americans in general are aware that pigmentation offers some protection from the sun. Many mistakenly think that the modest protection

**Table 17.1** African-American skin myths

| |
|---|
| Black skin does not burn |
| Black skin does not get skin caner |
| Black skin does not wrinkle |
| Cocoa butter fades dark spots |
| Black skin is oily and does not need moisturizer |

provided by brown skin compared to white skin is enough to eliminate the possibility of burning, wrinkling, or developing skin cancer. Consequently, sunscreen use is lower among African Americans, with one study reporting that 63% of African American adults never wear sunscreen [10]. Sunscreen use is also infrequent among adolescents, with a study by Hall et al. demonstrating significantly lower sunscreen use for African American high school students than for Caucasian high school students, with a frequent use rate of 4.8% compared to 16.5% [11]. Knowledge about melanoma among people of color in the US is low. In a recent study by Robinson et al., focus groups of African-Americans, Hispanics, and Asians revealed the common theme that skin cancer was not relevant to ethnic people [12]. This lack of information is particularly concerning given the fact that melanomas in Blacks and Hispanics are more likely to metastasize and have poorer outcomes than those in Caucasians [13, 14].

The author's recommendation is to raise the issues of sun protection and skin cancer prevention with patients of African descent and with all patients of color. A few minutes of education can be the key to early detection for at-risk patients and can ultimately be life-saving. To provide additional motivation to the patient, sunscreen's role in maintaining an even complexion can be discussed since this is an issue that often resonates more with people of African descent since they are prone to conditions like melasma and postinflammatory hyperpigmentation [15].

The prevalence of dyschromia in people of African descent gives rise to a number of folk remedies for treatment. Cocoa butter is at the top of the list. In addition to the belief that it treats discoloration, it is also believed to improve the appearance of scars and stretch marks. Hence, cocoa butter is an ingredient that is very popular in African-American skin care products. It is an excellent moisturizer for the skin and is prized for its rich, creamy texture and pleasant aroma. It is not, however, a significant skin lightening agent. And, two studies demonstrate no prevention of or improvement in stretch marks after utilizing a cocoa butter cream [16, 17]. Taking a thorough history of product use might reveal use of cocoa butter for dark spots and provide the opportunity for the physician to provide a more effective treatment. The same history might occasionally reveal use of less benign folk treatments as well. In many parts of Africa, and in African markets in the United States, high-potency topical steroids, prescription-strength hydroquinone, or mercury-containing products are used to fade dark spots, to even the complexion, or to lighten the skin.

As previously discussed in Chap. 1 on skin structure and function, there is conflicting data on sebaceous gland size and sebaceous excretion. In fact, some African American have oily skin, while others have dry skin. Given seasonal variations in the skin's needs and decreasing oil production as we age, the need for a moisturizer often changes over time for any given individual. Patients often are eager to accept suggestions for skin care products because of the confusion that arises from the number of products that are available.

## Hair Myths

The top five African-American hair myths are listed in Table 17.2. Three of the five myths are related to the issue of hair growth. In fact, African hair does not grow as quickly as Caucasian hair, and it breaks off more easily whether it is in its virgin state or chemically treated [18, 19]. So, the slower growth and easier breakage can make it seem as if the hair is not really growing. Styles like braids and twists are left in place for approximately 6–8 or more weeks. During that time, there is no heat styling, chemical application, or combing of the hair, so there is no weathering of the hair that leads to breakage of the ends of the hair. Hence, when the style is "taken down," the hair is noticeably longer. In fact, the braided style did not change the rate of hair growth, but rather it perceptibly reduced the amount of breakage. Of note, patients are sometimes concerned because of the amount of hair that is lost when their braids are taken down. Patients need to be reassured about normal hair loss, which is approximately 100 hairs per day. These hairs remain trapped in the braids for the duration of the hairstyle and are then all noticed at once when the braids are taken down. So for instance if braids were left in for 2 months, the patient would notice approximately 6,000 strands of hair in the comb and on the floor when the braids are removed. Patients sometimes need to be reassured about this normal hair loss.

Shampooing is intended to remove sebum and dirt from the hair. Some formulas are more aggressive than others. However, it is not the cleansing itself that provides the greatest vulnerability for African American hair. Rather, wet hair has lower tensile strength and is more easily broken than dry hair, so just combing the already fragile hair when it is wet can lead to breakage. In addition, the hottest styling implements, including blow dryers, cap dryers, curling irons, and flat irons, are used as part of styling recently shampooed hair and can cause additional breakage. Deep conditioners and leave-in conditioners can be used to decrease force needed to comb hair and provide protection from heat styling implements.

Many people do not realize that dermatologists treat hair and scalp conditions in addition to skin diseases. So, they may not realize that their provider is a resource for them. The physician should take the time to ask about hair-grooming practices as part of the medical history and be sure to examine patient's scalps during full-body skin exams.

**Table 17.2** African-American hair myths

| |
|---|
| Black hair doesn't grow |
| Trimming ends makes hair grow |
| Braids make hair grow |
| Washing your hair too much dries it out |
| It is necessary to grease the scalp |

## Caring for the African American Patient

Ultimately, caring for the African American patient is no different than caring for any other patient. It is incumbent on the physician to develop a respect for the culture of his or her patients, to listen to the patient's needs and concerns, and to be aware that there may be issues that the physician may need to raise because the patient may be reluctant to or may not realize that the physician is knowledgeable enough to answer their questions. Key areas for the physician to address include sun protection, skin cancer prevention, and hair-grooming practices, since these are areas where patients may have incomplete information or inaccurate beliefs.

## References


1. http://www.census.gov/main/www/popclock.html. Accessed 25 Sept 2011.
2. http://en.wikipedia.org/wiki/African_diaspora. Accessed 25 Sept 2011.
3. CIA World Factbook. https://www.cia.gov/library/publications/the-world-factbook/wfbExt/region_afr.html
4. http://en.wikipedia.org/wiki/North_Africa
5. http://en.wikipedia.org/wiki/African_diaspora
6. http://www.census.gov/prod/cen2010/briefs/c2010br-06.pdf
7. Alexis AF, Sergay AB, Taylor SC. Common dermatologic disorders in skin of color: a comparative practice survey. Cutis. 2007;80(5):387–94. Nov.
8. Dunwell P, Rose A. Study of the skin disease spectrum occurring in an Afro-Caribbean population. Int J Dermatol. 2003;42(4):287–9. Apr.
9. Arsouze A, Fitoussi C, Cabotin PP, Chaine B, Delebecque C, Raynaud E, Kornfeld S, Dehen L, Bafounta ML, Bourgeois-Droin C, Dubertret L, Dupuy A, Petit A. Presenting skin disorders in black Afro-Caribbean patients: a multicentre study conducted in the Paris region. Ann Dermatol Venereol. 2008;135(3):177–82. Mar.
10. Pichon LC, Corral I, Landrine H, Mayer JA, Norman GJ. Sun-protection behaviors among African Americans. Am J Prev Med. 2010;38(3):288–95. Mar.
11. Hall HI, Jones SE, Saraiya M. Prevalence and correlates of sunscreen use among US high school students. J Sch Health. 2001;71(9):453–7. Nov.
12. Robinson JK, Joshi KM, Ortiz S, Kundu RV. Melanoma knowledge, perception, and awareness in ethnic minorities in Chicago: recommendations regarding education. Psychooncology. 2011;20(3):313–20. Mar.
13. Hu S, Parmet Y, Allen G, Parker DF, Ma F, Rouhani P, Kirsner RS. Disparity in melanoma: a trend analysis of melanoma incidence and stage at diagnosis among whites, Hispanics, and blacks in Florida. Arch Dermatol. 2009;145(12):1369–74. Dec.
14. Rouhani P, Hu S, Kirsner RS. Melanoma in Hispanic and black Americans. Cancer Control. 2008;15(3):248–53. Jul.
15. Davis EC, Callender VD. Postinflammatory hyperpigmentation: a review of the epidemiology, clinical features, and treatment options in skin of color. J Clin Aesthet Dermatol. 2010;3(7):20–31. Jul.
16. Buchanan K, Fletcher HM, Reid M. Prevention of striae gravidarum with cocoa butter cream. Int J Gynaecol Obstet. 2010;108(1):65–8. Jan.
17. Osman H, Usta IM, Rubeiz N, Abu-Rustum R, Charara I, Nassar AH. Cocoa butter lotion for prevention of striae gravidarum: a double-blind, randomised and placebo-controlled trial. BJOG. 2008;115(9):1138–42. Aug.
18. Loussouarn G. African hair growth parameters. Br J Dermatol. 2001;145(2):294–7. Aug.
19. McMichael AJ. Hair breakage in normal and weathered hair: focus on the Black patient. J Investig Dermatol Symp Proc. 2007;12(2):6–9. Dec.

# Chapter 18
# Cultural Considerations in Asian Patients

**Chanisada Wongpraparut and Henry W. Lim**

Asia is the world's most populous continent, with over four billion people. According to geographic and cultural area, Asia is commonly divided into the Central Asia (Kazakhstan, Kyrgyzstan,Tajikistan, Turkmenistan, Uzbekistan), East Asia (including China, Japan, Korea), West Asia (including Armenia, Turkey, and the Middle East), North Asia (Asian part of Russia), South Asia (including India, Pakistan, Sri Lanka, Nepal, Bhutan), and Southeast Asia (including Myanmar, Thailand, Laos, Cambodia, Vietnam, Singapore, Indonesia, Malaysia, Philippines) [1]. However, some definitions exclude Turkey, the Middle East, Central Asia and Russia, while others refer to the Asia-Pacific region, which does not include the Middle East or Russia, but does include islands in the Pacific Ocean.

Asians have different cultural backgrounds and have a large range of skin types (from skin type II to VI) [2]. Certain skin diseases have different manifestations and prevalence among Asian patients. While in the West it is common for physicians to approach diseases by assuming they are due to external factors, degeneration of the body part/organ, or a combination of both, Asians believe the body is a whole, and each part of it is thoroughly interconnected in its health and in a diseased state [3]. People in Asia usually believe that diet plays an important role in disease, with some diets perceived to make the disease worse, while others would improve it. It is very common for Asians to ask for specific dietary restriction as a part of their treatments when they visit their physicians [4].

C. Wongpraparut, M.D.
Department of Dermatology, Faculty of Medicine Siriraj Hospital,
2 Prannok Street, Bangkok 10700, Thailand
e-mail: chanisada@hotmail.com

H.W. Lim, M.D. (✉)
Department of Dermatology, Henry Ford Medical Center, New Center One,
3031 W. Grand Boulevard, Suite 800, Detroit, MI 48202, USA
e-mail: hlim1@hfhs.org

A.F. Alexis and V.H. Barbosa (eds.), *Skin of Color: A Practical Guide to Dermatologic Diagnosis and Treatment*, DOI 10.1007/978-0-387-84929-4_18,

While tanning is considered to impart good health (and wealth) in the West, Asians prefer porcelain-white skin since fair-skinned individuals are perceived to be of a higher socioeconomic status. Some Asian cultural practices can leave skin marks that may be misinterpreted by unfamiliar physicians as physical abuse. To understand the sociocultural traditions and health beliefs among Asians, it is important for all physicians to be familiar with these practices; this is especially important with the changing demographics of the population in Western countries, including the United States. It will help cross-cultural communication and cooperation between healthcare professionals and patients, decrease unnecessary medical investigations and improve treatment outcomes.

This chapter will cover various traditional Asian practices for skin diseases, the Asian cultural practices that leave distinctive cutaneous signs or complications, and some of the commonly held beliefs among Asians.

## Traditional Asian Practice for Cutaneous Conditions

### *Herbal Medicine*

Herbal medicine is widely used in Asia. Most commonly, plants or parts of plants are used for therapeutic purposes. Herbs can come as fresh or dried plants, extracts, powders, tablets or capsules. Claims have been made that herbal medicine is useful as a treatment for a variety of skin conditions; however, only a few evidence-based studies showed its benefit.

The first double-blind study that was published in the English literature appeared in 1992. The investigator conducted a double-blind, placebo-controlled trial by using herbal medicine for atopic dermatitis. Patients were randomized to receive Dr. Luo's formulated mixture which contained ten herbs or placebo. The ten herbs were *Clematis armandii*, *Dictamnus dasycarpus*, *Glycyrrhiza glabra*, *Ledebouriella seseloides*, *Lophatherum gracile*, *Rehmannia glutinosa*, *Paeonia lactiflora*, *Potentilla chinensis*, *Tribulus terrestris*, and *Schizonepeta tenuifolia*. In 37 children that completed the study, clinical response in the herbal medicine group was significantly superior to that observed in the placebo group; no internal organ toxicity was noted [5]. A 1-year follow up study demonstrated that half of patients who continued using herbal medicine showed at least 90% reduction in clinical severity scores. By the end of the year, one-fifth of them were able to discontinue the therapy without a relapse [6]. The mechanism behind this ten-herbs formulation was thought to inhibit the expression of CD23 in the individual affected with atopic dermatitis.

In 2004, another study of herbal medicine for atopic dermatitis was conducted involving five herbal extracts: *Flos lonicerae (jinyinhua)*, *Herba menthae (bohe)*, *Cortex moutan (danpi)*, *Rhizoma atractylodis (cangzhu)*, and *Cortex phellodendri (huangbai)* [7]. There was no corticosteroid or corticosteroid-related compound found in this formulation [8]. Eighty-five children with moderate to severe atopic dermatitis were enrolled and randomized to receive capsules of traditional Chinese medicines or placebo for 12 weeks. In both groups, scoring of atopic dermatitis (SCORAD), children's dermatology life quality index (CDLQI), and the requirement of topical steroid and oral antihistamine were compared before, during, and after a course of therapy. Although there was no significant difference in the SCORAD between two groups, the CDLQI in actively treated group was significantly improved compared to the placebo group. Total amount of topical steroid used was also significantly reduced by one-third in the herbal medicine group [9].

Psoriasis is another skin disease that has been treated by herbs; the treatment used ranges from topical to systemic, as well as combination with ultraviolet therapy. In a multicenter study involving 13 hospitals, *Radix Angelicae dahuricae* (which contains furocoumarins) plus UVA was compared to PUVA therapy. There was no statistically significant difference in the efficacy between these two methods; however, most subjects preferred the use of *Radix Angelicae dahuricae* because of milder side effects [10].

Several reports describing the adverse effects from herbal drugs have been published. Serious adverse effects from Chinese herbal medicine included hypersensitivity, toxic epidermal necrolysis, hepatic toxicity, and renal damage, some of which can be fatal [11, 12]. Some of herbal medicines were reported to contain unwanted substances including corticosteroids, diazepam, lead, arsenic, and mercury [11, 13, 14]. An analysis of 11 Chinese herbal creams for treating eczema demonstrated that most of them (8 of 11) contained dexamethasone at a mean concentration of 456 μg/g (range: 64–1,500 μg/g) [15]. There are also other reports with similar results [16, 17]. Exposure to arsenic can occur from taking herbal medicine. Cutaneous signs of chronic arsenism include arsenical keratoses (punctate hyperkeratosis of palms and soles) and macular hypopigmentation and increase a risk to develop Bowen's disease and cutaneous and internal malignancies [18]. A patient who has cutaneous signs of chronic arsenic toxicity should be asked for a history of herbal drugs intake. Figures 18.1 and 18.2 demonstrate cutaneous signs in patients with chronic arsenism from taking herbal medicine.

## *Aromatherapy*

Volatile liquid plant materials, known as essential oil and other aromatic compounds from plants, can be used for therapeutic, psychological, and physiological purposes. Aromatherapy refers to a treatment that uses essential oils added to the bath, massaged into the skin, inhaled directly, or diffused to scent an entire room. Oils are extracts from several parts of plant such as flowers (e.g., lavender, rose), leaves (e.g., eucalyptus, peppermint), grasses (e.g., lemongrass), twigs (e.g., juniper), and roots (e.g., calamus, vetivert) [19].

Aromatherapy has been used for dermatological conditions [19]. Lemongrass is considered to have an anti-inflammatory property. Eucalyptus has anti-inflammatory and analgesic properties; it has been used for treatment of herpes zoster and candidiasis [20]. Jasmine is thought to have antiseptic and anti-inflammatory effects.

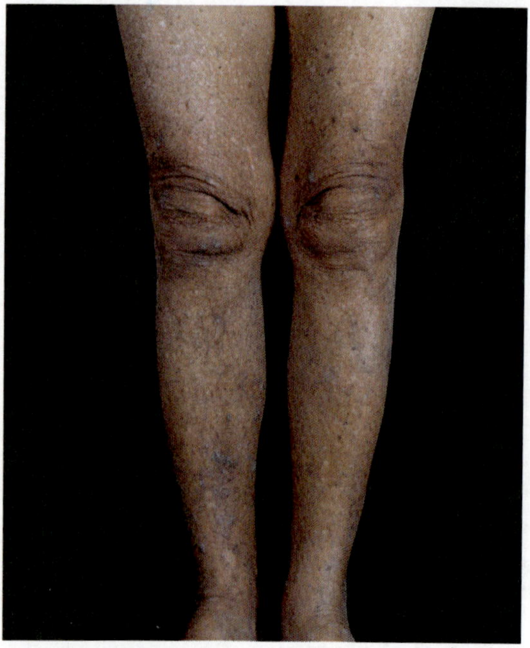

**Fig. 18.1** Macular hypopigmentation in a patient with chronic arsenism from taking herbal medicine

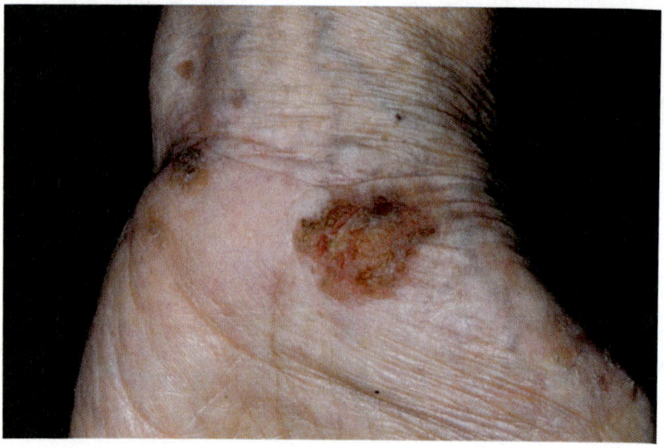

**Fig. 18.2** Bowen's disease in a patient with chronic arsenism from taking herbal medicine

True lavender has been used to promote wound healing; it also has analgesic property. Tea tree has antimicrobial effects and has been used for the treatment of acne and warts. Peppermint has been used for treatment of dermatitis and herpes infection, while benzoin for skin infections, acne, dermatitis, and psoriasis [19].

However, it should be noted there have been only limited studies done on aromatherapy for dermatological conditions. Tea tree (*Melaleuca alternifolia*) has long been used as antiseptic agent. A single-blinded trial of 124 patients with mild to moderate acne that compared 5% tea tree oil and 5% benzoyl peroxide was performed. Both groups had similar effects on clinical improvement. The onset of the beneficial effect of tea tree oil was slower; however, patients in tea tree oil group had fewer adverse effects [21]. Another study of tea tree oil was done comparing it with 1% tolnaftate and placebo for tinea pedis. Tolnaftate group had highest mycological cure, followed by tea tree group and placebo. Tea tree oil reduced the symptoms of tinea pedis as effectively as tolnaftate [22].

Aromatherapy was shown to be beneficial in alopecia areata. Eighty-six patients were randomized into two groups: the active group received essential oil (cedarwood, lavender, rosemary, thyme) in a mixture of carrier oils (jojoba and grape seed) for massaging into their scalp, while the control group received only carrier oils for their massage. Forty-four patients in the active group showed clinical improvement compared to 15% in the control group [23].

Several cases of contact dermatitis and phototoxic reaction from aromatherapy were reported [24–27]. A 33-year-old woman self-administered aromatherapy by adding six drops of oil of bergamot and six drops of geranium oil in her bath. After a bath, she then spent about half an hour on a sunbed. Within 48 h, she developed erythema and blistering on exposed areas and was admitted to a burn unit with superficial partial-thickness burns over 70% of her body [28]. It was then recognized that one of the ingredients in oil of bergamot is 5-methoxypsoralen, which is a potent phototoxic agent. Another two patients were reported with localized and disseminated bullous phototoxic reaction developing within 48–72 h after exposure to bergamot aromatherapy followed by subsequent ultraviolet irradiation [26]. This adverse effect should be noted by all because oil of bergamot has been gaining popularity in aromatherapy lately. Figure 18.3 demonstrates allergic contact dermatitis due to essential oil in an aromatherapy treatment.

## *Acupuncture*

Acupuncture is a term derived from the Latin word "acus" and "puncta," meaning puncture the body by needle. It is originally a technique of inserting and manipulating needles into specific points on the body for therapeutic purposes. At present, at least four kinds of needles are used in Asia. Filiform steel needle, the most popular one, is used to acupoint in the body. Other needles include the ear needle, the lancet or bloodletting needle, and the cutaneous needle [29]. The ear needle is used for microacupoint on the ear. The lancet is purposely used for puncture of superficial engorged veins [29]. The cutaneous needle is used to puncture superficial skin and has a role in the treatment of skin conditions such as psoriasis, atopic dermatitis, and neurodermatitis [29].

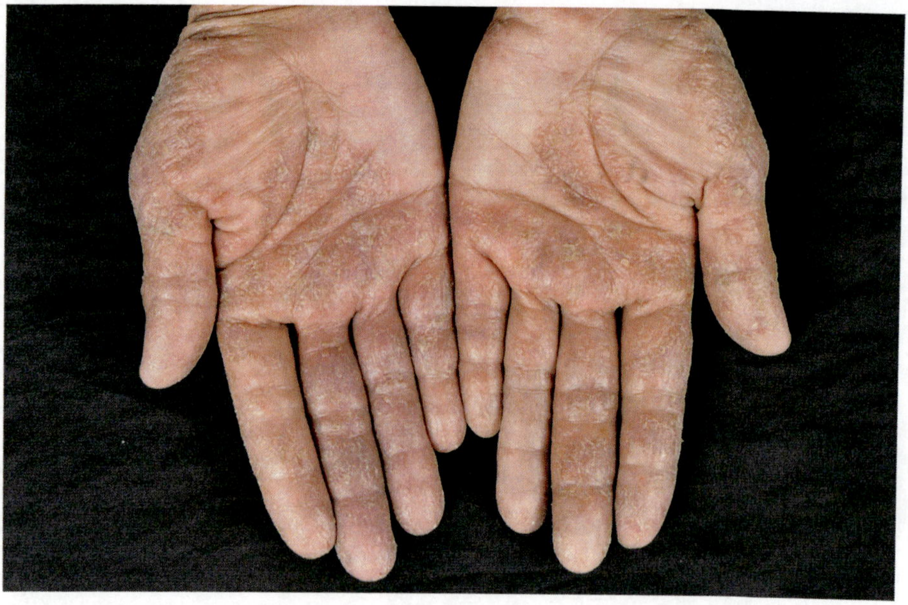

**Fig. 18.3** Allergic contact dermatitis from essential oil in aromatherapist (Courtesy of Dr. Waranya Boonchai)

According to traditional Chinese medicinal theory, acupuncture points are situated on meridians, along which *qi*, the vital energy, flows. There is no known anatomical or histological basis for the existence of acupuncture points or meridians, although detailed maps have been developed and used for centuries. Several basic evaluation processes are often required before making the diagnosis and treating the patient with acupuncture. These steps are comprised of taking a history of the illness, obtaining information about the patient's lifestyle, observing the skin and tongue color, palpating the pulse, listening to breath sounds, and smelling body and breath odors [30]. Currently, acupuncture remains a substantial part of the traditional Chinese medicine, is used as an anesthesia, and is administered to treat various medical conditions including dermatologic diseases. The skin diseases that have been treated with acupuncture include acne, alopecia, eczema, chicken pox, herpes zoster, psoriasis, rosacea, systemic lupus erythematosus, urticaria, and vitiligo [31].

The only controlled trial of acupuncture for psoriasis was performed in 56 patients. Half of the patients received the active therapy consisting of placement of needles with sufficient depth followed by proper electrical stimulation. In the other half of the group (the placebo group), the needles were purposely placed outside the recommended location without electrical stimulation. After 10 weeks of twice-weekly treatment, there was no demonstrable difference between the active treatment group and the placebo group [32].

Acupuncture is associated with some adverse effects such as transmission of infectious diseases due to unsterile technique, allergic contact dermatitis, panniculitis, localized argyria, and skin ulceration [33–37].

## Asian Cultural Practices That Leave Skin Changes and Complications

Some Asian traditional practices may leave unusual skin lesions, which may be mistaken for physical or child abuse. These will be discussed below.

### *Coin Rubbing, Coining*

Known by several different names, coining (cao giÓ in Vietnamese, gua sha in Chinese) is a dermabrasive therapy mostly practiced in Southeast Asia, especially Vietnam. The purpose is to relieve a variety of illnesses such as aches, pains, fevers, fatigue, flu, nausea, and abdominal pain. This technique involves the use of oil or ointment and a coin. Commonly used balms or oils include Tiger balm and liquid herbal medicines containing camphor, wintergreen oil, eucalyptus oil, peppermint oil, and cinnamon oil [38]. The procedure is done by lubricating the skin with a balm or oil followed by rubbing the coin firmly and repeatedly in a linear pattern until the ecchymosis appears under the skin. This technique, commonly applied to the back, lateral chest, and lateral and posterior neck, causes extravasation of blood from dermal capillaries which results in petechiae and ecchymosis, which usually last for 3–7 days [39]. Although the marks on the skin look painful, usually they are not. However, there was a case report of serious injury from a severe burn obtained during the coining treatment [40].

### *Cupping*

This is a form of traditional medicine practiced in several countries in Asia such as China and Vietnam. It is important for dermatologists to recognize this technique because it leaves a distinctive cutaneous lesion. In cupping, an alcohol-saturated cotton ball is placed on a small stand on the skin; the cotton ball is then lit, and a glass cup is place over the fire, flushed against the patient's skin. After the oxygen in the space is enclosed by the cup and the skin is exhausted, the fire extinguishes itself; as the air cools in the cup, a vacuum forms that pulls up the skin, causing a trauma to superficial blood vessels which results in circular-shaped purpura and ecchymosis [41]. Usually 4–8 cups, and up to 12 cups, are placed on each side of the back in vertical columns with 5–20 min for application time. As a cup is left on longer, a more prominent circular mark is produced. Cupping can be repeated every 4–6 months [41]. Patients may report a feeling of relaxation after the procedure. This technique is generally performed for chronic pain, headache, and stomach ailments. However, there are few reports of this practice for acne [42, 43]. The theory behind this procedure is to increase the circulation around the area of cupping and help in the elimination of trapped toxin in the tissue [44]. Nowadays, manual pumps and plastic cups are available in Asia, which avoid the difficulty and danger of using alcohol and fire.

## *Moxibustion*

Moxibustion is a technique using a stick or cone of burning mugwort herb placed over the affected body part. It is a traditional medicine practiced in China, Japan, Korea, Vietnam, Tibet, and Mongolia. Moxa can be either put directly on the skin (direct moxibustion) or insulated by a layer of garlic, ginger, salt, or aconite cake (indirect moxibustion) and lit. Moxibustion is also used in conjunction with acupuncture, as a complementary technique for warming an acupuncture point. The purpose is to stimulate circulation through the points and induce a smoother flow of blood and *qi* (the vital energy). In most cases, the burning moxa is placed indirectly on the skin, resulting in only local transient redness which is the expected result. However, if the moxa is burned directly on the skin, second-degree burns can occur [45]. Figure 18.4 demonstrates burns from direct moxibustion in a Vietnamese patient. Moxibustion is primarily used to relieve pain and as a treatment for asthma and low blood pressure [45]. There was a study of indirect moxibustion by herb cake for atopic dermatitis. It was done once a day for 7 days. Forty-five percent of patients were considered cleared, and 55% of patients had marked improvement [29, 46].

## *Tattoo and Henna*

Sak yant (yantra tattooing) is a form of sacred tattooing practiced in Southeast Asian countries. The ancient tradition of tattoo (sak yant) is normally done by monks but can also be performed by laypeople. The tattoos usually consist of sacred images (animal, buddhas, or temples) as well as written parts of holy script. The common tattoo locations are shoulders, arms, trunk, and back. The origins of sak yant and the magic lettering are derived from the ancient Khmer culture. The purpose of tattooing is believed to provide mystical powers and protect the individuals from danger.

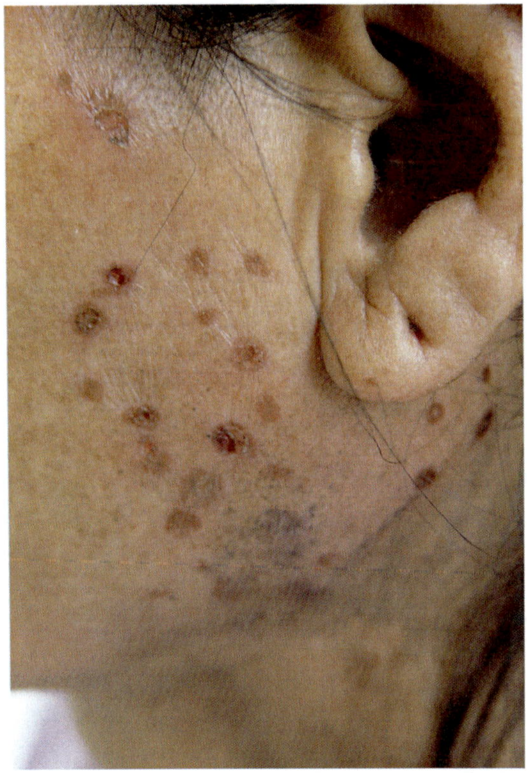

**Fig. 18.4** Skin burn from direct moxibustion in Vietnamese patient (Courtesy of Dr. Sasima Eimpunth). This is the work of Dr. Sasima Eimpunth while working at Naresuan University Hospital

There are case reports of HIV, hepatitis B, hepatitis C, and mycobacterium transmission from tattooing with unsterile techniques [47–50]. Figure 18.5 demonstrates *Mycobacterium fortuitum* infection from amateur tattooing.

Henna temporary tattooing has been used in South Asian countries and in the Middle East for a long time for hair dyeing, skin decoration, and social purposes. In India, there is a traditional prewedding ceremony called mehndi ceremony. The mehndi (henna paint) is applied on bride's hands, arms, feet, and legs with the belief that the darker the mehndi color, the more her husband will love her. It was estimated that at least half of Indians have been exposed to henna in their lifetime [51].

Henna is the Arabic name for the bush *Lawsonia* (*inermis, alba*); it is cultivated in India, Sri Lanka, the eastern Mediterranean region, and North Africa [52, 53]. The dark-green powder extracted from henna leaves contains naphthoquinone, an active substance which requires several hours after painting to get the color stain in the skin. Some substances are added to the tattoo mix including eucalyptus, essential oil, vinegar, and other secret additives [52]. For black henna, paraphenylenediamine (PPD) is often added to darken the color, to decrease the staining time, as well as to provide a longer lasting effect. While pure henna is considerably safe, the PPD contained in black henna is a common sensitizer [53, 54]. Several allergic reactions from PPD in black henna have been reported including allergic contact dermatitis,

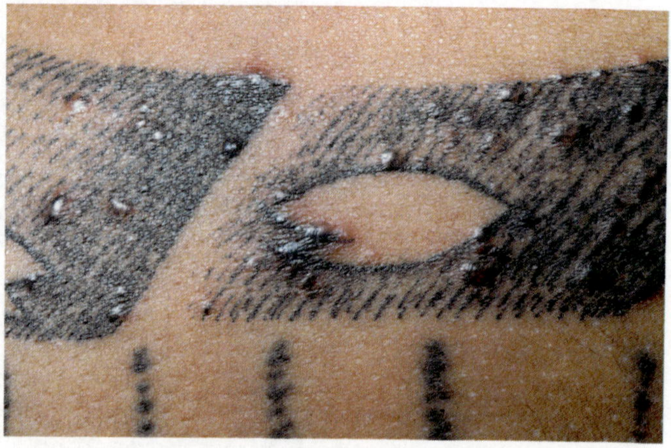

**Fig. 18.5** *Mycobacterium fortuitum* infection from amateur tattooing

vesicular erythema multiforme-like reaction, urticaria, and angioedema [55–57]. Recently, there was a study that analyzed the content of henna dyes available in Korea. From 15 henna dye samples, nickel, cobalt, and PPD were detected in 11, 4, and 3 samples, respectively [53]. Nowadays, henna temporary tattooing is gaining popularity worldwide as it is a painless procedure as well as temporary, and no precise skill is required to apply them. However, users should be aware of the unfavorable reaction from PPD and heavy metal contaminants that may be found in henna.

## Commonly Held Beliefs Among Asians

Because of the wide range of ethnic composition, religious beliefs, and cultural practices, Asians do have a wide range of perception on the appearance of their skin and different perceptions of skin diseases. For example, vitiligo, in addition to the obvious esthetic consideration, has extremely significant social impact among the South Asians; patients with vitiligo are considered to be afflicted with a highly undesirable disease, hence treated as outcasts. Many East Asians consider hot shower as the treatment of even minimally pruritic dermatoses, resulting in xerotic skin, hence exacerbating the pruritus and the excoriation. East Asian women consider porcelain-white facial skin to be the mark of beauty; tanning therefore is to be avoided, hence the widespread use of not only sunscreens but parasols on sunny days. For the same reason, much effort and expense are spent on the treatment of melasma. While age is considered to impart wisdom, dyeing of hair is commonly practiced among Asian men and women; therefore, similar to patients seen in the West, contact dermatitis to hair dye can frequently occur in these patients.

## Conclusion

The practice of Asian traditional medicine has spread globally. An understanding of cross-cultural tradition is crucial. Professional healthcare providers who treat Asians, especially those who are first generation, should be aware of and understand cultural practices in order to strengthen the doctor-patient relationship and help to improve treatment outcomes.

## References

1. Culture of Asia. http://en.wikipedia.org/wiki/culture_of_Asia. Accessed Aug 2009.
2. Taylor SC. Epidemiology of skin diseases in ethnic populations. Dermatol Clin. 2003;21:601–7.
3. Traditional Asian health beliefs and healing practices. http://www.dimensionsofculture.com/home/traditional_asian_health_beliefs_and_healing_practices. Accessed Aug 2009.
4. Moy JA, McKinley-Grant L, Sanchez MR. Cultural aspects in the treatment of patients with skin disease. Dermatol Clin. 2003;21:733–42.
5. Sheehan MP, Atherton DJ. A controlled trial of traditional Chinese medicinal plants in widespread non-exudative atopic eczema. Br J Dermatol. 1992;126:179–84.
6. Sheehan MP, Atherton DJ. One-year follow up of children treated with Chinese medicinal herbs for atopic eczema. Br J Dermatol. 1994;130:488–93.
7. Hon KL, Leung TF, Wong Y, et al. A pentaherbs capsule as a treatment option for atopic dermatitis in children: an open-labeled case series. Am J Chin Med. 2004;32:941–50.
8. Hon KL, Lee VW, Leung TF, et al. Corticosteroids are not present in a traditional Chinese medicine formulation for atopic dermatitis in children. Ann Acad Med Singapore. 2006;35:759–63.
9. Hon KL, Leung TF, Ng PC, et al. Efficacy and tolerability of a Chinese herbal medicine concoction for treatment of atopic dermatitis: a randomized, double-blind, placebo-controlled study. Br J Dermatol. 2007;157:357–63.
10. Zhang GW. Treatment of psoriasis by photochemotherapy: a comparison between the photosensitizing capsule of Angelica dahurica and 8-MOP. Zhonghua Yi Xue Za Zhi. 1983;63:16–9.
11. Koo J, Arain S. Traditional Chinese medicine in dermatology. Clin Dermatol. 1999;17:21–7.
12. Lim YL, Thirumoorthy T. Serious cutaneous adverse reactions to traditional Chinese medicines. Singapore Med J. 2005;46:714–7.
13. Kew J, Morris C, Aihie A, Fysh R, Jones S, Brooks D. Arsenic and mercury intoxication due to Indian ethnic remedies. BMJ. 1993;306:506–7.
14. Tay CH. Cutaneous manifestations of arsenic poisoning due to certain Chinese herbal medicine. Australas J Dermatol. 1974;15:121–31.
15. Keane FM, Munn SE, du Vivier AW, Taylor NF, Higgins EM. Analysis of Chinese herbal creams prescribed for dermatological conditions. BMJ. 1999;318:563–4.
16. Graham-Brown RA, Bourke JF, Bumphrey G. Chinese herbal remedies may contain steroids. BMJ. 1994;308:473.
17. Hughes JR, Higgins EM, Pembroke AC. Oral dexamethasone masquerading as a Chinese herbal remedy. Br J Dermatol. 1994;130:261.
18. Wong SS, Tan KC, Goh CL. Cutaneous manifestations of chronic arsenicism: review of seventeen cases. J Am Acad Dermatol. 1998;38:179–85.
19. Stevensen CJ. Aromatherapy in dermatology. Clin Dermatol. 1998;16:689–94.

20. Ashour HM. Antibacterial, antifungal, and anticancer activities of volatile oils and extracts from stems, leaves, and flowers of *Eucalyptus sideroxylon* and *Eucalyptus torquata*. Cancer Biol Ther. 2008;7(3):399–403.
21. Bassett IB, Pannowitz DL, Barnetson RS. A comparative study of tea-tree oil versus benzoylperoxide in the treatment of acne. Med J Aust. 1990;153:455–8.
22. Tong MM, Altman PM, Barnetson RS. Tea tree oil in the treatment of tinea pedis. Australas J Dermatol. 1992;33:145–9.
23. Hay IC, Jamieson M, Ormerod AD. Randomized trial of aromatherapy. Successful treatment for alopecia areata. Arch Dermatol. 1998;134:1349–52.
24. Boonchai W, Iamtharachai P, Sunthonpalin P. Occupational allergic contact dermatitis from essential oils in aromatherapists. Contact Dermatitis. 2007;56:181–2.
25. Crawford GH, Katz KA, Ellis E, James WD. Use of aromatherapy products and increased risk of hand dermatitis in massage therapists. Arch Dermatol. 2004;140:991–6.
26. Kaddu S, Kerl H, Wolf P. Accidental bullous phototoxic reactions to bergamot aromatherapy oil. J Am Acad Dermatol. 2001;45:458–61.
27. Trattner A, David M, Lazarov A. Occupational contact dermatitis due to essential oils. Contact Dermatitis. 2008;58:282–4.
28. Cocks H, Wilson D. Dangers of the intake of psoralens and subsequent UV exposure producing significant burns. Burns. 1998;24:82.
29. Chen CJ, Yu HS. Acupuncture, electrostimulation, and reflex therapy in dermatology. Dermatol Ther. 2003;16:87–92.
30. Tan EK, Millington GW, Levell NJ. Acupuncture in dermatology: an historical perspective. Int J Dermatol. 2009;48:648–52.
31. Iliev E. Acupuncture in dermatology. Clin Dermatol. 1998;16:659–88.
32. Jerner B, Skogh M, Vahlquist A. A controlled trial of acupuncture in psoriasis: no convincing effect. Acta Derm Venereol. 1997;77:154–6.
33. Koizumi H, Tomoyori T, Kumakiri M, Ohkawara A. Acupuncture needle dermatitis. Contact Dermatitis. 1989;21:352.
34. Ara M, de Santamaria CS, Zaballos P, Yus C, Lezcano MA. *Mycobacterium chelonae* infection with multiple cutaneous lesions after treatment with acupuncture. Int J Dermatol. 2003;42:642–4.
35. Jeong KH, Lee MH. Two cases of factitial panniculitis induced by electroacupuncture. Clin Exp Dermatol. 2009;34:e170–3.
36. Takeishi E, Hirose R, Hamasaki Y, Katayama I. Localized argyria 20-years after embedding of acupuncture needles. Eur J Dermatol. 2002;12:609–11.
37. Teo LH, Tang MB, Tan AW, Tan HH, Ng SK. Ulcers related to acupuncture and traditional Chinese medicine: a case series and review of the literature. Arch Dermatol. 2009;145:490–2.
38. Coining method. http://altmed.creighton.edu/coining/methods.htm. Accessed Aug 2009.
39. Gua Sha. http://en.wikipedia.org/wiki/gua_sha. Accessed Aug 2009.
40. Amshel CE, Caruso DM. Vietnamese "coining": a burn case report and literature review. J Burn Care Rehabil. 2000;21:112–4.
41. Yoo SS, Tausk F. Cupping: East meets West. Int J Dermatol. 2004;43:664–5.
42. Chen D, Jiang N, Cong X. 47 cases of acne treated by prick-bloodletting plus cupping. J Tradit Chin Med. 1993;13:185–6.
43. Ding LN. 50 cases of acne treated by puncturing acupoint dazhui in combination with cupping. J Tradit Chin Med. 1985;5:128.
44. Kouskoukis CE, Cupping LM. The art and the value. Am J Dermatopathol. 1983;5:235–9.
45. Lee CS, Lim HW. Cutaneous diseases in Asians. Dermatol Clin. 2003;21:669–77.
46. Wang D. Indirect moxibustion with herb cake for treatment of atopic dermatitis: dermatitis: 20 cases (in chinese). China Acupunct. 2000;20:612.
47. Ghorpade A. Tattoo inoculation lupus vulgaris in two Indian ladies. J Eur Acad Dermatol Venereol. 2006;20:476–7.

48. Kluger N, Muller C, Gral N. Atypical mycobacteria infection following tattooing: review of an outbreak in 8 patients in a French tattoo parlor. Arch Dermatol. 2008;144:941–2.
49. Ko YC, Ho MS, Chiang TA, Chang SJ, Chang PY. Tattooing as a risk of hepatitis C virus infection. J Med Virol. 1992;38:288–91.
50. Preda VA, Maley M, Sullivan JR. *Mycobacterium chelonae* infection in a tattoo site. Med J Aust. 2009;190:278–9.
51. Pasricha JS, Gupta R, Panjwani S. Contact dermatitis to henna (Lawsonia). Contact Dermatitis. 1980;6:288–9.
52. Wolf R, Wolf D, Matz H, Orion E. Cutaneous reactions to temporary tattoos. Dermatol Online J. 2003;9:3.
53. Kang IJ, Lee MH. Quantification of para-phenylenediamine and heavy metals in henna dye. Contact Dermatitis. 2006;55:26–9.
54. Jasim ZF, Darling JR, Handley JM. Severe allergic contact dermatitis to paraphenylene diamine in hair dye following sensitization to black henna tattoos. Contact Dermatitis. 2005;52:116–7.
55. Gulen F, Zeyrek D, Altinoz S, Peker E, Demir E, Tanac R. Urticaria and angioneurotic edema due to the temporary henna tattoo. Minerva Pediatr. 2006;58:583–5.
56. Jovanovic DL, Slavkovic-Jovanovic MR. Allergic contact dermatitis from temporary henna tattoo. J Dermatol. 2009;36:63–5.
57. Sidwell RU, Francis ND, Basarab T, Morar N. Vesicular erythema multiforme-like reaction to para-phenylenediamine in a henna tattoo. Pediatr Dermatol. 2008;25:201–4.

# Chapter 19
# Cultural Considerations in Latino Patients

**David Rodriguez**

Successfully treating the Hispanic dermatologic patient presents a worthwhile challenge for physicians. Sound clinical skills aside, a comprehensive understanding of Hispanic culture and attitude toward ethnicity and race are also fundamental in achieving the desired results. The terms Hispanic and Latino are closely related and often used interchangeably, but they are poorly understood. First and foremost, it would be important to note that the word Hispanic is *not* a racial moniker. In fact, the fabrication of the word is credited to Grace Flores-Hughes, a Mexican-American bureaucrat in the Nixon administration. During this time, the Department of Health, Education, and Welfare required an all-encompassing term that would create an acceptable label for Spanish-speaking individuals from the Caribbean and the Americas; thus, the term Hispanic was born [1]. It was first used in US census data in 1980 to identify individuals of Spanish ancestry [2], and for all intents and purposes, a person is considered Hispanic if they originate from *Hispania*, an old Latin word for what is present-day Spain, or are born in areas colonized by Spain and in which Spanish is the primary language.

The term *Latino* was first coined and used during the 1700s by the French. It served to differentiate new-world colonists who spoke Romance languages such as Spanish and French from individuals who spoke non-Romance languages such as English and Dutch. In the USA however, the term was not adopted by the government until 1997 and was not used in the US census until 2000 [3, 4]. While many of either Spanish or Portuguese ancestry use the terms Hispanic and Latino interchangeably, it would also be important to note that those who hail from former Portuguese and French colonies such as Brazil, French Guiana, and Suriname do not consider themselves Hispanic or Latino and might actually become offended if

D. Rodriguez, M.D. (✉)
Dermatology Associates and Research, 1301 Ponce de Leon Boulevard,
Coral Gables, FL 33134, USA
e-mail: darmd1@aol.com

A.F. Alexis and V.H. Barbosa (eds.), *Skin of Color: A Practical Guide to Dermatologic Diagnosis and Treatment*, DOI 10.1007/978-0-387-84929-4_19,

referred to as such; thus, clinician beware! These subtle differences, however trivial to the non-Hispanic, are essential in dealing effectively with the Hispanic patient.

Hispanics are not racially or ethnically homogenous nor is there a monolithic *Hispanic culture*. In the USA, Hispanics and Latinos have immigrated from over 23 different countries, and indeed most of these were former Spanish colonies. Unfortunately, Hispanic stereotypes have been perpetuated in the media, which has ignored the fact that Latin America is a vast place. The media has also ignored that a white Cuban, a Zapotec Amerindian from Southern Mexico, and an Afro-Colombian, while sharing a common language, are really three quite distinct individuals. It would therefore be wise to resist generalizations while treating these patients.

Originally, Latin America contained various ethnically and culturally distinct indigenous populations that were sometimes forcibly mixed with the colonizing European (mainly Spanish) conquistadors. There was a second wave of African peoples who were arriving in the new world as part of the slave trade that subsequently mixed with the indigenous and European populations. Out of this milieu arose a group of people that, while sharing a common language, are racially mixed by varying degrees from region to region. Racial variations within a country are also the norm, for example, in some parts of South America there are direct descendants of European immigrants without any mixed racial lineage live alongside Amerindian communities.

It is therefore important for the physician to understand that Hispanics can have blonde hair and blue eyes or, in contrast, be African in their phenotypic expression. Hispanics can also be of mixed heritage; *mulattos*, individuals with both African and European ancestry, are commonly found, especially in the Caribbean. Hispanics from Central and South America tend to express a mix of Amerindian and European features, so termed *mestizo*.

The Spanish-speaking world inherited from its colonial past a racial caste system that, while waning in influence, still shapes the attitudes of some Hispanics toward race today. Roughly speaking, this system places a premium on being white or having European features; unmixed whites are at the top of the social ladder, most of the population; being mixed is in the middle. Unmixed Amerindians and Afro-Hispanics occupy the lower rungs. In very general terms, the more *European* someone looks, the more socially accepted and thus upwardly mobile they tend to be. Thus, despite the great progress that has been made in the integration of all racial groups, there is still a great deal of prejudice and stigma among many Hispanics when it comes to their skin color, their hair, and many of their facial features.

When interacting with the Hispanic patient, the physician should acknowledge and try to comprehend what racial group he/she feels most comfortable in. This is especially true of the multiracial *mestizo* group which has emerged as a result of centuries of migration, assimilation, and intermarriage. To illustrate the point, many Hispanics that possess Fitzpatrick skin types IV or V describe themselves as white. While these self-descriptions might seem inaccurate, the physician should accept their *classification* and should educate and empower them with the tools necessary to understand their skin type and how to best treat their skin condition.

Familism and personalism are two essential concepts that must be understood in order to comprehend the Hispanic patient. Despite the aforementioned great variability within these groups, there are some similarities that hold true across most Hispanic populations. They share many things in common such as a close-knit family structure, common social mores, health beliefs, and practices. In some cases, they may consider their immediate family to include distant relatives such as favorite aunts and uncles along with *compadres,* close family friends. This is especially important because it is very common for an aunt, an uncle, or an older cousin to bring a child into a doctor's office. It is also common practice for elders in the family to provide childcare for many of the grandchildren, nieces, and nephews so that the younger adults may work. Therefore, familism refers to this expansive yet emotionally and economically cohesive unit that predominates in the Hispanic community. There may be a tendency for those of us who are not Hispanic to view this expanded family unit as an anomaly or even negatively, but this extended family is an essential component of the patients well-being.

It is quite common among Hispanics today to follow *traditional* gender roles, with the eldest male typically being the authority figure. The respect of the elders is very important among all generations, even though the eldest relatives may be a great aunt or a second cousin. The manner in which we direct the questions and the formality in which we speak to Hispanic patients should show the respect toward the elder patient or an elder family member that may be present. This is especially true during the first few visits to the office or clinic setting.

While respect for the elders is expected in many cases, Hispanics also tend to favor *personalism*. This is defined as a preference for face-to-face interaction of a friendly and familial nature [5]. One example of personalism is not only addressing the patient formally but also asking personal questions, such as "How are your kids doing?" etc. Anecdotal exchanges pertaining to certain foods or other interests are also very important in this regard. It is of course imperative to gather a good medical history and be able to assess the skin problem, but it is arguably just as important to inquire about personal details such as family, place of origin, etc., and insert these questions at some point during the office visit. Techniques such as these will help forge a strong bond with this patient population that will more than likely translate to a higher rate of compliance and a reduction in absenteeism.

Many Hispanic health beliefs are derived from a variety of sources. They may be a mixture of anachronisms such as medieval Spanish medicine or a combination of indigenous remedies with currently accepted medical knowledge. Curiously, certain health beliefs in the form of folk illnesses have transcended the ethnic, racial, and spatial divide of the Spanish-speaking world and are commonly referenced to by a multitude of Hispanics. Some of these are:

- *Ataque de nervios*: episodic, dramatic outbursts of negative emotion – usually in response to a current stressor (but often related to a significant childhood stressor).
- *Bilis:* bile is thought to flow into the blood stream after a traumatic event, with the end result of nervousness.

- *Decaiminientos*: fatigue and listlessness from a spiritual cause.
- *Empacho*: an intestinal obstruction characterized by abdominal pain, vomiting, constipation, anorexia, or gas and bloating. Postpartum women and infants and children are most susceptible.
- *Mal de ojo*: the *evil eye* that may affect infants or women. It is caused by a person with a *strong eye* (especially green or blue) looking with admiration or jealousy at another person. *Mal de ojo* is avoided by touching an infant when admiring or complimenting it.
- *Nerviosimo*: *sickness of the nerves,* which is common and may be treated spiritually and/or medicinally.
- *Pasmo*: paralysis or paresis of extremities or face and is treated with massage.
- *Susto*: fright resulting in *soul loss*. Susto may be acute or chronic and includes a variety of vague complaints. Women are affected more than men [6].

It is therefore understandable that many Hispanics have a tendency not to believe doctors; 33% of Hispanics believe that the use of home remedies is more effective in treating illness that prescribed medications [7]. This, of course, varies by degree of acculturation, education, and socioeconomic level but is pervasive to a significant degree. A study found that of 51 Mexican mothers living in the USA, 70% believed in folk illnesses and 20% had taken their children for treatment by a *curandero* or traditional folk healer [8]. Therefore, several useful tips have been suggested:

- Understand (and be sensitive to) the role folk medicine may play in patients one encounters.
- Practice delivering messages of tolerance and respect – "the art of medicine."
- During the interview, ask "What do you think caused your illness?" and "We all have favorite remedies that we use when we are sick. What have you done to treat this condition?"
- When appropriate, and not contraindicated, incorporate some benign folk medicine remedies into one's advice to the patient to improve the compliance and trust [6].

In the year 2000, the largest of the minority groups in the United States was the Hispanic. In 1990, there were 21.9 million Hispanics in the USA. This number increased by 61% in 2000, making Hispanics 35.2 million, 12.6% of the US population [9]. In 2008, 15.4% of the US population was reported to be Hispanic. It is estimated that by 2050, they will account for 24.4% of the population, rising from 35.6 million people to 102.6 million, an increase of 188% [9]. Hispanics in the USA are mainly from Mexico, standing at 20.9 million in 2000 [9]. These exponentially growing numbers highlight the fact that it is essential to understand the idiosyncrasies and health beliefs of this ever more influential population.

Current census data shows that the population of Mexico is over 106.4 million people [10]. Of these people, the percentage of 60% is mestizo, 30% Amerindian or largely Amerindian, 9% white, and 1% is classified as other. As reported in 2002, the Mexicans account for 66.9% of all Hispanics in the USA [11]. However, Mexican people have been in the USA for centuries throughout the various parts of the country, most abundantly in California, New Mexico, and Arizona. Yet, some Hispanics in New Mexico are direct descendants of the Spanish who settled in the area over 400 years ago!

The next largest groups of Hispanics in the USA are from the Caribbean Islands, which include Puerto Rican (9.1%), Cuban (3.5%), and Dominican (2.6%) [12]. Both Puerto Rico and Cuba were the last two colonies that achieved independence from Spain after the Spanish-American War of 1898. The similarity of this group of Hispanics is found both in their culture and in their ethnic composition, as Hispanics in the Caribbean have a much more pronounced African influence than Hispanics in Central or South America. The ethnic composition of Cuba is as follows: white 65.1%, mulatto and mestizo 24.8%, and black 10.1%. The ethnic composition of Puerto Rico is similar with white (mostly Spanish origin) 76.2%, black 6.9%, Asian 0.3%, Amerindian 0.2%, mixed 4.4%, and other ethnicities comprising 12%. Dominican society is even more mixed with mixed (mulatto) 73%, white 16%, and black at 11% [13, 14].

The next most common group of Hispanics comes from Central and South America. They comprise 14.3% of the US Hispanic population [1]. In this group of nations, we find a very high percentage of mestizo or indigenous populations – indeed, many regions retain a strong Amerindian influence with some nations comprised of 90% mestizos [13]. However, South American includes a great variability of races and ethnicities. One can have indigenous populations of the Amazon basin and the Andes, as well as remnants of colonial regions with African slaves, as found in the Bahia area of Brazil. In the areas of Argentina, Chile, and Southern Brazil, the vast majority of the population is of European ancestry which arrived anywhere from 200 to less than 60 years ago. To elegantly summarize the above demographic data, the coming years will see the dermatologist treating more and more people of color in their practice and must be prepared.

Figure 19.1 shows the distribution of the Hispanic population in the USA with the majority of patients residing within a handful of regions. Certain urban populations have a large minority of Hispanics: Miami-Dade County, Florida (62.4%), Los Angeles, California (47.7%), Chicago, Illinois (26.0%), and New York City (16.7%) [5]. Most Hispanics are concentrated in these areas, but as the population continues to grow and job opportunities arise, more and more Hispanics will move to new areas of the USA.

It is noteworthy that of all immigrant populations, the Hispanic is the *least likely* to have health care coverage. As reported in by the US government in 2007, there was a noted discrepancy between the Hispanic population and the non-Hispanic population in health insurance coverage. Within the non-Hispanic population, 10.4% did not receive health insurance coverage; this is relatively low in comparison to 32.1% of the Hispanic population that did not receive coverage [6]. Lack of health insurance plays an enormous role in the treatment and methods we select for Hispanic patients. Despite this lack of insurance, the Hispanic population spends a substantial amount of money on products and procedures to improve their appearance and *youthfulness* and are considered brand loyal as a whole. According to the American Society of Plastic Surgeons, the number of patients who received

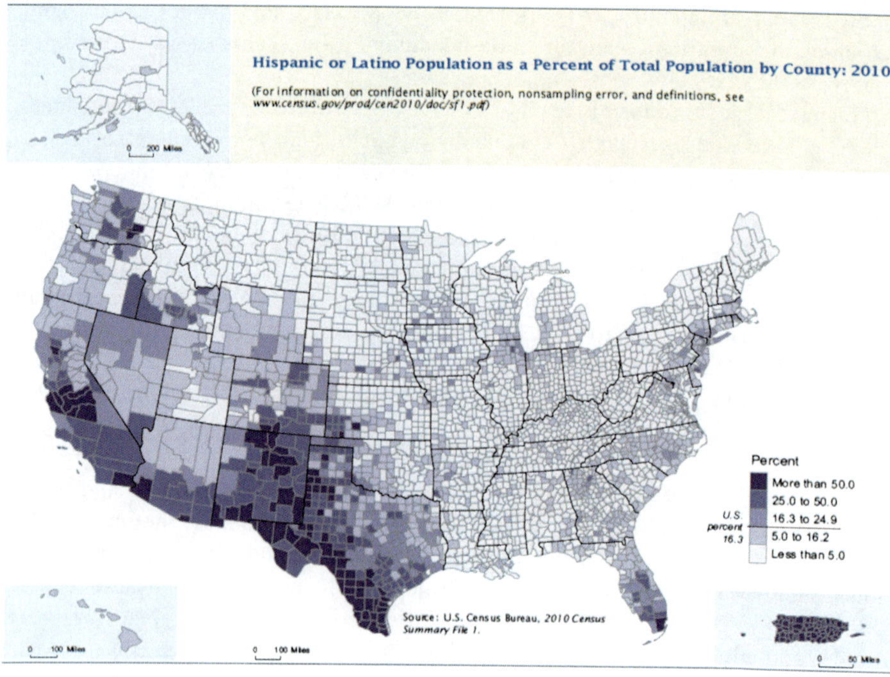


**Fig. 19.1** The Hispanic population in the USA is distributed throughout a handful of states with the majority of patients residing within the colored regions. (Source http://www.census.gov/prod/cen2010/briefs/c2010br-04.pdf)

cosmetic procedures declined 2% in 2008; however, the number of procedures among Hispanics increased by 18%. The average Hispanic female applies approximately four creams a day! This has enormous implications in clinical practices as it points to a greater than expected demand for cosmetic procedures and products.

As demographic changes occur in the USA and the Hispanic population continues to rise, physicians must be intimately aware of the differences among this minority population. By understanding the overt differences and subtle similarities within the Hispanic population, we will be able to more effectively treat and educate these patients and, therefore, be more able to improve their disease state. We know that patients are more at ease with their physician if they perceive the physician understands them well; thus, we will be more effective in treating their illness if we do. It is also well-known that the more culturally sensitive we are to our patients, the less of a chance there is for misinterpretation and discord. In turn, this significantly decreases the risk of a malpractice claim.

Before concluding, it must be said that this is an at-risk segment of society for various reasons. From a purely dermatologic perspective, many Hispanics view being healthy as being and looking clean; they engage excessive use of soaps, perfumes, colognes, and pomades damaging their skin through unnecessary cleansing or washing. As mentioned above, they tend to lack health and insurance and may arrive in the office with already advanced disease. A recent study found that diseases of the skin are common in Hispanic farm workers and that they are lacking in preventative education [15]. Moreover, the incidence of melanoma is on the rise in Hispanics, and education and screening are therefore sorely needed [14].

What we are seeing in the USA is a growing kaleidoscope of people that have been labeled Hispanic, yet phenotypically, they can be extremely diverse; in this case, one size does not truly fit all. Dermatologists must be able to understand these differences and respect the patient's preconceived identity. A critical challenge with treating Hispanic patients is reeducating the patient on dermatologic care given to them previously within the context of their culture. Of paramount concern is the reeducation of issues dealing with sun protection, skin malignancy, and aging. If population trends continue, all parameters show that Hispanic patients will make up a very large percentage of our patients – whether we are in Seattle, Washington, or Miami, Florida!

## References


1. Grace Flores-Hughes Interview – She Made 'Hispanic' Official, The Washington Post, July 26, 2009. http://www.washingtonpost.com/wp-dyn/content/article/2009/07/24/AR2009072402091.html.
2. Gibson C, Jung K. Historical census statistics on population totals by race, 1790 to 1990, and by Hispanic origin, 1970 to 1990, for the United States, regions, divisions, and states. Working paper series No. 56, 2002.
3. Office of Management and Budget. Revisions to the standards for the classification of federal data on race and ethnicity. Federal register notice 30 Oct 1997.
4. Grieco EM, Cassidy RC. Overview of race and Hispanic origin: 2000. United States Census Bureau.
5. Hispanic/Latina women: cultural norms and prevention. FADAA. http://www.fadaa.org/services/resource_center/resources/JTF/hispanic.asp. Accessed 24 May 2010.
6. Kemp C. Mexican & Mexican-Americans: health beliefs & practices. http://bearspace.baylor.edu/Charles_Kemp/www/hispanic_health.htm. Accessed 13 May 2010.
7. Molina,CW, Marilyn A, eds. Latino health in the US: a growing challenge. American public health association 1994;4:25–34.
8. Risser AL, Mazur LJ. Use of folk remedies in a Hispanic population. Arch Pediatr Adolesc Med. 1995;149(9):978–81.
9. Ramirez RR. We the people: Hispanics in the US, Census 2000, special report. US Census Bureau. Dec 2004.
10. World Bank, world development indicator 2010. Data from World Bank estimates from census reports.
11. U.S. Census Bureau, annual demographic supplement to the March 2002. Current population survey.
12. Pew Hispanic Center Tabulations of 2007 American Community Survey. Table 5. Detailed Hispanic Origin: 2007. http://pewhispanic.org/files/factsheets/hispanics2007/2007_Hispanic%20 Profile_Final.pdf.
13. Cuba. Puerto Rico. Dominican Republic. CIA world factbook. https://www.cia.gov/library/publications/the-world-factbook/fields/2075.html. Accessed 13 May 2010.
14. Ellis M. Melanoma incidence and survival rates vary among racial and ethnic groups. http://www.healthnews.com/medical-updates/melanoma-incidence-and-survival-rates-vary-among-racial-and-ethnic-groups-3989.html. Accessed 24 May 2010.
15. Wake Forest University Baptist Medical Center (2006, April 26). Skin disease common among hispanic farmworkers in North Carolina, research shows. Science Daily. http://www.sciencedaily.com/releases/2006/04/060426000625.htm. Accessed 18 May 2010.

# Chapter 20
# Dermatologic Disorders in Children of Color

**Nanette B. Silverberg**

## Pediatric Skin and Hair Disorders

Children of color constitute non-Caucasian children of various racial and ethnic backgrounds who have darker skin tones, including African American, Asian, Hispanic and Latino, and Middle Eastern extractions. Children of color come from a different genetic pool than Caucasian children and therefore have different biological responses [1].

Global immigration has been responsible for alterations in the demographics of skin of color in many locations. In Asia, the population is more homogeneous than in the United States, where the "melting pot" effect has brought broad shifts in skin disease. One such shift was the introduction of *Trichophyton tonsurans* into the United States by immigrant Hispanics, currently the major etiologic agent in cases of tinea capitis in both Caucasian and African American children. More recently, white piedra has been noted to be on the rise in the United States, again noted in immigrant children from both Middle Eastern and Mexican backgrounds. Another type of effect noted with immigration is that children of immigrants have an incidence of atopic dermatitis more closely resembling their new country than the country of parental origin.

This chapter provides an overview of pediatric dermatologic diseases as they pertain to skin of color. The first section looks at the development of skin and soft tissue structures in children of color, the second examines the presentation of common childhood diseases in children of color, and the third looks specifically at diseases genetically limited to children of color. Table 20.1 broadly reviews disorders with pigmentary alteration seen in children of color.

N.B. Silverberg, M.D. (✉)
Pediatric and Adolescent Dermatology, St. Luke's Roosevelt Hospital Center and Columbia University College of Physicians and Surgeons, New York, NY, USA
e-mail: nsilverberg@juno.com

A.F. Alexis and V.H. Barbosa (eds.), *Skin of Color: A Practical Guide to Dermatologic Diagnosis and Treatment*, DOI 10.1007/978-0-387-84929-4_20,

**Table 20.1** Common causes of pigmentary alterations in children of color

| | | | |
|---|---|---|---|
| Lesions < 6mm | | | |
| | Facial localization | | |
| | | Hyperpigmentation | |
| | | | Acne/postinflammatory pigmentary alteration |
| | | | Dermatosis papulosa nigra |
| | | | Eccentric tinea versicolor |
| | | | Seborrheic dermatitis |
| | | Hypopigmentation | |
| | | | Seborrheic dermatitis |
| | | | Tinea Versicolor (Eccentric location) |
| | | | Vitiligo |
| | Trunk | | |
| | | Hyperpigmentation | |
| | | | Acne/postinflammatory pigmentary alterations |
| | | | Eruptive vellus hair cysts (lightly palpable) |
| | | | Erythema dyschromicum perstans |
| | | | Lichen planus (usually raised and pruritic) |
| | | | Pityriasis rosea |
| | | | Syringomas (usually raised) |
| | | | Tinea versicolor |
| | | Hypopigmentation | |
| | | | Lichen sclerosus et atrophicus |
| | | | Tuberous sclerosis (confetti-like hypopigmentation) |
| | | | Vitiligo |
| Lesions > 6mm | | | |
| | Facial localization | | |
| | | Hyperpigmentation | |
| | | | Café au lait macules/ speckled lentiginous nevus |
| | | | Congenital melanocytic nevi |
| | | | Epidermal nevi |
| | | | Melasma |
| | | | Nevus of Ota |
| | | | Smooth muscle hamartomas |
| | | Hypopigmentation | |
| | | | Nevus depigmentosus |
| | | | Pityriasis alba |
| | | | Postinflammatory pigmentary alteration |
| | | | Vitiligo, including segmental |
| | Trunk | | |
| | | Hyperpigmentation | |
| | | | Becker's nevus |
| | | | Café au lait macule |
| | | | Erythema dyschromicum perstans |
| | | | Nevus of Ito |
| | | | Tinea versicolor |

(continued)

**Table 20.1** (continued)

| |
|---|
| Hypopigmentation |
| Hypomelanosis of Ito |
| Mycosis fungoides |
| Nevus depigmentosus |
| Pityriasis alba |
| Pityriasis lichenoides |
| Progressive macular hypomelanosis |
| Tinea versicolor |
| Vitiligo vulgaris |
| Generalized |
| Hyperpigmentation |
| Argyria |
| Bronze diabetes |
| Carotenemia |
| Medication-induced |
| Hypopigmentation |
| Albinism |
| Vitiligo vulgaris |

## Differences in Skin Development Noted in Skin of Color

Pigmentation in the skin begins in utero with the migration of melanocytes from week 8 through birth. Melanocytes originate in the neural crest and move from the ventral neural tube toward the dorsal surfaces overlying the abdomen and then downward over the extremities. These migration patterns are governed by genes such as the homeobox genes, which may be aberrant in disorders such as Waardenburg syndrome [2]. Dermal movement and migration of melanocytes are followed by late gestational movement upward into the epidermis. Melanocytes then integrate into the basal layer of the epidermis. Skin tone is created when melanosomes are transferred to the surrounding keratinocytes. Melanocyte quantity is essentially the same across all races and ethnicities; however, melanosome packaging and contents allow for functional or qualitative differences in skin tone and response to UV light. Melanosomes in darker-skinned children are larger in size with having larger packets of melanin in comparison to a Caucasian patient, who generally would have individual, small melanosomes [3]. Asians may have a mixture of clustered and individual melanosomes, a hybrid of Caucasian and Black melanosome distributions [3]. Larger melanosomes act as a large reservoir of color in darker children; these larger reservoirs can be easily disrupted causing epidermal or dermal pigmentary release or postinflammatory pigmentary alteration.

Melanocyte migration is rarely complete at birth. Even when complete, it is uncommon for mature melanosome production and transfer to be complete. In newborns of color, scrotal and labial pigmentation can be observed. Incidence of newborn scrotal pigmentation ranges from 31.3% of Asian [3] and a majority of Black male infants. Skin tone may not be fully established until the latter half of the first

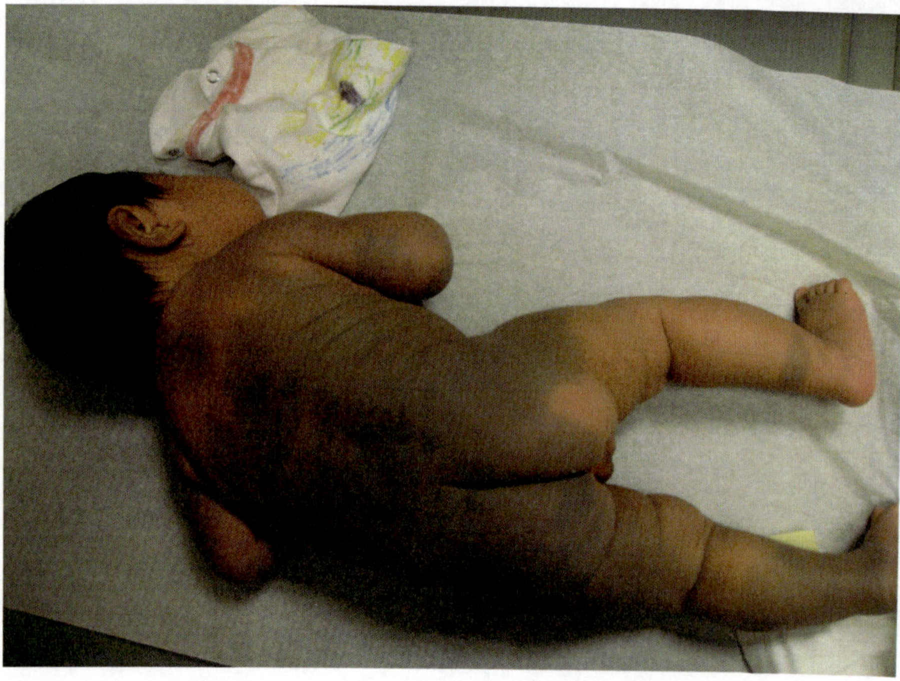

**Fig. 20.1** Mongolian spots

year of life [1]. Another illness noted in newborns of color is transient neonatal pustular melanosis. This benign disorder is present at birth and can affect any part of the body. The lesions progress from small pustules full of neutrophils to small collarettes of scale around hyperpigmented macules. Hyperpigmentation can take weeks to months to resolve but requires no therapy.

When melanocytes have not completely migrated into the epidermis, they reflect a blue color, i.e., the Tyndall effect, referred to as a Mongolian spot (Fig. 20.1). Mongolian spots are noted in most Black children (96%) and in a large proportion of Hispanic (46%) and Asian children (83.6%) [4, 5]. The sacral spine is the most common location in all skin tones; however, eccentric Mongolian spots are often noted over the hip and shoulder girdles in Black children [1]. Resolution of Mongolian spots is usual by the end of the first year of life. Resolution is nearly universal by age 6 years. Nonresolving congenital blue skin pigmentation, i.e., dermal melanocytosis, is referred to as nevus of Ota on the face (V1, V2) or on the chin (V3), neck, shoulders or upper chest, nevus of Ito. Typically, nevus of Ota will have ocular involvement with or without a blue discoloration of the sclera. Dermal melanocytosis may be treated with a Nd:YAG 1,064-nm laser [1, 6].

Melanocytes can also be found in the oral mucosa, hair bulbs, and nail beds. Melanocytes may form benign localized pockets of pigment referred to as orolabial melanotic macules [7]. Linear pigmentation of the nail bed is termed melanonychia striata and can be caused by medications, trauma, irritation or idiopathic [8].

While pigmentation has global in utero genetic influences, localized genetic alterations in pigment production occur as postzygotic changes. These can generate localized hyper- or hypopigmented macules and patches. Ovoid patches following embryological lines of development are referred to as café au lait or nevus depigmentosus. Linear pigmentation along these embryological lines is globally termed pigmentary mosaicism. Many children of color will have a single area of pigmentary alteration. Multiple areas of pigmentary alteration require genetic work-up for genetic and/or chromosomal abnormalities, including neurofibromatosis (multiple café au lait), hypomelanosis of Ito (hypopigmented pigmentary mosaicism involving multiple segments of the skin), or tuberous sclerosis (ash leaf macules, confetti- and thumbprint-like hypopigmentation) [1, 9].

In patients of color, an enhancement of the pigmentary differences between the ventral and dorsal surfaces of the arms may be noted, termed Voight's or Futcher's lines. Other benign pigmentations include the linea alba noted as a central area of lighter pigmentation over the lower chest and abdomen [10].

## Common Pediatric Diseases in Children of Color

The most common disorder seen in a pediatric dermatology clinic dealing with patients of any color is atopic dermatitis (AD) [11]. AD is best diagnosed by the presence of a recurrent pruritic eruption in typical distribution, with family history of atopy in the majority of cases; however, formal diagnosis can be made using the criteria of Hanifin and Rajka (Table 20.2). Seventy percent of children with AD have a family history of atopy [12]. For infants, typical distribution is on the face, especially the cheeks, and the extensor surfaces of the extremities, while school-age children are affected by flexural dermatitis of the neck, antecubital, and popliteal regions. Teenagers and adults may find hand dermatitis, typified by hyperkeratotic, erythematous plaques with overlying small papules along the finger margins, to be the remnant of an atopic tendency. AD is the cutaneous form of atopic disease, which also includes asthma, seasonal allergies, and food allergies.

Atopic dermatitis certainly seems more common and more severe in children of color. Patients of color from a Caribbean background are at twice the risk of developing atopic dermatitis than Caucasian London-born children [13]. In addition, atopic dermatitis in Black children is six times more likely to be rated as "severe" than in white children in the United Kingdom [14].

Certain features of AD are altered in children of color. Facial atopic dermatitis is particularly intractable and severe in Asian infants and young children. In all darker patients, erythema can be masked by pigmentation, and this may cause an artificial reduction in severity scores of atopic dermatitis in children of color [11]. Postinflammatory pigmentary alterations, especially hypopigmentation, are more common in infants of color but can be seen in any age group [8]. Follicular eczema is a form of atopic dermatitis manifested by truncal follicular prominence. Despite the lack of lichenification and erythema in this variant, pruritus can be quite severe.

**Table 20.2** The criteria for atopic dermatitis

| |
|---|
| *Diagnosis requires three major criteria and three minor criteria:* |
| Major criteria: |
| Pruritus |
| Dermatitis affecting the flexural surfaces in adults and the face or extensors in infants |
| Chronic or relapsing dermatitis |
| Personal or family history of cutaneous or respiratory atopy |
| Minor criteria: |
| Early age of onset |
| Keratosis pilaris |
| Ichthyosis |
| Hyperlinear palms |
| Dry skin |
| Hand and foot dermatitis |
| Perifollicular accentuation |
| Circumoral pallor |
| Facial hypopigmentation |
| Cheilitis |
| Infraorbital darkening |
| Infraorbital folds (Dennie-Morgan lines) |
| Recurrent conjunctivitis |
| Anterior neck folds |
| Nipple eczema |
| Triggers including foods, emotional factors, environmental factors, and irritants (e.g., wool, solvents, sweat) |
| Susceptibility to cutaneous viral and bacterial infections |
| Impaired cell-mediated immunity |
| Immediate skin-test reactivity |
| White dermographism |
| Raised serum IgE |
| Keratoconus |
| Anterior subcapsular cataracts |

Adapted from Hanifin JM, Rajka G. Diagnostic features of atopic dermatitis. Acta Derm Venereol (Stockh) 1980;92 (Suppl.):44–7; and Rothe MJ, Grant-Kels JM. Diagnostic criteria for atopic dermatitis. Lancet 1996;348:769–770

Lichenification of the dorsal hands and ankles is generally prominent in severe disease in patients of color (Fig. 20.2). Pityriasis alba, manifesting as asymptomatic areas of annular hypopigmentation that do not highlight with Wood's lamp, is a minor criterion of AD. Pityriasis alba is more obvious in populations of color. Other facial stigmata of atopic dermatitis are more commonly noted in children of color, particularly in Black and Hispanic children. This includes Dennie-Morgan folds under the eyes (Fig. 20.3), which are common in children of color even in the absence of atopic dermatitis (49% of Black children vs. 25% of Caucasian children without atopic dermatitis) [15], circumoral pallor, and the "allergic salute" (a prominent ridge over the nasal bridge caused by the upward movement of the hand against the nose due to nasal pruritus seen in children with allergic rhinoconjunctivitis, i.e., the saluting posture), which can be very dark in Black children.

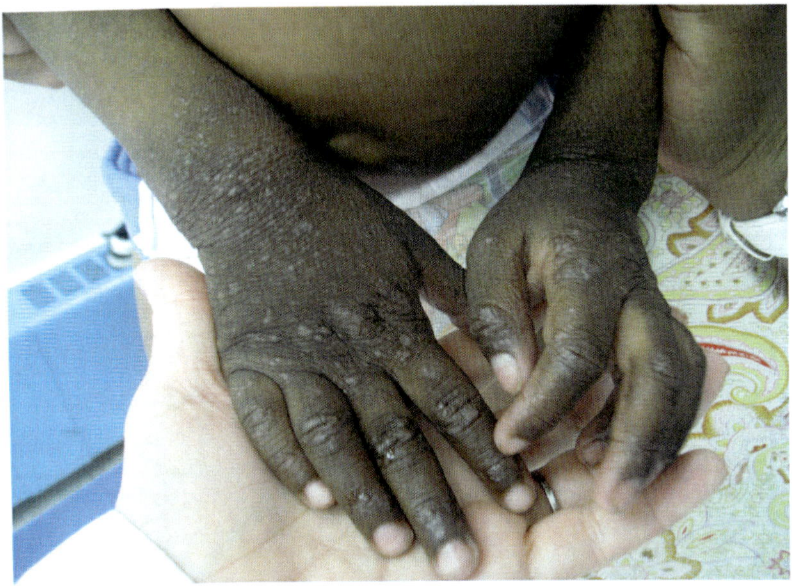

**Fig. 20.2** Lichenification and lichenoid atopic dermatitis lesions in a Black toddler

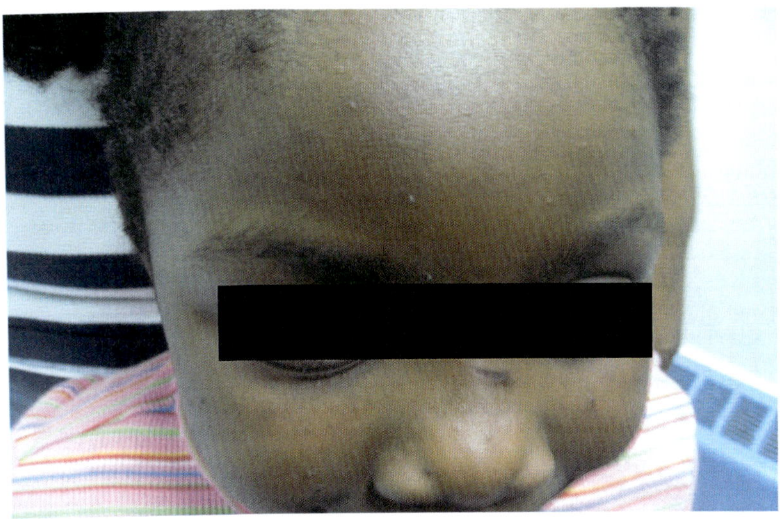

**Fig. 20.3** Dennie-Morgan folds in a patient with atopic dermatitis and allergic salute

Treatment of atopic dermatitis in children of color is very similar to the standard principles of therapy; however, the overrepresentation of moderate to severe disease in children of color often requires prolonged or alternative therapies.

General recommendations for skin care of atopic dermatitis in children of color are summarized in Table 20.3. Notably, certain differences in pigmentation need to be addressed in children of color with AD. First, patients and parents should be made

**Table 20.3** Skin care of children of color with atopic dermatitis[a]

| |
|---|
| **Bathing modification** |
| Fragrance-free, gentle cleansers |
| Syndets and fragrance-free soaps mixed with emollients |
| Gentle bathing |
| Bathtub soaks when skin disease is active |
| Limit bathing to 15 min or less |
| Avoid very hot bathwater |
| Bath additives |
| Addition of oils or oatmeal to the bath for rapid relief of pruritus |
| Addition of bleach (see header on recurrent bacterial superinfection of atopic dermatitis) |
| **Moisturization and barrier repair** |
| Lotions for summer |
| Creams and petrolatum products for winter |
| Patients from the near East and Middle East may have preference for oil-based emollients |
| Topical "devices," i.e., emollients with anti-inflammatory additives |
| To be used adjunctively to other topical agents to reduce the need for topical corticosteroids |
| **Lifestyle alteration** |
| Soft fabrics, especially cotton |
| Detergents without added fragrance or dyes |
| Reduce allergen exposure in individuals with proven allergic diathesis, e.g., dust mite allergy |
| **Topical medicaments** |
| Topical corticosteroids |
| Low potency (class 5–7) for facial and intertriginous lesions |
| Mid-potency products applied after bath for moderate to severe disease |
| Soak and slather techniques – generalized application after bath for extensive body surface areas |
| Topical calcineurin inhibitors[a] for topical corticosteroid failures; intertriginous, genital, or facial disease; and/or pityriasis alba |
| Pimecrolimus 1% cream for mild to moderate atopic dermatitis, ages 2 years and over |
| Tacrolimus 0.03% ointment for moderate to severe atopic dermatitis ages 2–15 years |
| Tacrolimus 0.1% ointment for moderate to severe atopic dermatitis ages 16 and older or for children of color who have fair but incomplete response to 0.03% ointment |
| **Pruritus care/relief of sleep disturbance** |
| Oral antihistamines at bedtime |
| Wet pajamas covered by dry pajamas |
| Silver-impregnated silk pajamas |
| **Therapy of severe or recalcitrant atopic dermatitis** (for large body surface area, erythroderma, and/ or intractable symptomatology) |
| Oral immunosuppressants (all require screening blood counts, chemistries, and liver function testing) |
| Cyclosporine A |
| Requires monitoring of blood pressure and renal function Mycophenelate Mofitil |
| Methotrexate |

(continued)

**Table 20.3** (continued)

| |
|---|
| Ultraviolet light therapy (not for patients with lupus or other forms of photosensitivity) |
| Narrowband UVB |
| Generalized (for extensive disease) |
| Hand-foot unit (for palmoplantar disease) |
| **Special situations** |
| Recurrent bacterial superinfection of atopic dermatitis |
| Oral antibiotics 1–2 weeks |
| Mupirocin for the 3 N's: nares, navel, and nails (optional: anus) |
| Bleach bathes |
| Household usage of ethyl alcohol handrubs |
| Culture and treat household *Staph* carriers |
| Food allergies |
| Avoidance of the allergen both as an ingested food and in topical preparations |
| When suspected in early infancy, empiric shifting of formula from milk or soy-based to alimental formulations may be needed |
| Prescribe epinephrine autoinjector for anaphylactic reactions (weight-based dosing) |
| Refer for allergy testing for high body surface areas, intractable disease, and history of allergic-type symptoms with food ingestion |
| Wintertime |
| Vitamin D supplementation, 400 IU |
| Cool-mist humidifier |

[a] Topical calcineurin inhibitors have a black-box warning on their label that states they are not for children under the age of 2 years, and they may be linked to lymphomas or skin cancers

Modified from [1] with permission

aware that pigmentary alterations are common as a result of the illness, and, second, that these are not caused by therapy but rather prevented by early institution of therapy [16]. Another issue in children of color is the higher rate of xerosis, requiring ointment medicaments and petrolatum-based products in most cases. Additionally, it has been noted that African American children, ages 2–15 years, may require tacrolimus 0.1% ointment, rather than 0.03% ointment, in order to achieve therapeutic response; despite this, usage of tacrolimus 0.03% ointment is the first-line tacrolimus prescription in this age group. Furthermore, the entity of follicular eczema is deceptive. Though it looks mild due to the lesions being nearly flush with the skin surface, the level of pruritus associated is often severe, and the therapy requires mid-potency topical corticosteroids. In the case of pityriasis alba, both low-potency topical corticosteroids and pimecrolimus have been reported to be effective in open-label nonrandomized trial, however, only topical tacrolimus twice daily (6–9 weeks) has been demonstrated to be superior to placebo for clearance of pityriasis alba lesions [17]. One special location of atopic dermatitis, the scalp, is very tricky. The background incidence of tinea capitis and seborrheic dermatitis and the close clinical mimicry make diagnostic separation difficult. The differential diagnosis of scalp atopic dermatitis is listed in Table 20.4 with comparative features used to differentiate each illness.

**Table 20.4** The differential diagnosis of atopic dermatitis of the scalp with comparative features

| Diagnosis | Morphology of lesions | Onset | Diagnostic laboratory testing | In-office testing |
|---|---|---|---|---|
| Atopic dermatitis | Erythema and fine scale, often nuchal localization, no lymphadenopathy | 90% by 5 years of age | Biopsy for H&E<br>Rule out tinea capitis by fungal culture | Potassium hydroxide preparation to rule out Tinea capitis |
| Seborrheic dermatitis | Erythema and hyperkeratosis, infants with thick yellow-brown hyperkeratosis (i.e., cradle cap) | Infantile and pubescent | Rule out tinea capitis by fungal culture | Potassium hydroxide preparation to rule out Tinea capitis |
| Psoriasis | Erythematous plaques with micaceous scale, rare tinea amiantacea with thick hyperkeratosis stuck to hair shafts | Any age | Biopsy can be performed in cases not able to be diagnosed clinically | Potassium hydroxide preparation to rule out Tinea capitis |
| Tinea capitis | Diffuse fine scale, thick hyperkeratosis with or without alopecia, often black dot type; inflammatory type with boggy erythematous plaques, pustules | School-aged children | Fungal culture is most definitive | Potassium hydroxide preparation to rule out Tinea capitis |
| White piedra | White concretions attached to the hairs with or without fine scalp hyperkeratosis | School-aged children on scalp<br>Adults with sexual transmission in groin | Fungal culture is definitive | Potassium hydroxide demonstrates concretions of spores around the hairs |
| | Excoriated erythematous papules of the scalp, especially nuchal | School-aged children with straight hair | Live louses may be observed or more commonly residual ova or nits | Wet prep of hairs |
| Lice | White concretions that can be sheared off of hairs | | | Potassium hydroxide preparation to rule out Tinea capitis |

## Seborrheic Dermatitis

Seborrheic dermatitis is an immunological response to normal or excess levels of natural yeast species (*Malassezia*) present at the surface of the sebaceous hair follicle. While common in all infants and teenagers, seborrheic dermatitis has specific nuances in children of color. In infancy, seborrheic dermatitis manifests with erythema and hyperkeratosis of the scalp. Greasy erythematous plaques of the face and intertriginous skin are noted. Lesions generally fade off after early infancy. In infants, seborrhea is of concern in darker skin tones due to extensive pigmentary alteration of the facial and intertriginous skin. In preschoolers, seborrheic dermatitis resembles tinea capitis. School-age children with seborrhea warrant fungal cultures of the scalp to determine etiology of scalp hyperkeratosis [18]. Teenagers with seborrheic dermatitis generally have disease limited to the scalp. However, eyebrow, perinasal, and petaloid lesions of the face can be observed. These lesions can leave significant postinflammatory pigmentary changes. Therapy includes usage of selenium sulfide shampoos, low-potency topical corticosteroids, and antifungal creams and shampoos [19]. Usage of pimecrolimus for facial-hypopigmented seborrheic dermatitis in adult Black Americans has demonstrated good results within 2 weeks, but usage in childhood has not been described, and usage for infants is not recommended [20].

### *Pityriasis Rosea*

Pityriasis rosea, a common disorder of childhood, is a papulosquamous disorder in which lesions begin with a single relatively large herald patch on the trunk or proximal extremities, followed by smaller lesions in a Christmas tree pattern over the trunk and back. While traditional appearance of salmon-colored plaques with collarettes of scale is described in textbooks, skin of color patients typically have dark brown to violaceous plaques with a collarette of scale. Other features that differ from the traditional appearance of pityriasis rosea in Caucasians are unusual or "atypical" distribution or type of lesions; in Black American children, sites include the face in 30% and scalp in 8% of children. One-third of Black American children had papular lesions. Appearance and clearance are often within 2 weeks; however, postinflammatory hyperpigmentation is seen in 48% of Black children at 4 weeks, and hypopigmentation can be seen in 29% with purely papular lesions. Postinflammatory pigmentary changes can persist far beyond 6 weeks in patients of color. Therapy includes topical corticosteroids and oral antihistamines as needed for reduction of pruritus. However, there is no published data on whether postinflammatory changes are minimized with this therapy [21]. Narrowband UVB can be used for prolonged disease course and to promote repigmentation in the setting of postinflammatory hypopigmentation. Oral erythromycin has been found to be ineffective in a trial of 184 Iranian children and adults in a head-to-head a trial of four times daily erythromycin for up to 8 weeks vs. placebo cream [22].

## Nickel Allergic Contact Dermatitis

Nickel allergy is no more common in patients of color than in the rest of the population; however, chronic and severe nickel allergy in the United States has been reported to occur predominantly in children of color in some studies [22], while another study in a predominantly Caucasian populus demonstrated 11% of children with patch test proven nickel allergy were African American [21]. Lesions are generally a result of style-related wearing of nickel-laden jeans and belt buckles, which result in progressive intensification of cutaneous allergy and often a widespread id reaction. Typical locations of skin lesions are in the infraumbilical and periumbilical regions, where very lichenified plaques are noted [23]. Extensor surface papules overlying the elbows and knees are id reaction associated with the allergy [24]. Newer reported sources of nickel exposure include cell phones which can lead to facial contact dermatitis [25]. Complete removal of nickel-laden clothes and accessories from the wardrobe is generally curative. Dimethylglyoxime test kits can also be purchased to test clothing and accessories for nickel content. In addition, dietary modifications, such as avoiding canned foods, to reduce oral ingestion, may enhance long-term clearance of nickel contact symptoms. Topical corticosteroids of mid to high potency and topical calcineurin inhibitors can be used to clear lesions of contact dermatitis and are superior to emollients alone [26].

## Psoriasis

Psoriasis affects 2.5% of the Caucasian American population and 1.3% of the African American population [27]. Despite the reduced prevalence in darkly pigmented patients, symptomatology including pigmentary alterations including the hypopigmented Woronoff's rings that sometimes surround plaques of psoriasis and postinflammatory hyperpigmentation may be more visible in patients of color. Micaceous scale is often noted, especially on the scalp, and tinea capitis should be excluded prior to therapy of scalp psoriasis in children of color. On the body and extremities, inflammation can occasionally appear violaceous, mimicking lichen planus. Therapy of psoriasis vulgaris of childhood includes usage of keratolytic emollients to remove hyperkeratosis, topical corticosteroids of mid-potency (with or without calcipotriene), calcipotriene, and for extensive body surface area of disease – methotrexate and etanercept (off-label) [28]. One common problem in children of color is the difficulty of using shampoo-based formulations on the scalp, due to drying of hairs with frequent shampooing. Consequently leave-in oil-based topical fluocinonide has been a helpful adjunct to hydrating the hair while softening the hyperkeratosis [29].

## Confluent and Reticulated Papillomatosis of Gougerot and Carteaud

Confluent and reticulated papillomatosis of Gougerot and Carteaud is a velvety reticulate pigmentation with central chest confluence, generally affecting the trunk, and most cosmetically obvious in patients of color due to increased pigmentation. Recently, linkage to *Dietzia papillomatosis*, an *Actinomycete* species overgrowth [30] and associatied disorder of cornification induced by this overgrowth, has prevailed as the pathogenesis; however, in the past pityrosporum overgrowth has been suspected as well. Treatment does not vary from skin of color to Caucasian patients. Topical calcipotriene twice daily in combination with topical ammonium lactate 12% lotion can be used to clear lesions over a few months in teenagers and young adults of color [31]. Oral minocycline and, anecdotally, doxycycline (Riaux A) are effective therapies [32], but isotretinoin has been described as well [33].

## Follicular Disorders

Disorders of the follicular unit are more prevalent in children of color [8]. Hairs in Black and some Hispanic children are elliptical on cross section and spiral on light microscopy due to a curved hair follicle. The shape of the hair prevents sebum from moving along the shaft, making hairs dryer and requiring less frequent washing than Caucasian hair and more usage of pomades. Asian hair shafts are round on cross section and are not as susceptible to traction as the hair of Black children. The follicular diseases of children of color vary from susceptibility to traction-induced hair loss [34, 35] to a greater degree of hypertrichosis in renal transplant patients of color placed on oral cyclosporine American [36] to acneiform diseases induced by hair removal. Notable upper lip hair is more common in Black female adolescents 2 years after menarche than in Caucasian patients but may ameliorate with age [37].

Traction alopecia (Fig. 20.4) in childhood is a form of hair loss noted primarily at the frontal hairline which is the result of tightly pulled hairstyles. The rudiments of chronic alopecia in adulthood can begin in children by hairstyles that involve tight traction, thermal straightening, hair extensions that are glued on or sewn-in, and chemical straightening in Black patients, especially in Black teenage girls. For a more in-depth review of follicular damage and degeneration in patients of color, please see Chap. 21. Individuals with traction-related hair loss should avoid frequent hair processing and traction. Therapeutic interventions that may aid in hair regrowth or slow hair loss include topical and injectable corticosteroids, oral antibiotics or immunosuppressives, and/or topical minoxidil [38].

Trichorrhexis nodosa can be an acquired form of hair fragility in Black children due to thermal and/or chemical straightening techniques or prolonged helmet wear. Clinically, hair appears lusterless and white beading can be noted. Avoidance of traction processing and occlusion may reverse acquired disease [39].

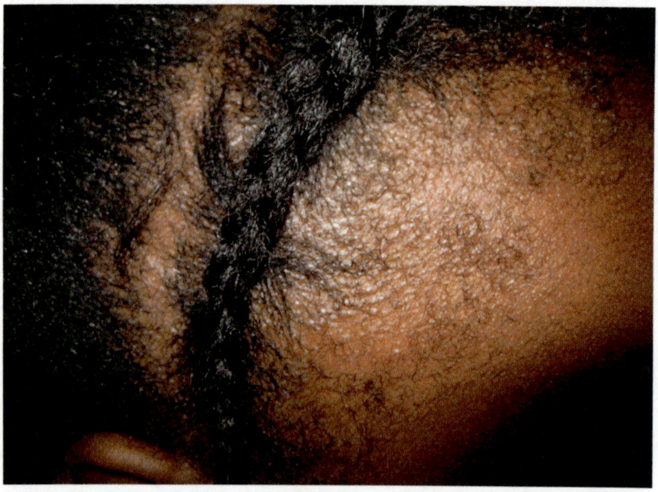

**Fig. 20.4** Traction alopecia of the scalp secondary to chronic tight braiding (Permission from Figure 20.4 which is figure 11.8 in Silverberg Atlas of Pediatric Cutaneous Biodiversity)

Acneiform disorders are another common form of follicular disease in pediatric patients of color. Acne vulgaris is a common disorder of adolescents of all ethnicities. Pomade acne in patients of color is a form of acne in the scalp, face, and neck areas marginal to the scalp induced by usage of thick pomades to hydrate dry hair shafts [40]. Postinflammatory changes after can to acne lesions heal, which can be worsened by picking, are noted more frequently in patients of color and are often a significant complaint long after acne has cleared. Therapies and skin care advice for acne vulgaris in children of color are summarized in Table 20.5. Of note, usage of retinoids, azelaic acid, and sun protection can aid in resolution of hyperpigmentation along with judicious usage of hydroquinones [4, 8, 41]. Pseudofolliculitis barbae is a form of inflammatory acne induced by shaving or plucking hairs in Black patients, both male and female. Polymorphisms of the gene for hair keratin 6 have been noted in susceptible individuals. Topical acne therapy, clipping rather than shaving, and, in specific situations, hair removal laser can be used to alleviate symptomatology [42]. Acne keloidalis nuchae is a disorder of the hair follicle of the nuchal scalp that is associated with posthaircut papule formation, followed by keloidal scar formation (Fig. 20.5) [25]. Reduction in skin lesions and prevention of scarring require a combination of avoidance of shaving of the nuchal scalp and therapies including topical acne therapy, oral antibiotics in severe cases, corticosteroid injections for keloidal lesions and scars, and excision of persistent scars [3]. One treatment pearl in the therapy of PFB and AKN of childhood is that prior to age 9 years oral erythromycin is the antibiotic of choice; oral tetracyclines can only be prescribed for children ages 9 years or older [3]. The readers are referred to Chap. 2 for further details on the therapy of acneiform disorders.

Periorificial (perioral) dermatitis is a rosacea-like inflammatory disorder of the hair follicles of the face in which monomorphic papules form periorificially around the eyes, nose, and lips. Topical corticosteroid usage can induce onset of lesions.

**Table 20.5** Therapy of acne in children of color

- Education
  - Dietary education
    - Low-glycemic index diet
    - Avoidance of dairy
  - Avoidance of comedogenic agents
    - No thick pomades including cocoa butter, petrolatum, and unrefined mineral oil products on the face or anterior scalp/hair
  - Sunscreen usage
    - To reduce postinflammatory changes
    - To counteract drug-induced dryness or photosensitivity
  - Avoidance of products recommended by nonprofessionals
    - E.g., toothpaste and baking soda, as these enhance dyspigmentation
- Medications
  - Topical medicaments (mechanism of activity)
  - Salicylic acid (0.5–2%) (comedolytic, enhances normal pigmentation)
  - Benzoyl peroxide (antibacterial for *P. acnes* by a nonantibiotic mechanism of killing and reduces risk of oral and topical antibiotic resistance)
  - Topical erythromycin or clindamycin (anti-inflammatory, enhances clearance when used with benzoyl peroxide. N.B. Combination products often look white on dark patients and should be prescribed for after-school usage or at bedtime.)
  - Topical dapsone (anti-inflammatory agent, a nonantibiotic mechanism data for age 12 and over)
  - Topical azelaic acid (comedolytic, antibacterial, reduces hyperpigmentation)
  - Topical retinoids, e.g., tretinoin, adapalene, and tazarotene (comedolytic, anti-inflammatory)
  - Oral medications (mechanism/ side effects)
    - Subantimicrobial doxycycline (anti-inflammatory mechanism/less gastrointestinal and phototoxicity side effects than full dosage)
    - Oral tetracyclines, e.g., minocycline, doxycycline, and tetracycline (anti-inflammatory/newer formulations with slow-release capsules can be given once daily, improving compliance and reducing risk of stomach upset and headaches/dizziness seen with minocycline; not for usage for ages under 9 years secondary to effects on dentition)
    - Oral erythromycin (anti-inflammatory/reserved for oral usage in patients age 8 or under, or for tetracycline allergic individuals; stomach upset is not uncommon on this medication, and some formulations can cause chemical hepatitis)
    - Oral trimethoprim-sulfamethoxazole or amoxicillin (anti-inflammatory and antibacterial; reserved for patient with severe facial pustules who have cultures demonstrating gram-negative bacteria, i.e., comorbid gram-negative folliculitis due to risks of allergy and severe drug reactions including toxic epidermal necrolysis as seen with trimethoprim-sulfamethoxazole)
    - Oral isotretinoin (anti-inflammatory, comedolytic, and reduces sebum production, all of which contribute to less bacterial overgrowth; drug is heavily regulated due to teratogenicity and reports of suicidality on the drug. Usage is limited to scarring acne or acne unresponsive to multiple courses (2+) of oral antibiotics)
    - Oral zinc supplementation has been described to reduce resistance to antibiotic agents
  - Cosmetic interventions
    - Topical agents
      - Topical soybean trypsin inhibitor, contained in sunscreens reduces appearance of facial dyspigmentation
      - Hydroquinones over the counter and prescription reduce appearance of hyperpigmentation
    - Procedures
      - Chemical peels using glycolic acid or salicylic acid can be performed safely if concentrations and times of exposure are increased gradually and conservatively; usage of hydroquinones in advance of the procedure reduces risk of adverse pigmentary changes
      - Microdermabrasion can be used at lower settings on patients of all ages and skin types to enhance clearance of dyspigmentation
      - Fraxel laser has been used in patients of color for reduction of dyspigmentation and acne scars
      - Avoid dermabrasion, $CO_2$ laser, and photodynamic therapy in patients of color as modalities of acne therapy

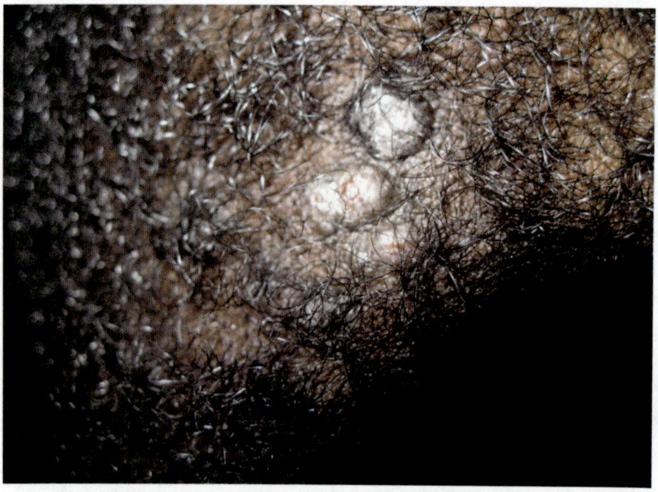

**Fig. 20.5** Acne keloidalis nuchae in a 15-year-old after a short haircut (Permission from figure 20.5 from Silverberg Atlas of pediatric Cutaneous Biodiversity Figure 2.28)

A similar, if not identical, disorder of Black children has been termed FACE – facial Afro-Caribbean eruption [43]. Clearance of lesions can be achieved with topical metronidazole or oral antibiotics, especially erythromycin. Removal of precipitants and revision of skin care regimens to usage of noncomedogenic products are beneficial in prevention of new lesions [44].

Scars are common in patients of color, especially adolescents and adults of Asian, Hispanic, and African descent. Temporary scarring such as hyperpigmentation or hypopigmentation is common after injury and arthropod bites in children of color. Follicular ice-pick scarring and keloidal scars after acne can be noted. Keloid formation over the upper chest, at sites of recent ear piercing, and after surgery or trauma can be noted. Onset after puberty is usual, but prepubertal keloids do occur. Family history of keloids is not uncommon in patients with keloids. Intralesional triamcinolone and topical silicone gel sheeting [8] can be used to reduce keloid size. Shave excision of earlobe keloids paired with postoperative intralesional kenalog injections can be performed in teenagers. In needle-phobic children, usage of corticosteroid impregnated tape overlying keloids can be beneficial at reducing lesion size and pruritus. Keloid-prone children should avoid trauma to the skin where possible, including piercings, tattooing, and elective surgeries [45].

Infections of the hair follicle include dermatophyte infection, causing tinea capitis and superficial yeast overgrowth with *Malassezia* species, which causes tinea versicolor, the former a disease of school-aged children and the latter a disease of adolescence.

Tinea capitis is an infection of the hair follicle, the perifollicular skin, and the hairs, caused in the United States mostly by *Trichophyton tonsurans*, an endothrix infection that does not fluoresce with Wood's lamp. Tinea capitis is common in all demographic groups but is most common in children of color, representing the

**Table 20.6** Dosing and duration of oral antifungals for tinea capitis

| | |
|---|---|
| Griseofulvin (125 mg/5ml micronized suspension, 125- or 250-mg tab ultramicronized scored tablets) | |
| 20–25 mg/kg/day suspension with fatty foods for 6–8 weeks | |
| Children weighing 35–60 pounds – 125-mg tab to 187.5 mg daily | |
| Pediatric patients weighing over 60 pounds – 187.5 to 375 mg daily | |
| Children and infants 2 years of age and younger – dosage has not been established 6–8 weeks | |
| Terbinafine sprinkles[a] | |
| <25 kg | 125 mg/day for 6 weeks |
| 25–35 kg | 187.5 mg/day for 6 weeks |
| 35 kg | 250 mg/day for 6 weeks |

[a]Sprinkle each packet on soft nonacidic food and eat without chewing
Diflucan (10, 40mg/1ml, or 200-mg tabs) 6–9mg/kg per day for 3–6 weeks
Modified from [1], with permission

second most common skin disease in a London-based pediatric dermatology clinic survey [9]. Noninflammatory tinea in the United States is called black dot tinea, primarily due to the fact that Black children with black hairs are the major group affected by tinea capitis [46, 47]. Hair care practices such as shared combs and brushes, shared pillows, and household contact are the leading source of contagion [48]. Adults in the same household can become infected [49], but children seem to be the main group infected. Oral griseofulvin remains the gold standard of therapy and is dosed at 20–25 mg/kg/day [50]. Terbinafine is approved for tinea capitis in the United States as a granule formulation, sprinkled on food once daily for 6 weeks. Dosing of oral antifungals for tinea capitis is reviewed in Table 20.6. Topical antifungal shampoos can be used to reduce contagion and aid in lesional clearance [32, 51].

Tinea versicolor is a *Malassezia* species overgrowth of the superficial follicle. The yeast releases azelaic acid, causing localized hypopigmentation and also causes inflammation which may alternatively produce hyperpigmentation. Although the illness is common to all skin tones and ethnicities after onset of puberty, pigmentary disturbances initiated by the illness are clearly more cosmetically noticeable in patients of color and may recur a few times per year, exacerbating cosmetic defects [52].

## *Pigmentary Disorders*

Disorders of pigmentation and pigment cells have nuances in patients of color. Vitiligo affects 0.4–1% of the worldwide population causing depigmentation that is either localized or generalized. Localized disease of childhood is often linear, affecting a segment of Blaschko. Generalized disease is either intertriginous, acrofacial, or universal, the latter being very rare. A genetic association with the NALP1 gene has been seen in Caucasian patients, but an association with the same gene has not yet been shown in patients of color [53]. Due to the extensive color differential between dark skin and depigmentation, cosmetic defects are very prominent in patients of color. Repigmentation can be effected with topical corticosteroids with

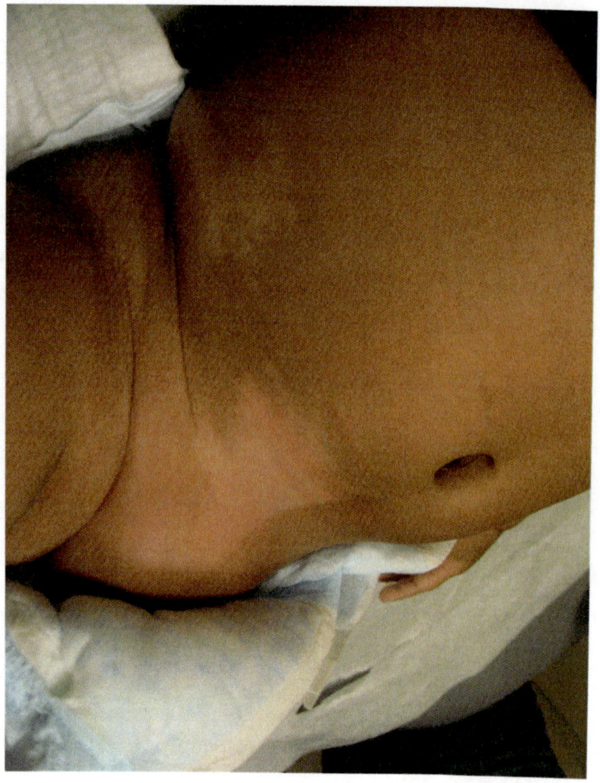

**Fig. 20.6** Nevus depigmentosus of the lower abdomen in an otherwise healthy Hispanic child

or without calcipotriene, topical calcineurin inhibitors, phototherapy using PUVA or narrowband UVB, or through excimer laser therapy. Grafting techniques using melanocyte suspensions or skin grafts can be attempted in medical therapy-resistant cases [54]. Thyroid screening is needed in children with generalized disease but not with segmental vitiligo [55].

Erythema dyschromicum perstans (EDP), otherwise known as ashy dermatosis, is a chronic pigmentary disorder in which gray macules, rarely preceded by inflammatory symptoms, spread across the trunk. This disease can be induced by drug ingestion or allergic contact allergy. Melanophages (macrophages laden with pigment granules) will be demonstrated on histology. Spontaneous remission is common in prepubertal children. Clofazimine has been reported to be effective in adults with EDP [56, 57].

Nevoid pigmentation is common in individuals of all skin tones. The distribution of pigmentation can be along the lines of Blaschko or in annular distribution as either café au lait spots or nevus depigmentosus, which is actually a localized area of hypo-rather than depigmentation. Nevus depigmentosus can be seen in 0.4% of Asian children; the incidence in other pigmented skin types is unknown (Fig. 20.6) [58]. Other forms of benign pigmentation include pigmentation of the sclera, oral and/or genital mucosal skin, and nails (melanonychia striata). Trauma can induce melanonychia

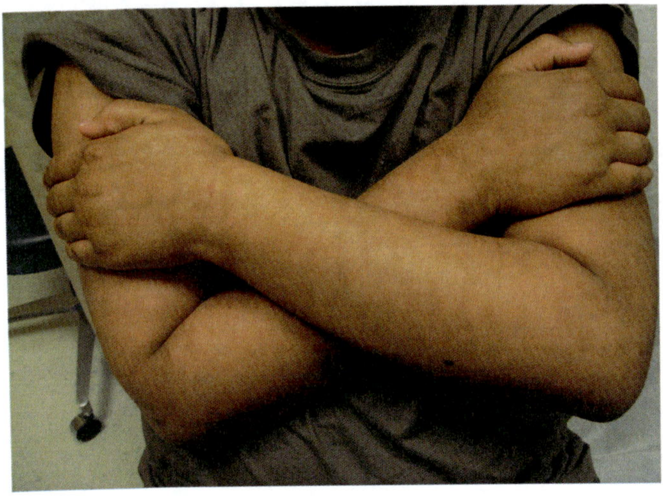

**Fig. 20.7** Pityriasis lichenoides in a 9 year-old Hispanic boy (Permission from Silverberg Atlas of pediatric Cutaneous Biodiversity Figure 15.2)

striata, as can some oral medications. Although melanonychia striata is common, some pigmented lesions of the nail bed may be indicative of melanoma of the nail unit (bed or matrix); suspicious features include width of the lesion of greater than 3 mm and pigmentation of the proximal nail bed, the Hutchinson's sign [6].

It is unknown as to the true incidence of melanoma in congenital nevi in children of color, but it seems lower than that noted in Caucasian children, making prophylactic removal unnecessary, unless clinically warranted by alterations in shape, size, or pigmentation [8]. Melanocytic nevi are far less common in patients of color [59]. In the differential of facial nevi in darkly pigmented individuals are dermatosis papulosa nigra, familial benign pigmented papules of the face and upper body seen in Black and Hispanic patients [60]. Syringomas also appear to be more common in children of color, especially Asian teenage females, appearing primarily in the periocular location [61].

## *Inflammatory Diseases*

Lymphocytic infiltrates of the skin can cause hypopigmented or violaceous skin lesions in children of color. Hypopigmented mycosis fungoides is a form of mycosis fungoides that presents as annular hypopigmented lesions. The trunk and extremities are the most common sites. Lesions may mimic pityriasis lichenoides chronica (Fig. 20.7), which may also be hypopigmented in children of color. Early onset and limitation to patients of color are characteristic. Multiple biopsies may be required to establish the diagnosis of mycosis fungoides. Involvement of the buttocks is common in mycosis fungoides of childhood and can aid in diagnosis. Wood's lamp fluorescence may be positive in mycosis fungoides and cannot be used to distinguish vitiligo from mycosis fungoides. Biopsy should be performed in all cases of suspected mycosis fungoides. Topical corticosteroids and narrowband UVB therapy [62] can help clear skin lesions but do not clear the disease permanently. The prognosis is a normal life span in most cases. Phototherapy is not ideal in younger children of color; the exposure times are longer for darker skin types and are difficult for younger children. Examination for lymph node enlargement and Sezary cells on blood smear should be performed intermittently to screen for disease progression [63].

Another common inflammatory skin disease seen in male infants and toddlers of color is infantile acropustulosis which can be secondary to scabies infection in up to half of cases. Potent topical corticosteroids and oral dapsone can be beneficial. Dapsone usage requires frequent blood counts due to dose-dependent hemolysis [8, 63].

Kawasaki disease was originally described in Japan and is a disease noted most commonly in children of color. Hospitalization rates for children in the United States are highest in Asian/Pacific islanders (39 per 100,000) or Black (19.7 per 100,000) children [3, 64].

Kawasaki disease is diagnosed by the presence of fever for 5 days or more, associated with four of the following five features: mucosal erythema of the lips with red strawberry tongue, conjunctival erythema, palmoplantar symptomatology including erythema and edema of the extremities, cervical lymph nodes, and a generalized rash. This illness can be associated with coronary artery inflammation and or cardiac artery dilatation in about 25% of untreated children (either acute or late onset), resulting in chronic heart disease or death. Prompt recognition of the disease and therapy with intravenous gamma globulin (2 mg/kg) may reduce long-term cardiac risk. Echocardiograms and electrocardiograms are required in all diagnosed or suspected cases of Kawasaki disease. Diagnostic clues include elevated CRP (>3) and desquamation of the diaper and acral areas. These clues can aid in delineating the diagnosis in cases where only two criteria are present in addition to persistent fever. Incomplete features are more common in children under the age of 1 year. The therapy of choice is a combination of intravenous gamma globulin and high-dose aspirin [65]. For cases that do not defervesce on IVIG and aspirin, intravenous methylprednisolone, infliximab, or methotrexate may be initiated. All children with Kawasaki disease require initial and long-term cardiac monitoring.

## *Metabolic Syndrome and Autoimmunity*

The metabolic syndrome of hypertension, hyperlipidemia, diabetes, and the prediabetic state are common in children of color in the United States due to an epidemic of obesity in children in the US, especially Black and Hispanic children of all ages [66]. By age 9 years, the appearance of acanthosis nigricans will be a reflection of high body mass index/obesity and associated abnormal fasting glucose and insulin tests in 90% of children. Acanthosis nigricans is noted in 19% of African American, 23% of Hispanic, and 4% of Caucasian children [67]. Forty-nine percent of fifth graders with acanthosis nigricans have the metabolic syndrome [68]. Dietary modification through calorie restriction and low glycemic index diets can be helpful and should be recommended in obese children with acanthosis nigricans.

Autoimmune diseases are a broad spectrum of illnesses in which the body attacks its own tissues. Some immune diseases are more common in patients of color, particularly lupus erythematosus and its cutaneous variants, including discoid lupus erythematosus. 23.5% of children with discoid lupus will have systemic lupus erythematosus, a higher percentage than adults. Generalized discoid lesions are strongly associated with systemic lupus, as opposed to localized lesions [69]. Given the high background incidence of lupus in women of color, children born or developing infantile facial erythematous plaques, atrophic or hypopigmented lesions in a raccoon eyes distribution should be worked up for neonatal lupus erythematosus through antibody testing for anti-Ro, anti-La, and U1RNP antibodies. Screening for neonatal heart block is required in children with neonatal lupus skin lesions, and careful sun protection is required until transplacentally transferred antibodies disappear from the child's circulation [70]. Additionally, photosensitivity such as polymorphous light eruption is more common in Blacks [71].

## *Genetic Disorders Seen Commonly in Patients of Color*

A few genetic disorders are noted more frequently in children of color. Albinism has a few distinctive subtypes in children of color. First, oculocutaneous albinism type 2 (OCA2) is the most common in African children. Less common variants in children of color include OCA 3/Rufous, in which a partial albinism is noted with a red hair tone. This type is often noted in South African Black children and is caused by a mutation in TRP-1 [72]. Oculocutaneous albinism type 4 (OCA 4) results from mutations of the MATP gene and is considered one of the most common forms of OCA in Japan. MATP is a melanosomal trafficking protein [73]. Hermansky-Pudlak type albinism is a partial albinism associated with prolonged bleeding, which currently has 8 different subtypes (HPS 1-8) with 8 different genes, and as many as 14 genes in mouse models [74]. The HPS genes are genes encoding lysosome-related organelles found in melanocytes, retinal pigment epithelial cells, platelets, T cells, neutrophils, and lung type II epithelial cells. Mutations of HPS-1 are noted in patients of Puerto Rican descent. HPS patients have an increased tendency to bleed and lysosomal dysfunction and depositional buildup, leading to end organ dysfunction (e.g., lungs and colon).

## Conclusions

Children of color have some innate differences in pigmentation, pigment lability, response to injury and trauma, and hair follicle configuration. These biological differences combined with stylistic hair and skincare practices result in a host of biologically different diseases and phenotypic appearance of skin disease.

## References


1. Silverberg NB. Pediatric dermatology in children of color. Access Dermatol, posten online 17 Aug 2010. Accessed 15 March, 2011.
2. Morell R, Carey ML, Lalwani AK, Friedman TB, Asher Jr JH. Three mutations in the paired homeodomain of PAX3 that cause Waardenburg syndrome type 1. Hum Hered. 1997;47:38–41.
3. Thong HY, Jee SH, Sun CC, Boissy RE. The patterns of melanosome distribution in keratinocytes of human skin as one determining factor of skin colour. Br J Dermatol. 2003;149:498–505.
4. Tsai FJ, Tsai CH. Birthmarks and congenital skin lesions in Chinese newborns. J Formos Med Assoc. 1993;92:838–41.
5. Cordova A. The Mongolian spot: a study of ethnic differences and a literature review. Clin Pediatr. 1981;20:714–9.
6. Ho SG, Chan HH. The Asian dermatologic patient: review of common pigmentary disorders and cutaneous diseases. Am J Clin Dermatol. 2009;10:153–68.
7. Meleti M, Vescovi P, Mooi WJ, van der Waal I. Pigmented lesions of the oral mucosa and perioral tissues: a flow-chart for the diagnosis and some recommendations for the management. Oral Surg Oral Med Oral Pathol Oral Radiol Endod. 2008;105:606–16.
8. Buka R, Friedman KA, Phelps RG, Silver L, Calero F, Rudikoff D. Childhood longitudinal melanonychia: case reports and review of the literature. Mt Sinai J Med. 2001;68:331–5.
9. Dessinioti C, Stratigos AJ, Rigopoulos D, Katsambas AD. A review of genetic disorders of hypopigmentation: lessons learned from the biology of melanocytes. Exp Dermatol. 2009;18(9):741–9.
10. Laude TA. Skin disorders in black children. Curr Opin Pediatr. 1996;8:381–5.
11. Child FJ, Fuller LC, Higgins EM, Du Vivier AW. A study of the spectrum of skin disease occurring in a black population in south-east London. Br J Dermatol. 1999;141:512–7.
12. Kiken DA, Silverberg NB. Atopic dermatitis in children, part 1: epidemiology, clinical features, and complications. Cutis. 2006;78:241–7.
13. Williams HC, Pembroke AC, Forsdyke H, Boodoo G, Hay RJ, Burney PG. London-born black Caribbean children are at increased risk of atopic dermatitis. J Am Acad Dermatol. 1995;32 (2 Pt 1):212–7.
14. Ben-Gashir MA, Hay RJ. Reliance on erythema scores may mask severe atopic dermatitis in black children compared with their white counterparts. Br J Dermatol. 2002;147(5):920–5.
15. Williams HC, Pembroke AC. Infraorbital crease, ethnic group, and atopic dermatitis. Arch Dermatol. 1996;132:51–4.
16. Kiken DA, Silverberg NB. Atopic dermatitis in children, part 2: treatment options. Cutis. 2006;78:401–6.
17. Rigopoulos D, Gregoriou S, Charissi C, Kontochristopoulos G, Kalogeromitros D, Georgala S. Tacrolimus ointment 0.1% in pityriasis alba: an open-label, randomized, placebo-controlled study. Br J Dermatol. 2006;155:152–5.
18. Williams JV, Eichenfield LF, Burke BL, Barnes-Eley M, Friedlander SF. Prevalence of scalp scaling in prepubertal children. Pediatrics. 2005;115:e1–6.
19. Elish D, Silverberg NB. Infantile seborrheic dermatitis. Cutis. 2006;77:297–300.
20. High WA, Pandya AG. Pilot trial of 1 % pimecrolimus cream in the treatment of seborrheic dermatitis in African American adults with associated hypopigmentation. J Am Acad Dermatol. 2006;54:1083–8.
21. Amer A, Fischer H, Li X. The natural history of pityriasis rosea in black American children: how correct is the "classic" description? Arch Pediatr Adolesc Med. 2007;161:503–6.
22. Rasi A, Tajziehchi L, Savabi-Nasab S. Oral erythromycin is ineffective in the treatment of pityriasis rosea. J Drugs Dermatol. 2008;7(1):35–8.
23. Sharma V, Beyer DJ, Paruthi S, Nopper AJ. Prominent pruritic periumbilical papules: allergic contact dermatitis to nickel. Pediatr Dermatol. 2002;19:106–9.
24. Silverberg NB, Licht J, Friedler S, Sethi S, Laude TA. Nickel contact hypersensitivity in children. Pediatr Dermatol. 2002;19:110–3.

25. Moennich JN, Zirwas M, Jacob SE. Nickel-induced facial dermatitis: adolescents beware of the cell phone. Cutis. 2009;84(4):199–200.
26. Bhardwaj SS, Jaimes JP, Liu A, Warshaw EM. A double-blind randomized placebo-controlled pilot study comparing topical immunomodulating agents and corticosteroids for treatment of experimentally induced nickel contact dermatitis. Dermatitis. 2007;18(1):26–31.
27. Gelfand JM, Stern RS, Nijsten T, Feldman SR, Thomas J, Kist J, Rolstad T, Margolis DJ. The prevalence of psoriasis in African Americans: results from a population-based study. J Am Acad Dermatol. 2005;52:23–6.
28. Paller AS, Siegfried EC, Langley RG, Gottlieb AB, Pariser D, Landells I, Hebert AA, Eichenfield LF, Patel V, Creamer K, Jahreis A. Etanercept pediatric psoriasis study group. Etanercept treatment for children and adolescents with plaque psoriasis. N Engl J Med. 2008;358(3):241–51.
29. Pauporte M, Maibach H, Lowe N, Pugliese M, Friedman DJ, Mendelsohn H, Cargill I, Ramirez R. Fluocinolone acetonide topical oil for scalp psoriasis. J Dermatol Treat. 2004;15(6):360–4.
30. Natarajan S, Milne D, Jones AL, Goodfellow M, Perry J, Koerner RJ. Dietzia strain X: a newly described *Actinomycete* isolated from confluent and reticulated papillomatosis. Br J Dermatol. 2005;153:825–7.
31. Silverberg NB, Heilman ER. Calcipotriene in the therapy of confluent and reticulated papillomatosis of Gougererot and Carteaud. J Clin Derm. 1998;1(4):12–4.
32. Davis MD, Weenig RH, Camilleri MJ. Confluent and reticulate papillomatosis (Gougerot-Carteaud syndrome): a minocycline-responsive dermatosis without evidence for yeast in pathogenesis. A study of 39 patients and a proposal of diagnostic criteria. Br J Dermatol. 2006;154:287–93.
33. Solomon BA, Laude TA. Two patients with confluent and reticulated papillomatosis: response to oral isotretinoin and 10 % lactic acid lotion. J Am Acad Dermatol. 1996;35:645–6.
34. Khumalo NP, Jessop S, Gumedze F, Ehrlich R. Hairdressing and the prevalence of scalp disease in African adults. Br J Dermatol. 2007;157:981–8.
35. Khumalo NP, Jessop S, Gumedze F, Ehrlich R. Determinants of marginal traction alopecia in African girls and women. J Am Acad Dermatol. 2008;59:432–8.
36. Silverberg NB, Singh A, Laude TA. Cutaneous manifestations of chronic renal failure in children of color. Pediatr Dermatol. 2001;18:199–204.
37. Lucky AW, Biro FM, Daniels SR, Cedars MI, Khoury PR, Morrison JA. The prevalence of upper lip hair in black and white girls during puberty: a new standard. J Pediatr. 2001;138:134–6.
38. Gathers RC, Lim HW. Central centrifugal cicatricial alopecia: past, present, and future. J Am Acad Dermatol. 2009;60:660–8.
39. Miyamoto M, Tsuboi R, Oh-I T. Case of acquired trichorrhexis nodosa: scanning electron microscopic observation. J Dermatol. 2009;36:109–10.
40. Bari AU, Khan MB. Dermatological disorders related to cultural practices in black Africans of Sierra Leone. J Coll Physicians Surg Pak. 2007;17:249–52.
41. Quarles FN, Johnson BA, Badreshia S, Vause SE, Brauner G, Breadon JY, Swinehart J, Lupo MP. Acne vulgaris in richly pigmented patients. Dermatol Ther. 2007;20:122–7.
42. Quarles FN, Brody H, Johnson BA, Badreshia S, Vause SE, Brauner G, Breadon JY, Swinehart J, Callendar V. Pseudofolliculitis barbae. Dermatol Ther. 2007;20:133–6.
43. Williams HC, Ashworth J, Pembroke AC, Breathnach SM. FACE-facial Afro-Caribbean childhood eruption. Clin Exp Dermatol. 1990;15:163–6.
44. Laude TA, Salvemini JN. Perioral dermatitis in children. Semin Cutan Med Surg. 1999;18:206–9.
45. Rauscher GE, Kolmer WL. Treatment of recurrent earlobe keloids. Cutis. 1986;37(1):67–8.
46. Alvarez MS, Silverberg NB. Tinea capitis. Cutis. 2006;78:189–96.
47. Sharma V, Silverberg NB, Howard R, Tran CT, Laude TA, Frieden IJ. Do hair care practices affect the acquisition of tinea capitis? A case-control study. Arch Pediatr Adolesc Med. 2001;155:818–21.
48. Silverberg NB, Weinberg JM, DeLeo VA. Tinea capitis: focus on African American women. J Am Acad Dermatol. 2002;46:S120–4.

49. Lorch Dauk KC, Comrov E, Blumer JL, O'Riordan MA, Furman LM. Tinea capitis: predictive value of symptoms and time to cure with Griseofulvin treatment. Clin Pediatr (Phila). 2009 1 Jun. Epub ahead of print, Accessed 21Dec 2009.
50. Silverberg NB. Easy griseofulvin dosing. Pediatr Dermatol. 2008;25:577.
51. Levin NA. Beyond spaghetti and meatballs: skin diseases associated with the Malassezia yeasts. Dermatol Nurs. 2009;21:7–13, 51.
52. Jin Y, Birlea SA, Fain PR, Spritz RA. Genetic variations in NALP1 are associated with generalized vitiligo in a Romanian population. J Investig Dermatol. 2007;127:2558–62.
53. Silverberg NB, Travis L. Childhood vitiligo. Cutis. 2006;77(6):370–5.
54. Pagovich OE, Silverberg JI, Freilich E, Silverberg NB. Thyroid abnormalities in pediatric patients with vitiligo in New York City. Cutis. 2008;81:463–6.
55. Silverberg NB, Herz J, Wagner A, Paller AS. Erythema dyschromicum perstans in prepubertal children. Pediatr Dermatol. 2003;20:398–403.
56. Torrelo A, Zaballos P, Colmenero I, Mediero IG, de Prada I, Zambrano A. Erythema dyschromicum perstans in children: a report of 14 cases. J Eur Acad Dermatol Venereol. 2005;19:422–6.
57. Shih IH, Lin JY, Chen CH, Hong HS. A birthmark survey in 500 newborns: clinical observation in two northern Taiwan medical center nurseries. Chang Gung Med J. 2007;30:220–5.
58. Rampen FH, de Wit PE. Racial differences in mole proneness. Acta Derm Venereol. 1989;69:234–6.
59. Hairston Jr MA, Reed RJ, Derbes VJ. Dermatosis papulosa nigra. Arch Dermatol. 1964;89:655–8.
60. Yesudian P, Thambiah A. Familial syringoma. Dermatologica. 1975;150(1):32–5.
61. Ferahbas A, Utas S, Ulas Y, Kontas O, Karakukcu M, Arseven V. Narrow band UVB treatment for a child with mycosis fungoides. Pediatr Dermatol. 2006;23:302–3.
62. Akaraphanth R, Douglass MC, Lim HW. Hypopigmented mycosis fungoides: treatment and a 6(1/2)-year follow-up of 9 patients. J Am Acad Dermatol. 2000;42:33–9.
63. Mancini AJ, Frieden IJ, Paller AS. Infantile acropustulosis revisited: history of scabies and response to topical corticosteroids. Pediatr Dermatol. 1998;15:337–41.
64. Holman RC, Curns AT, Belay ED, Steiner CA, Schonberger LB. Kawasaki syndrome hospitalizations in the United States, 1997 and 2000. Pediatrics. 2003;112(3 Pt 1):495–501.
65. Epps RE. Case reports: selected dermatoses in children of color. J Drugs Dermatol. 2007;6:78–82.
66. Chang Y, Woo HY, Sung E, Kim CH, Kang H, Ju YS, Park KH. Prevalence of acanthosis nigricans in relation to anthropometric measures: community-based cross-sectional study in Korean pre-adolescent school children. Pediatr Int. 2008;50:667–73.
67. Brickman WJ, Binns HJ, Jovanovic BD, Kolesky S, Mancini AJ, Metzger BE. Acanthosis nigricans: a common finding in overweight youth. Pediatr Dermatol. 2007;24:601–6.
68. Ice CL, Murphy E, Minor VE, Neal WA. Metabolic syndrome in fifth grade children with acanthosis nigricans: results from the CARDIAC project. World J Pediatr. 2009;5:23–30.
69. Sampaio MC, de Oliveira ZN, Machado MC, dos Reis VM, Vilela MA. Discoid lupus erythematosus in children–a retrospective study of 34 patients. Pediatr Dermatol. 2008;25:163–7.
70. Elish D, Silverberg NB. Neonatal lupus erythematosus. Cutis. 2006;77:82–6.
71. Kerr HA, Lim HW. Photodermatoses in African Americans: a retrospective analysis of 135 patients over a 7-year period. J Am Acad Dermatol. 2007;57:638–43.
72. Marneros AG, Norris JE, Olsen BR, Reichenberger E. Clinical genetics of familial keloids. Arch Dermatol. 2001;137:1429–34.
73. Dessinioti C, Stratigos AJ, Rigopoulos D, Katsambas AD. A review of genetic disorders of hypopigmentation: lessons learned from the biology of melanocytes. Exp Dermatol. 2009;18(9):741–9.
74. Santiago Borrero PJ, Rodríguez-Pérez Y, Renta JY, Izquierdo NJ, Del Fierro L, Muñoz D, Molina NL, Ramírez S, Pagán-Mercado G, Ortíz I, Rivera-Caragol E, Spritz RA, Cadilla CL. Genetic testing for oculocutaneous albinism type 1 and 2 and Hermansky-Pudlak syndrome type 1 and 3 mutations in Puerto Rico. J Investig Dermatol. 2006;126:85–90.

# Chapter 21
# Hair Transplantation

**Valerie D. Callender and Erica C. Davis**

The International Society of Hair Restoration Surgery (ISHRS)'s practice census survey reports that in 2010 there were approximately 279,381 hair transplant surgeries worldwide, which include surgeons from the United States, Canada, Mexico/Central and South America, Europe, Asia, Australia, and Middle East [1]. The majority of these procedures were performed in men (86%), and the number of racial or ethnic patients were not available. There are several surgical procedures available to treat hair loss in men and women. These include follicular unit transplantation (FUT), follicular unit extraction (FUE), scalp reduction, and scalp flaps. The latter two methods are not commonly performed and will not be discussed in this chapter.

## Ethnic Differences in Hair Characteristics

Although the biochemical composition of hair is generally consistent among all racial/ethnic groups, clinical hair characteristics certainly differ between various populations as numerous studies have shown [2–4]. Some tend to classify human hair into three subtypes based on race – African (Table 21.1), Asian (Table 21.2), and Caucasian (Table 21.3) – but in general, there are four different types of hair structure: straight, wavy, helical, and spiral [5] arising from either straight or curved hair follicles. Overall, blacks tend to have spiraled or helical hair structure that

V.D. Callender, M.D. (✉)
Callender Dermatology and Cosmetic Center, 12200 Annapolis Road, Suite 315, Glenn Dale, MD 20769, USA

Department of Dermatology, Howard University College of Medicine, Washington, DC, USA
e-mail: drcallender@callenderskin.com

E.C. Davis, M.D.
Callender Dermatology and Cosmetic Center, 12200 Annapolis Road, Suite 315, Glenn Dale, MD 20769, USA
e-mail: ericadavis2@hotmail.com

A.F. Alexis and V.H. Barbosa (eds.), *Skin of Color: A Practical Guide to Dermatologic Diagnosis and Treatment*, DOI 10.1007/978-0-387-84929-4_21,

**Table 21.1** Common[a] hair characteristics among populations of African ancestry

| *Hair features* |
|---|
| • Coiled, helical, or spiraled hair structure |
| • Elliptical, flattened in cross section |
| • Curved hair follicle |

[a]The above represents the most common features of hair in this population but significant individual variation (i.e., straight hair structure) does occur

**Table 21.2** Common hair characteristics among Asian populations

| *Hair features* |
|---|
| • Straight hair structure |
| • Round in cross section with greater diameter |
| • Straight hair follicle |

**Table 21.3** Common hair characteristics among Caucasians

| *Hair features* |
|---|
| • Straight, wavy, or helical hair structure |
| • Round or oval in cross section |
| • Straight hair follicle |

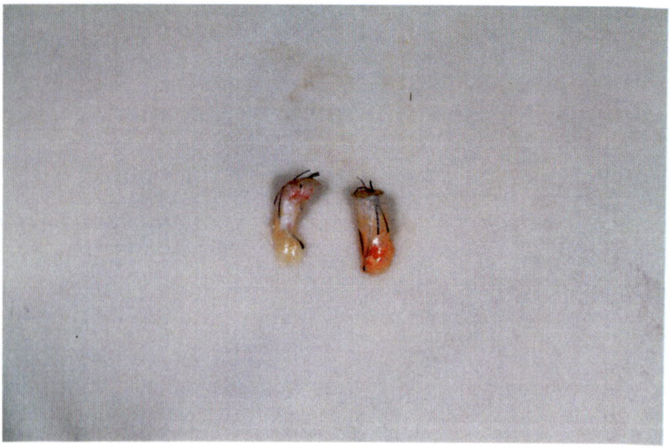

**Fig. 21.1** Curved hair follicle

appears clinically as tightly coiled, while Asian hair is on the opposite end of the hair spectrum and is very straight in structure, although there is considerable individual variation particularly among African Americans [6]. Caucasians tend to lie on the hair spectrum between blacks and Asians and can have anywhere from straight to wavy to even helical hair structure [6]. And of particular importance to hair restoration surgeons is the knowledge of hair follicle morphology as black patients typically have curved hair follicles (Fig. 21.1) compared to the straight hair follicles

**Table 21.4** Comparison of certain hair characteristics among racial/ethnic populations

| Hair features | Highest to lowest in numerical value |
|---|---|
| Follicular units/mm$^2$ | Asian[a] = Caucasian > Black |
| Average density (hairs/cm$^2$) | Caucasian > Asian[a] ≈ Black |
| Growth rate (μm/day) | Asian > Caucasian > Black |
| Telogen hairs (%) | Asian ≈ Caucasian ≈ Black |
| Predominant hair grouping | Black > Asian = Caucasian |
| Terminal follicles | Caucasian > Black |
| Anagen hairs | Caucasian > Black |

[a]Includes most nationalities in Asia with the exception of possibly the Chinese. One study found that follicular units/mm$^2$ in three Chinese women to be only slightly higher than that of blacks but lower than most other Asians and Caucasians. Average density of hairs/mm$^2$ in these women was also lowest of all study populations (Data from [70–73])

seen in white and Asian patients. The curved nature of the hair follicle can cause hair transplantation in blacks to be somewhat more challenging in donor harvesting and preparing viable grafts due to the increased risk of follicular transection [7].

Table 21.4 compares the results of various clinical studies that evaluated certain hair characteristics among black, white, and Asian populations. Overall, black patients were found to have a lower average hair density than whites; however, the curly morphology of the hair follicle, a slightly higher number of hair groupings in each follicular unit, and less contrast between scalp skin color and hair color may all work together to create the appearance of fullness and more coverage in black patients after hair transplantation [8, 9]. Hair growth rate was also lower in blacks [10]. Dominant trends among Asian subjects were a somewhat lower hair density, but a fast rate of hair growth and white subjects were found to have the highest hair density of all populations studied and a fast hair growth rate although not as rapid as seen in some Asian studies [10].

## Hair Transplants in Ethnic Populations: A Historical Perspective

The *father* of hair restoration surgery specifically for androgenetic alopecia (AGA) is without a doubt Dr. Norman Orentreich, who first reported the use of punch grafts in hair transplantation for AGA in men and the concept of donor dominance in 1959 [11]. However, there were a few who actually preceded him in the concept of transplanting autologous hair grafts using the punch graft technique. In 1939, Dr. Shoji Okuda (Fig. 21.2), a Japanese physician, published a report in the Japanese literature of 30 cases in which hair transplantation using punch grafting was used to successfully treat cicatricial alopecia, alopecia areata and leprosy involving the eyebrows, and atrichosis or hypotrichosis in the pubic area [12].

In respect to hair transplantation in blacks, one would be remiss not to mention the late Dr. Harold E. Pierce (Fig. 21.3), a Brigadier General in the US Air Force

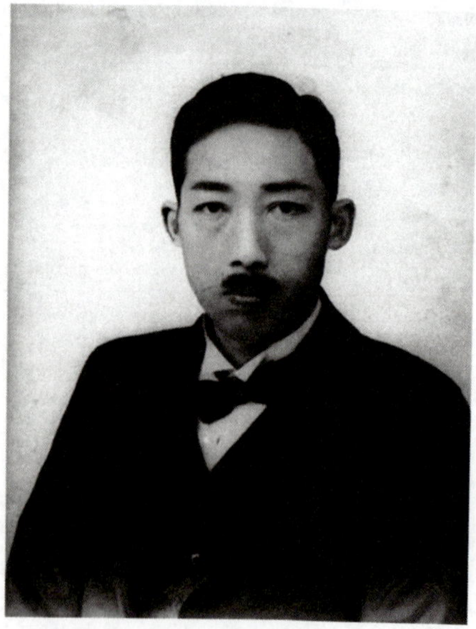

**Fig. 21.2** Dr. Shoji Okuda, Japanese physician and pioneer in autologous hair transplantation (From [12], with permission)

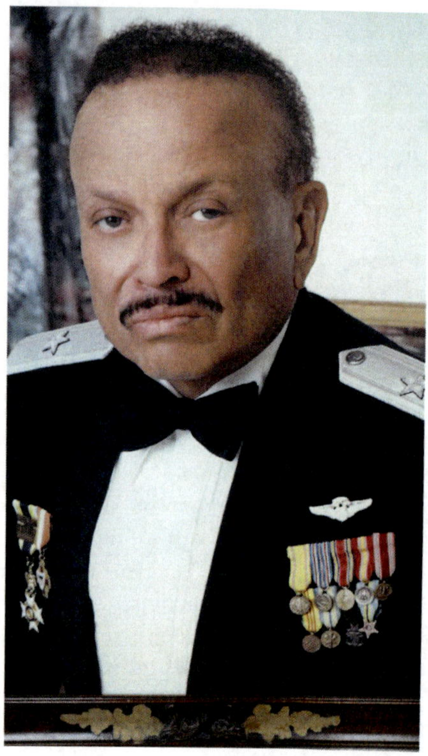

**Fig. 21.3** Dr. Harold E. Pierce, a pioneer in the field of cosmetic surgery in blacks (From [74], with permission)

and pioneer not only in hair transplantation in blacks but also in other cosmetic surgeries in darker-skinned individuals such as the laminar dermal reticulotomy, chemical peels, dermabrasion, and the treatment of keloids. Dr. Pierce published numerous articles and book chapters on hair restoration surgery in blacks, detailing its distinctions from those with straighter hair and also reporting innovations and modifications to standard techniques and instrumentation [9, 13, 14]. Dr. R. Martin Earles, trained in both general surgery and dermatology, has also led the way in developing innovative new methods in hair transplantation for African Americans. Dr. Earles pioneered the use of scalp reduction and flap rotation during hair transplantation in blacks as well as surgical treatment for traction alopecia in women [15, 16].

## Indications

### *Androgenetic Alopecia*

Androgenetic alopecia (AGA), also known as male or female pattern hair loss (MPHL/FPHL) (Fig. 21.4), is a type of hair loss seen in populations worldwide that develops in response to changing androgens levels as well as to genetic factors [17]. Table 21.5 compares the overall prevalence rates of AGA in male and female

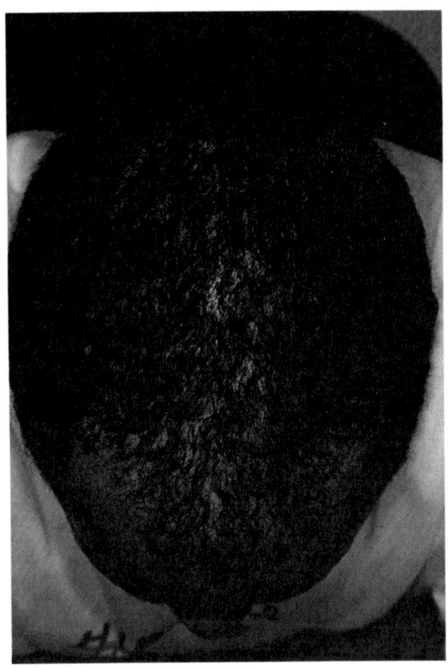

**Fig. 21.4** Male pattern hair loss

**Table 21.5** Prevalence rates of androgenetic alopecia among various racial/ethnic populations

| Population | Prevalence in males (%) | Prevalence in females (%) |
|---|---|---|
| Caucasian [75, 76] | 50 | 19 |
| South African [77] | 14.5 | 3.5 |
| Chinese [78] | 21.3 | 6 |
| Chinese [79] | 19.9 | 3.1 |
| Korean (18) | 14.1 | 5.6 |
| Singaporean [80] | Overall – 63<br>Chinese – 61<br>Malay – 65<br>Indian – 87 | NS |
| Thai [81] | 38.5 | NS |

*NS* Not studied

Caucasian patients to rates found in studies conducted in ethnic patients. Not only is there significant variation in prevalence rates between races but there is also sizable intraracial differences as Chinese and Korean patients have considerably lower rates than Singaporean and Thai patients as compared to Caucasians. Korean men may also have a more preserved frontal hair line than men of other races/ethnicities [18]. Native Americans and men with African ancestry also tend to have lower prevalence rates of frontal AGA and less severe hair loss than Caucasians [19–22].

Overall, AGA occurs more commonly in men than women, and more is known about the condition in the male population [23]. Unlike their male counterparts in which hair loss is undoubtedly androgen dependent, the role of androgens in all cases of FPHL in women is less clear, and therefore FPHL is the preferred term over female AGA by some authors [23]. Clinical exam and laboratory analysis may show that some women with FPHL have hyperandrogenemia and even display a pattern of hair loss typically found in males, but most women will not [24]. Although the morphologic changes to the hair follicle (i.e., miniaturization) are the same between male and female patients, the pattern of hair loss does show gender differences. Typically, men will experience hair loss in the bitemporal, frontal, midscalp, and vertex regions and can be categorized based on pattern and severity by the Hamilton-Norwood classification system [25]. Hair loss in women is categorized by the Ludwig pattern and typically manifests as diffuse central thinning of the crown with preservation of the frontal hairline or there can also be frontal accentuation of hair loss resembling a Christmas tree [26]. Many times, patients with mild hair loss (Norwood I–II or early Ludwig 1) are not optimal surgical candidates as further improvement may be limited and difficult to appreciate, and patients with diffuse hair loss or limited hair in the donor region make poor surgical candidates as well [23]. The ideal candidate for hair transplantation for men and women are those with adequate density in the donor region and extensive hair loss or thinning in the frontal region, which for men creates the most dramatic improvement [23].

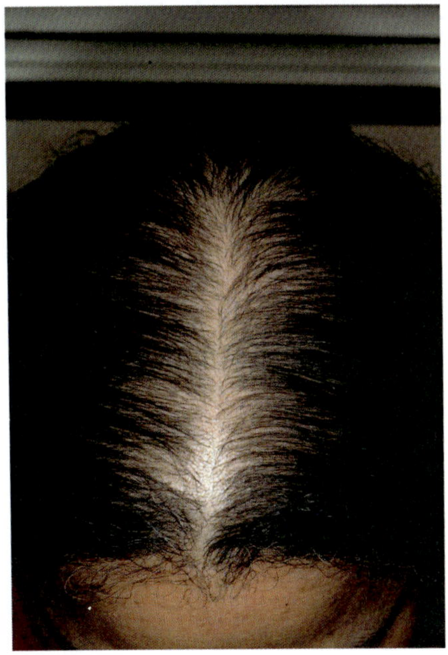

**Fig. 21.5** Female pattern hair loss

## *Traction Alopecia*

Traction alopecia (TA) (Fig. 21.5) is thought to occur from a mechanical loosening of the hairs from the follicle and perifolliculitis secondary to the chronic use of hairstyles or styling aids that increase tensile forces on scalp hairs such as tight ponytails [27], hair rollers [28], braids [5, 29, 30], and hair weaves [29]. TA is a common form of hair loss in women and children of African ancestry [31] but can also be seen in other populations such as practicing Sikh males who tie their scalp or beard hair very tightly under a turban or the chin, respectively [32–34], and South Korean nurses who develop TA from prolonged traction exerted at the point of attachment of the nurse's cap [35]. Clinically, TA appears as symmetrical hair loss most commonly localized to the temporal regions but can extend along the frontal and occipital hairlines in severe cases [7]. Histologically, in chronic TA, follicles and terminal hairs are markedly decreased although vellus hairs remain and follicles are replaced with fibrous tracts [36]. Sebaceous glands remain intact and there is generally very little inflammation [36, 37]. In the early stages of TA, hair loss is usually reversible and hair will begin to grow with discontinuation of the offending hairstyle. However, prolonged wear of tight hairstyles will eventually lead to irreversible hair loss. With the exception of those with significant occipital hair loss, patients with TA are generally very good candidates for hair transplantation; however, patient counseling regarding hair grooming practices is vital.

**Fig. 21.6** Traction alopecia

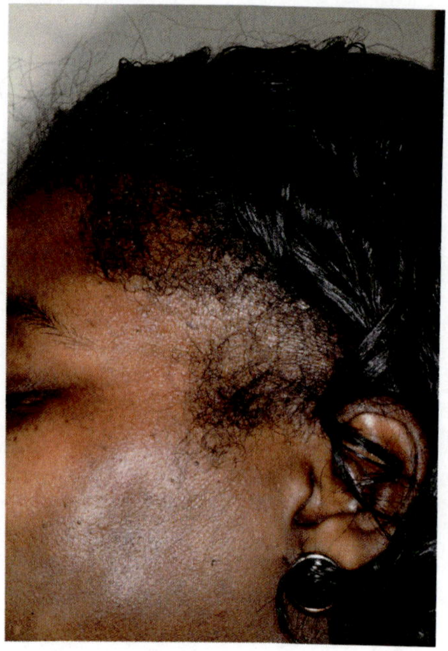

## *Central Centrifugal Cicatricial Alopecia*

Central centrifugal cicatricial alopecia (CCCA) (Fig. 21.6) is a progressive scarring alopecia centered over the vertex or mid scalp region that seems to disproportionately affect women of African descent, although the exact prevalence is unknown [7, 38]. A typical patient would be a black female in the second to fourth decade of life although CCCA can occur in men albeit less commonly [39, 40]. CCCA has also been previously referred to as *hot comb alopecia* [41], *chemical alopecia* [5], *chemically induced cosmetic alopecia* [42], *pseudopelade* [43], and *follicular degeneration syndrome* [44]. Usage of the current term, CCCA, is recommended by the North American Hair Research Society, which has worked to further classify cicatricial alopecias based on clinical and pathologic findings [45]. The etiology of CCCA is unclear at present, but contributing factors to its development may involve an interplay of genetic factors [44] and injurious hair care practices such as the use of chemical relaxers [7, 37] or even certain hairstyles [39].

Clinically, CCCA has a progressive course beginning with an early active inflammatory phase and over time eventually leading to the terminal stage of the disease characterized by scarring [7]. In early CCCA, the crown or vertex region of the scalp may appear (1) normal on clinical exam; (2) with discreet areas of short, broken hairs (author's personal observation); or (3) with small patches of hair loss [7, 46]. Over the course of the disease, hair loss progresses radially in a semisymmetric fashion [47]. Other signs and symptoms can include pruritus, erythema,

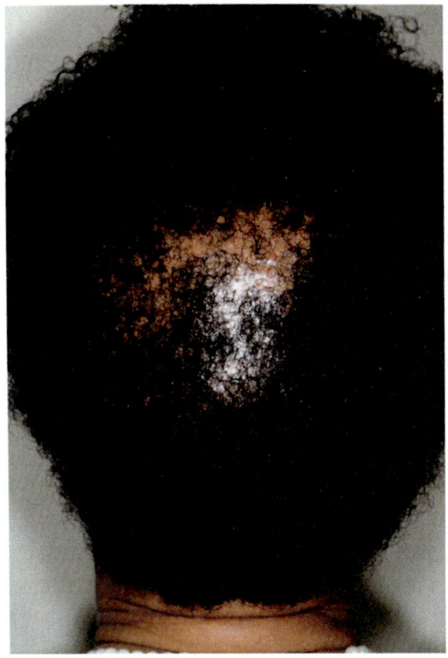

**Fig. 21.7** Central centrifugal cicatricial alopecia

scaling, scalp tenderness, or even sporadic follicular pustules [7]. Patients with chronic CCCA will present with loss of follicular openings and permanent hair loss. On histologic exam, early CCCA will show a perifollicular lymphocytic infiltrate and fibroplasia [37]. Some vellus-like hairs may persist but terminal hair follicles are increasingly replaced with fibrous tracts [37]. As the disease progresses, there is premature desquamation of the inner root sheath; however, controversy exists over whether this finding is exclusive to CCCA [48–50]. Advanced CCCA shows destruction of pilosebaceous units and dermal lymphohistiocytic infiltration and fibrosis [38].

Difficult therapeutic challenges may arise when performing hair restoration surgery for CCCA when compared to transplanting in nonscarring alopecias, such as AGA, FPHL, and traction alopecia. The procedure should only be considered for cases in which CCCA progression has been stabilized for at least 6 months with medical treatment [8]. In addition, graft survival rates are lower because of the limited blood supply in scar tissue, which may necessitate larger grafts and multiple smaller sessions [8]. A test session may also be necessary prior to the procedure to monitor for graft survival and hair growth. This involves transplanting four to six 4-mm round grafts from the donor site into 3.5-mm recipient sites typically in the vertex on the fringe of the area of hair loss (Fig. 21.7) [7]. A biopsy is taken from the recipient area to determine if any inflammation is present. Hair restoration surgery can then proceed if the scalp biopsy shows no inflammation and the test site demonstrates successful growth after 4–6 months [7].

## Contraindications

Hair type and follicle structure do not prevent patients from being acceptable candidates for hair transplantation. Contraindications for the procedure, however, do include patients with limited hair at the donor site (<40 follicular units/$cm^2$) [23], active scalp inflammation such as seen with CCCA, other concurrent scalp disorders like acne keloidalis and dissecting cellulitis, or a history of keloidal scarring [7]. However, the diagnosis of CCCA is not an absolute contraindication to hair transplantation. As stated above, if aggressive medical management with anti-inflammatory agents can stabilize the disease for at least 6 months, then hair restoration surgery can be considered for areas of permanent hair loss [8].

## Consultation

The importance of the consultation session should not be underestimated. It is during this time that the physician should assess the patient's desires and expectations and address any unrealistic goals before surgery is performed. In addition, this is also an opportunity to explain what is required of the patient such as changes in certain hair grooming practices and determine their level of commitment. During the consultation, a medical history including an in-depth history of allergies, medical illnesses, hair loss, scalp diseases, oral and topical medications, and hair grooming practices should be obtained. The amount of time and rate at which hair loss has occurred may help estimate the eventual degree of expected hair loss with AGA, which is important to communicate to the patient [51]. In general, patients in their late teens or 20s with thinning hair are more likely to experience complete hair loss than those with gradual thinning which becomes clinically evident in the third or fourth decade of life [51]. By first explaining the progressive nature of AGA, the younger patient can then understand why creating a wide, rounded, youthful hairline, which is permanent after transplantation, may not be appropriate [52]. The goal is to create a natural-appearing hairline that is age-appropriate but at the same time keeping in mind future hair loss [52]. The same reasoning can also be applied to the surgeon's decision to forego transplanting the ever-thinning vertex region [51].

A history of hair grooming practices is particularly important to obtain as these will frequently vary by race or ethnicity as well as gender. Men with a short haircut or "fade" in the donor area must be informed that a scar in that area will be noticeable. Usage and frequency should be obtained regarding permanents, chemical relaxers, texturizers, hair dyes, heat styling with curling irons or blow dryers, other hair care products (e.g., gel, hair spray), and very tight hairstyles such ponytails, cornrows, or braiding. Prior to surgery, patients with TA and CCCA should be informed of the importance of changing harmful hair care practices. In addition, patients with CCCA must also be aware of the possibility of disease recurrence and the decreased rate of graft survival in scar tissue [7].

**Table 21.6** Characteristics of appropriate candidates for hair transplantation

| Good candidates | Poor candidates |
|---|---|
| Male AGA (III–V) | Male AGA (VI–VII) |
| Female pattern hair loss (Ludwig 2–3) | Diffuse female pattern hair loss |
| Permanent TA (frontal) | Permanent TA (occipital) |
| Stable CCCA[a] | Active CCCA |

[a]CCCA is considered stable if there has been no progression of hair loss and no scalp inflammation present for 6 months or more
*AGA* Androgenetic alopecia, *TA* Traction alopecia, *CCCA* Central centrifugal cicatricial alopecia

The physical exam can also determine whether patients are adequate candidates for hair transplantation (Table 21.6). Patients with thinning hair at the donor site (<40 follicular units/cm$^2$) are poor candidates for surgery [23]. Signs of active inflammation and the presence of other scalp diseases as listed above (see *Contraindications*) can also preclude certain patients either temporarily or indefinitely from hair restoration surgery [7, 8].

## Instrumentation

Typically, the surgical instrumentation used for Asian patients with straight hair follicles does not differ from that used in surgery for Caucasians. However, Table 21.7 lists the surgical supplies and instrumentation recommended for follicular unit transplantation in patients with curved hair follicles. This particular follicular structure will typically require the use of larger surgical instrumentation in donor harvesting during FUE (1.5–2 mm rather than the standard 1 mm size) to avoid transecting the hair follicle (Fig. 21.8) and in the creation of acceptable recipient sites [7]. Generally, recipient sites greater than 1.5 mm in size are able to accommodate larger grafts containing follicles with a greater degree of curvature [7]. Another measure to help avoid damage to curved hair follicles would be the use of curved blades instead of the traditional straight blades used to prepare the grafts [53].

## Anesthesia

Most commonly, 1–2% lidocaine with epinephrine is used for analgesia during hair restoration surgery [54]. Bupivacaine is also a commonly used alternative with the added benefits of longer duration of action and greater potency than lidocaine; however, its onset of action is slower, and more importantly, bupivacaine is arrhythmogenic and should be used with caution [54]. Tumescence anesthesia with epinephrine in a saline solution will help to reduce bleeding during the procedure and maximize skin turgor, which facilitates donor strip excision and straightens the curved hair follicle [7]. The latter benefit also helps to avoid transection of the hair follicle.

**Table 21.7** Surgical supplies and instrumentation recommended for follicular unit transplantation in patients with curved hair follicles

| Surgical supplies and instrumentation for follicular unit transplantation in patients with tight curl pattern |
|---|
| *Donor harvesting* |
| • Loupe magnification |
| • Hair clips |
| • Electrical trimmer |
| • Single bladed scalpel |
| • Curved no.10 or 15 blade |
| • Tissue clamps |
| • 3-0 or 4-0 Prolene (blue) suture |
| *Graft preparation* |
| • Stereomicroscope |
| • Fiber optic box lighting |
| • Straight or curved Personna blade (DermaBlade) |
| • Petri dishes |
| • Saline solution |
| *Recipient site creation* |
| • Curved or straight microvascular forceps |
| • Spear point (SP) blades – 90 and 91 |
| • Mende knife – 1.3 mm, 1.5 mm |
| • Nokor needles – 16 and 18 gauge |
| • Punches – 2 mm through 4 mm |

Adapted from [82], with permission of Lippincott Williams & Wilkins

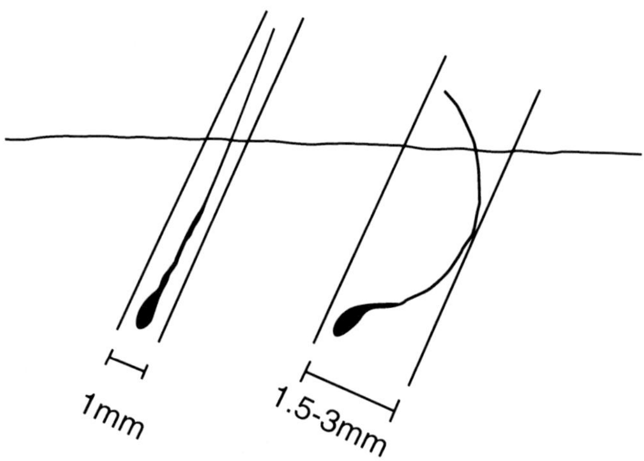


**Fig. 21.8** Schematic showing the potential for transection of straight versus curved hair follicles during donor harvesting. Note the necessity for larger instruments to harvest intact grafts

## Donor Harvesting

Hair for transplantation is typically harvested from the area of the occipital protuberance. This region is generally unaffected by male and female AGA, CCCA, and traction alopecia and will provide hair that is an exact physical match for the missing hair in the areas of hair loss [51]. Donor hair grafts can be harvested by numerous techniques (Table 21.8). As mentioned above, hair transplantation for AGA using punch grafting was popularized by Dr. Norman Orentreich beginning in the 1950s [55]. For patients with AGA, FPHL, and traction alopecia, newer surgical techniques in hair restoration (Follicular unit transplantation, FUT) produce more aesthetically pleasing results; however, these larger, round grafts typically 3–4 mm in size may still be appropriate for CCCA patients. Larger grafts containing hairs with a high degree of follicular curvature and very tight curl pattern would still produce a cosmetically appealing outcome as the curly hair provides greater scalp coverage [8].

More advanced techniques in donor harvesting include follicular unit transplantation (FUT) and follicular unit extraction (FUE). FUT is considered by some to be the current gold standard in hair transplantation and involves harvesting a single donor strip from the posterior scalp [56]. Typically, the width of the strip should be 1 cm or less but the size (width and length) of the strip depends on the number of hair follicles needed for the recipient site and the hair density of the donor region [7]. A densitometer can be helpful for this purpose. Wider strips can cause greater wound tension upon closure, which may not be prudent for populations that are more prone to develop hypertrophic scars and keloids (i.e., blacks and Asians) [57]. The use of loupe magnification and tumescence anesthesia is also recommended for curlier hair to better visualize the follicle and straighten the hairs, respectively, to avoid transection of the hair shaft and/or follicle. In contrast to the strip excision in FUT, FUE uses very small punch excisions (1 mm) to harvest individual follicular units directly from the donor site [58]. This technique was developed in response to concerns regarding donor site complications like scarring after conventional strip harvest [58] and may be a better option for patients who wear very short haircuts [51]. Although the scarring may be less apparent with FUE, disadvantages with this technique include a lower number of intact grafts (higher transection rate) and longer length of time to harvest donor hairs per procedure [51].

**Table 21.8** Donor hair grafts can be harvested by numerous techniques

| Donor harvesting techniques |
|---|
| *Extraction* |
| • Punch extraction |
| • Donor strip excision[a] |
| • Follicular unit extraction |
| *Closure* |
| • Standard reapproximation of wound edges |
| • Trichophytic closure |

[a]Used in follicular unit transplantation

The resultant scar at the donor site can be an important concern for patients, particularly for those with short haircuts. For example, many men of African descent wear their haircut very short in which the scalp is clearly visible. Therefore, the aesthetic appearance of the scar or lack thereof can be of significant importance to these patients who not only want a cosmetically pleasing result but may also want to maintain privacy regarding their hair transplant procedure. Strip excision sites can be closed in the standard fashion or with a newer technique called trichophytic closure, which is thought to produce a minimal scar [59]. Trichophytic closure involves de-epithelializing 1 mm of epidermis on the inferior wound edge prior to closure. With time, hairs will grow through the scar and camouflage any scar tissue formed in that area. Gaviria [60] conducted a study comparing the standard method of closure to trichophytic closure in 987 patients (67% skin of color) and found the new technique to produce better cosmetic results. Some patients did experience ingrown hairs among other complications. However, more clinical studies are needed to further evaluate this technique, particularly in blacks who tend to have a tighter curl pattern and are more prone to diseases of ingrown hairs such as pseudofolliculitis barbae [61].

## Graft Preparation

Knowledge of the hair morphology and meticulous dissection techniques are two components to executing a successful hair transplant in patients with tight curl patterns. Preparing follicular units and multifollicular unit grafts should be performed using a stereomicroscope with backlighting or loupe magnification to increase visibility and decrease the chance of inadvertent follicular transection [7]. The use of a bendable Personna® blade (DermaBlade™) (Fig. 21.9) during dissection of

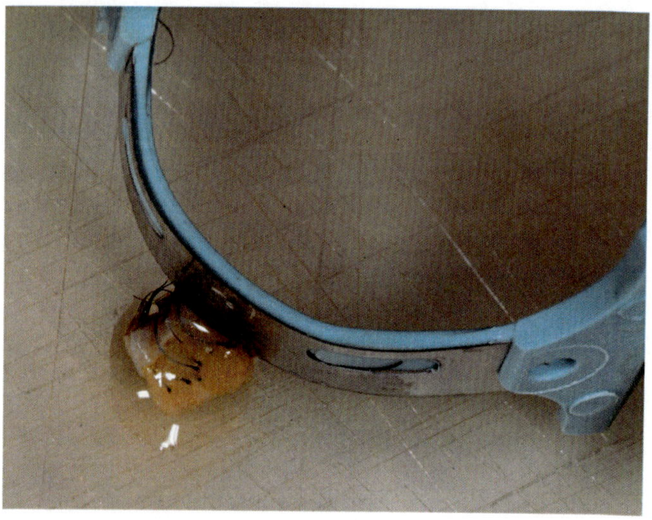

**Fig. 21.9** Bendable blades can conform to the curvature of the hair follicle to help avoid transection

individual grafts can also help minimize damage as the blade can bend to match the degree of curvature of the hair follicle [7, 53]. A traditional straight blade can be used for Asian patients given the straight nature of the hair follicle. Typically, each graft contains between 1 and 4 follicular units and should be placed into a saline solution to avoid desiccation until they are ready to be implanted into the recipient sites.

## Recipient Site Creation

There are several different surgical instruments that can be used to create graft recipient sites. Although the surgeon's preference may play a part in the decision, the surgical tool used should mostly be determined by the size of the recipient site needed. Available options include fine blades, needles, or punches. In patients with curved hair follicles, recipient sites tend to be larger in order to accommodate a larger graft with a higher degree of curl, and these sites can range from 1.2 to 2.0 mm in diameter. Hair transplantation and test sessions in patients with cicatricial alopecias such as CCCA will also use larger grafts for which punches are generally used to create larger recipient sites [7]. The usual aesthetic complaints associated with the use of punch grafts or *plugs* are generally not an issue with this method for CCCA because (1) the grafts are placed in the vertex or crown and not in the more visible anterior hairline, (2) curlier hair provides greater coverage, and (3) for darker-skinned patients, less contrast between dark scalp skin and dark hair can make thinner areas less noticeable [8]. In nonscarring alopecias such FPHL or traction alopecia, smaller grafts are generally used such as for follicular unit transplantation in which Nokor needles or flat blades (Spearpoint, Mende) are sufficient for recipient site creation [7]. When inserting hair grafts into the recipient sites, it is vitally important to place grafts in the appropriate orientation of normal hair growth for that particular patient in order to avoid an unnatural-appearing result.

## Complications

Table 21.9 lists the possible complications associated with hair restoration surgery [52]. Of particular concern for patients of African or Asian descent is postoperative keloid formation, given that these two populations are more prone to develop these benign masses [57]. Typically, the donor site experiences more complications with keloidal or hypertrophic scarring, which can occur in patients with no prior history of abnormal scarring [7]. However, a thorough medical history and physical exam including the scalp and sites that are more prone to keloid formation such as earlobes, shoulders, chest, and back [57], if necessary, prior to the procedure, may be helpful in the prevention of possible complications. Keloids and hypertrophic scars can be treated with a combination of class I topical corticosteroids twice daily for 2–4 weeks and intralesional triamcinolone 20–30 mg/ml injected every 2–4 weeks until the area flattens out or with injectable steroids alone [7]. Cobblestoning at punch graft sites in the recipient site area should be treated immediately with topical or intralesional corticosteroids [8].

**Table 21.9** Possible complications associated with hair restoration surgery

| Possible complications with hair transplantation |
|---|
| • Postoperative bleeding (<0.5%) |
| • Infection (<0.5%) |
| • Edema (5%) |
| • Temporary scalp numbness |
| • Folliculitis |
| • Persistent scalp pain |
| • Telogen effluvium |
| • Cobblestoning |
| • Keloid formation |
| • Hypertrophic scarring |
| • Data from [52] Arteriovenous fistula formation |

## Postoperative Counseling

Successful hair transplantation depends, in part, on adequate postoperative counseling, particularly for ethnic patients. It is important to discuss with the patient which hair care practices and products are acceptable and those to avoid in the immediate postoperative period as well as long term. The cosmetic surgeon should be familiarized particularly with ethnic hair care practices and products since their use can impact the overall outcome of surgery. For example, many African American women tend to wash their hair once a week compared to daily as in other racial/ethnic groups and have hair care practices, such as chemical or heat straightening and hair braiding, with the potential to cause hair loss or damage [7]. After hair transplantation, patients should be instructed to wash their hair gently and avoid all chemicals that could potentially cause scalp irritation or injury such as chemical hair relaxers, hair dyes, and excessive use of other hair products such as gel or hair spray. Patients can resume normal hair grooming 10–14 days postoperatively once the sutures are removed. For patients with TA, certain hairstyles such as tight braiding should be avoided indefinitely. Some patients may find it easier to wear a wig during the first 2 weeks postoperatively to avoid excessive hair grooming [7].

## Special Considerations

Today, hair transplantation is not limited to the scalp region alone. Cosmetic surgeons are transplanting hair to the eyebrows, eyelashes, beard, mustache, chest, and pubic area [62, 63]. Although just a small feature of the face, the absence of eyebrows can create an unnatural look and can make conveying certain facial expressions such as surprise and anger difficult [63]. Eyelashes, on the other hand, also have their place in determining facial aesthetics but more importantly functions to help protect the eye from dust and other foreign bodies [63]. Facial hair can be lost secondary to trauma, surgery, alopecia areata, endocrinopathies, and chronic plucking [63, 64].

There is no sufficient donor source that has the same caliber and growth rate as eyebrows; therefore, the patient must understand that the cosmetic result may never appear completely natural [62]. Posterior scalp hair is the best option but transplanted hair must be trimmed every 2 weeks [62]. The female eyebrow has a more arched shape with the most superior point above the lateral limbus, while the male eyebrow is typically lower and less arched with a straighter appearance [63]. Follicular unit transplantation for the eyebrows is performed in the same manner as for the scalp with the exception of the follicular units being separated into single hair follicles [62]. Patients will begin to see growth after 3–4 months but full growth is not expected until 6–8 months after surgery [62].

Given their similarities, hairs from the eyebrow can be a suitable option for eyelash transplantation. With a well-executed and meticulous technique, a strip composite eyebrow graft can be successfully transplanted at the eyelash line with good cosmetic results [65]. However, drawbacks include scarring at the donor site, limited donor supply, and significant differences in hair length [65].

## Emerging Technologies

Although excellent clinical results in hair restoration can be obtained with today's current methods, new and innovative techniques are still being developed. Low-level laser light therapy delivers 650–800-nm light at low power through an at-home comb (HairMax) or in-office hood unit to the scalp to stimulate hair growth [51]. Other devices aim to convert follicular unit transplantation or extraction into faster, more efficient processes by automating both graft extraction and recipient site creation [51, 66]. Even traditional lasers such as the carbon dioxide and erbium:YAG (yttrium aluminum garnet) lasers have been suggested as possible alternatives to manual recipient site creation [67, 68]. Finally, research is also under way to bioengineer hair follicles. This future technology would revolutionize hair restoration surgery by creating an unlimited donor supply and eliminating the creation of large scars [51, 69].

## References

1. 2011 Practice Census Statistics. International society of hair restoration surgery. http://www.ishrs.org/PDF/FinalPracticeCensusReport7_11_11.pdf. Accessed June 2012.
2. Rook A. Hair II Racial and other genetic variations in hair form. Br J Dermatol. 1975;92:599–600.
3. Wolfram LJ. Human hair: a unique physiochemical composite. J Am Acad Dermatol. 2003;48((6 Suppl)):S106–14.
4. Gold RJ, Scriver CG. The amino acid composition of hair from different racial origins. Clin Chim Acta. 1971;33:465–6.
5. Halder RM. Hair and scalp disorders in blacks. Cutis. 1983;32:378–80.

6. McMichael AJ. Hair and scalp disorders in ethnic populations. Dermatol Clin. 2003;21: 629–44.
7. Callender VD, Young CM. Alopecias and hair restoration in women. In: Soriano T, Hexsel DM, Grimes PE Kim J, editors. Aesthetics and cosmetic surgery for darker skin types. Philadelphia: Lippincott Williams & Wilkins; 2008. p. 287–95.
8. Callender VD. Hair transplantation for pigmented skins. In: Halder RM, editor. Dermatology and dermatological therapy of pigmented skins. Boca Raton: Taylor & Francis; 2006. p. 245–57.
9. Pierce HE. The uniqueness of hair transplantation in black patients. J Natl Med Assoc. 1976;68:343.
10. Loussouarn G. Diversity of hair growth parameters. In: Leveque JL, Maibach HI, Berardesca E, editors. Ethnic skin and hair. New York: Informa Healthcare; 2007. p. 245–62.
11. Unger WP. The history of hair transplantation. Dermatol Surg. 2000;26:181–9.
12. Inui S, Itami S. Dr. Shoji Okuda (1886–1962): the great pioneer of punch graft hair transplantation. J Dermatol. 2009;36:561–2.
13. Pierce HE. Modifications designed to assure the success of the strip graft hair transplant technique. J Natl Med Assoc. 1976;68:387–8.
14. Pierce HE. An improved method of closure of donor sites in hair transplantation. J Dermatol Surg Oncol. 1979;5:475–6.
15. Earles RM. Hair transplantation, scalp reduction, and flap rotation in black men. J Dermatol Surg Oncol. 1986;12:87–91. 95–6.
16. Earles RM. Surgical correction of traumatic alopecia marginalis or traction alopecia in black women. J Dermatol Surg Oncol. 1986;12:78–82.
17. Sperling LC. Alopecias. In: Jorrizzo JL, Rapini RP, Bolognia JL, editors. Dermatology. 2nd ed. St. Louis: Elsevier/Mosby; 2009.
18. Paik JH, Yoon JB, Sim WY, et al. The prevalence and types of androgenetic alopecia in Korean men and women. Br J Dermatol. 2001;145:95–9.
19. Muller SA. Alopecia: syndromes of genetic significance. J Invest Dermatol. 1973;60:475–92.
20. Hamilton JB. Age, sex, and genetic factors in the regulation of hair growth in man: a comparison of Caucasian and Japanese populations. In: Ellis RA, Montagna W, editors. The biology of hair growth. New York: Academic; 1958. p. 399–433.
21. Setty LR. Hair patterns of the scalp of white and Negro males. Am J Phys Anthropol. 1970;33:49–55.
22. Buechner HA, Brown M, Tretola RJ. Baldness and emphysema. J La State Med Soc. 1964;116:329–32.
23. Olsen EA, Messenger AG, Shapiro J, et al. Evaluation and treatment of male and female pattern hair loss. J Am Acad Dermatol. 2005;52:301–11.
24. Futterweit MD, Dunaif A, Yeh HC, et al. The prevalence of hyperandrogenism in 109 consecutive female patients with diffuse alopecia. J Am Acad Dermatol. 1988;19:831–6.
25. Norwood OT. Male pattern baldness: classification and incidence. South Med J. 1975;68: 1359–65.
26. Olsen EA. Female pattern hair loss. J Am Acad Dermatol. 2001;45((3 Suppl)):S70–80.
27. Ozcelik D. Extensive traction alopecia attributable to ponytail hairstyle and its treatment with hair transplantation. Aesthetic Plast Surg. 2005;29:325–7.
28. Lipnik MJ. Traumatic alopecia from brush rollers. Arch Dermatol. 1961;84:183–5.
29. Grimes PE, Davis LT. Cosmetics in blacks. Dermatol Clin. 1991;9:53–68.
30. Rudolph RI, Klein AW, Decherd JW. Corn-row alopecia. Arch Dermatol. 1973;108:134.
31. Callender VD, McMichael AJ, Cohen GF. Medical and surgical therapies for alopecias in black women. Dermatol Ther. 2004;17:164–76.
32. James J, Saladi RN, Fox JL. Traction alopecia in Sikh male patients. J Am Board Fam Med. 2007;20:497–8.
33. Kanwar AJ, Kaur S, Basak P, et al. Traction alopecia in Sikh males. Arch Dermatol. 1989;125:1587.

34. Singh G. Letter: traction alopecia in Sikh boys. Br J Dermatol. 1975;92:232–3.
35. Hwang SM, Lee WS, Choi EH, et al. Nurse's cap alopecia. Int J Dermatol. 1999;38:187–91.
36. Sperling LC. Traction alopecia. In: An Atlas of hair pathology with clinical correlations. New York: Parthenon Publishing Group; 2003. p. 51–7.
37. Whiting DA, Olsen EA. Central centrifugal cicatricial alopecia. Dermatol Ther. 2008;21:268–78.
38. Gathers RC, Lim HW. Central centrifugal cicatricial alopecia: past, present, and future. J Am Acad Dermatol. 2009;60:660–8.
39. Gathers RC, Jankowski M, Eide M, et al. Hair grooming practices and central centrifugal cicatricial alopecia. J Am Acad Dermatol. 2009;60:574–8.
40. Sperling LC, Shelton III HG, Smith KJ, et al. Follicular degeneration syndrome in men. Arch Dermatol. 1994;130:763–9.
41. LoPresti P, Papa CM, Kligman AM. Hot comb alopecia. Arch Dermatol. 1968;98:234–8.
42. Nicholson AG, Harland CC, Bull RH, et al. Chemically induced cosmetic alopecia. Br J Dermatol. 1993;128:537–41.
43. Dawber R. What is pseudopelade? Clin Exp Dermatol. 1992;17:305–6.
44. Sperling LC. The follicular degeneration syndrome in black patients: 'Hot Comb Alopecia' revisited and revised. Arch Dermatol. 1992;128:68–74.
45. Olsen EA, Bergfeld WF, Cotsarelis G, et al. Summary of North American hair research society (NAHRS)-sponsored workshop on cicatricial alopecia. Duke University Medical Center, 10, 11 Feb 2001. J Am Acad Dermatol. 2003;48:103–10.
46. Sperling LC. Central centrifugal scarring alopecia. An Atlas of hair pathology with clinical correlations. New York: The Parthenon Publishing Group; 2003. p. 91–100.
47. Sperling LC, Cowper SE. The histopathology of primary cicatricial alopecia. Semin Cutan Med Surg. 2006;25:41–50.
48. Sperling LC, Sau P. The follicular degeneration syndrome in black patients. Arch Dermatol. 1992;128:68–74.
49. Whiting DA. Cicatrial alopecia: clinicopathological findings and treatment. Clin Dermatol. 2001;19:211–25.
50. Headington JT. Cicatricial alopecia. Dermatol Clin. 1996;14:773–82.
51. Avram M, Rogers N. Contemporary hair transplantation. Dermatol Surg. 2009;35:1705–19.
52. Stough DB, Whitworth JM, Seager DJ. Hair restoration. In: Jorrizzo JL, Rapini RP Bolognia JL, editors. Dermatology. 2nd ed. St. Louis: Elsevier/Mosby; 2009.
53. Callender VD, Davis EC. Hair transplant technique: a flexible blade for preparing curly hair grafts. Dermatol Surg. 2011;37:1032–4.
54. Seager DJ, Simmons C. Local anesthesia in hair transplantation. Dermatol Surg. 2002;28:320–8.
55. Orentreich N. Autografts in alopecias and other selected dermatological conditions. Ann N Y Acad Sci. 1959;83:463–79.
56. Lee TS, Minton TJ. An update on hair restoration therapy. Curr Opin Otolaryngol Head Neck Surg. 2009;17:287–94.
57. Kelly AP. Update on the management of keloids. Semin Cutan Med Surg. 2009;28:71–6.
58. Rassman WR, Bernstein RM, McClellan R, et al. Follicular unit extraction: minimally invasive surgery in hair transplantation. Dermatol Surg. 2002;28:720–8.
59. Shapiro R, Callender VD. Hair transplantation. In: Hordinsky M, McMichael A, editors. Hair and scalp diseases: medical, surgical, and cosmetic treatments. New York: Informa Healthcare; 2008.
60. Gaviria JI. Trichophytic closure in ethnic hair [Abstract 139]. Presented at the ISHRS 17th Annual Scientific Meeting, Amsterdam, 22–26 July 2009, p. 124–6.
61. Perry PK, Cook-Bolden FE, Rahman Z, et al. Defining pseudofolliculitis barbae in 2001: a review of the literature and current trends. J Am Acad Dermatol. 2002;46((2 Suppl)):S113–9.
62. Avram M. Follicular unit transplantation for male and female pattern hair loss and restoring eyebrows. Ophthalmol Clin North Am. 2005;18:319–23.

63. Gandelman M, Epstein JS. Hair transplantation to the eyebrow, eyelashes, and other parts of the body. Facial Plast Surg Clin North Am. 2004;12:253–61.
64. Goldman GD. Eyebrow transplantation. Dermatol Surg. 2001;27:352–4.
65. Kasai K. Eyelash reconstruction with strip composite eyebrow graft. Ann Plast Surg. 2008;60:649–51.
66. Bauman AJ. Follicular unit extraction using a novel self-rotating instrument (Rotocore). Presented at the ISHRS 17th Annual Scientific Meeting, Amsterdam, 22–26 July, 2009, p. 108–9.
67. Grevelink JM. Laser hair transplantation. Dermatol Clin. 1997;15:479–86.
68. Neidel FG, Fuchs M, Krahl D. Laser-assisted autologous hair transplantation with the Er:YAG laser. J Cutan Laser Ther. 1999;1:229–31.
69. Stenn K, Parimoo S, Zheng Y, et al. Bioengineering the hair follicle. Organogenesis. 2007;3:6–13.
70. Cottington E, Kissinger R, Tolgyesi W. Observations on female scalp hair population, distribution and diameter. J Soc Cosmet Chem. 1977;28:219–29.
71. Bernstein RM. The aesthetics of follicular transplantation. Dermatol Surg. 1997;23:785–99.
72. Sperling LC. Hair density in African Americans. Arch Dermatol. 1999;135:656–8.
73. Loussouarn G. Diversity of hair growth parameters. In: Berardesca E, Leveque JL, Maibach HI, editors. Ethnic skin and hair. New York: Informa Healthcare; 1997. p. 245–62.
74. Kelly Paul A, Taylor SC. Dermatology for skin of color. New York: McGraw-Hill; 2009.
75. Hamilton JB. Patterned loss of hair in man: types and incidence. Ann NY Acad Sci. 1951; 53:708–28.
76. Norwood OT. Incidence of female androgenetic alopecia (female pattern alopecia). Dermatol Surg. 2001;27:53–4.
77. Khumalo NP, Jessop S, Gumedze F, et al. Hairdressing and the prevalence of scalp disease in African adults. Br J Dermatol. 2007;157:981–8.
78. Wang TL, Zhou C, Shen YW, et al. Prevalence of androgenetic alopecia in China: a community-based study in six cities. Br J Dermatol. 2010;162:843–7.
79. Xu F, Sheng YY, Mu ZL, et al. Prevalence and types of androgenetic alopecia in Shanghai, China: a community-based study. Br J Dermatol. 2009;160:629–32.
80. Tang PH, Chia HP, Cheong LL, et al. A community study of male androgenetic alopecia in Bishan, Singapore. Singapore Med J. 2000;41:202–5.
81. Pathomvanich D, Pongratananukul S, Thienthaworn P, et al. A random study of Asian male androgenetic alopecia in Bangkok, Thailand. Dermatol Surg. 2002;28:804–7.
82. Callender VD, Young CM. Alopecia and hair restoration in women. In: Grimes PE, editor. Aesthetics and cosmetic surgery for darker skin types. Philadelphia: Lippincott Williams & Wilkins; 2008. p. 293.

# Index



A.F. Alexis and V.H. Barbosa (eds.), *Skin of Color: A Practical Guide to Dermatologic Diagnosis and Treatment*, DOI 10.1007/978-0-387-84929-4,

**D**

**M**